W9-CUC-500

*f*P

SUSPICIOUS MINDS

HOW CULTURE SHAPES MADNESS

Joel Gold and Ian Gold

FREE PRESS

New York   London   Toronto   Sydney   New Delhi

Free Press
An imprint of Simon & Schuster, Inc.
1230 Avenue of the Americas
New York, NY 10020

Copyright 2014 by Ian Gold, Ph.D., and Joel Gold, M.D.

First Free Press hardcover edition July 2014

FREE PRESS and colophon are trademarks of Simon & Schuster, Inc.

For information about special discounts for bulk purchases,
please contact Simon & Schuster Special Sales at 1-866-506-1949
or business@simonandschuster.com.

The Simon & Schuster Speakers Bureau can bring authors to your live event.
For more information or to book an event contact the Simon & Schuster Speakers Bureau
at 1-866-248-3049 or visit our website at www.simonspeakers.com.

Interior design by Erich Hobbing
Jacket design by Oliver Munday

Manufactured in the United States of America

1   3   5   7   9   10   8   6   4   2

Library of Congress Cataloging-in-Publication Data
Gold, Joel (Joel Todd).
Suspicious minds : how culture shapes madness / Joel Gold and Ian Gold.
pages   cm
Includes bibliographical references and index.
1. Cultural psychiatry. 2. Social psychiatry. 3. Mental illness I. Gold, Ian, 1962– II. Title.
RC455.4.E8G65 2014
362.2'042—dc23   2014010820

ISBN 978-1-4391-8155-3
ISBN 978-1-4391-8157-7 (ebook)

For our parents

פֿאָר קינדער צעריַיסט מען אַ וועלט.

And for Jos

CONTENTS

CONTENTS

PART II
THE SOCIAL LIFE OF MADNESS

ACKNOWLEDGMENTS

A great many people helped us with this book. More than anyone, we owe a debt of gratitude to Derek Webster, who helped us to find the contours of our ideas and showed us how to express them more clearly and effectively. This book is incomparably better than it would have been if we hadn't had the benefit of his insight, experience, and support.

Many friends and colleagues offered valuable suggestions and advice on our work. We're particularly grateful to James Kirkbride and Ned Shorter, who gave us a great deal of feedback on parts of the manuscript.

We're also very grateful for the help given to us by Ralph Adolphs, Alia Al-Saji, Tim Bayne, Carol Bernstein, Marie-Eve Carrier, Suparna Choudhury, Max Coltheart, Mylissa Falkner, Lisa Fielding, Cordelia Fine, Glen O. Gabbard, Sandro Galea, Michael Garrett, Brad Goodman, Edward Hagen, Mike Jay, Lawrence Joseph, Joshua Karpati, Jay S. Kwawer, Robyn Langdon, Jesse Laz, Eric Lewis, Dolores Malaspina, Eric Marcus, Janet McTeer, Nancy McWilliams, Alessandra Miklavçic, Kengo Miyazono, Donatella Moltisanti, Joel Paris, Dan Posner, Benjamin J. Sadock, Jack Sava, Gilda Sherwin, Rob Stephens, and Gabrielle Weiner.

We've been helped enormously by our research assistants Tessa Blanchfield, Alison Bruni, Emma Cusumano, Devon Kapoor, Leah Katzman, Marie Prévost, Elizabeth Scott, Brooke Struck, Judy Yeh, and Anna Zuckerman. We owe a special debt to Karina Vold. We're also very grateful to Yvan Tétreault for his work on producing the excellent figures.

We could not have finished—or even started—this book without the help and support given to us by our agent, Max Brockman, and our editors Nick Greene, Karyn Marcus, Leah Miller, Sydney Tanigawa, and

ACKNOWLEDGMENTS

Webb Younce. Thanks are also due to all of the people at Free Press and Simon & Schuster, especially Patty Romanowski, who helped bring this book to life.

To any friends, family, or colleagues we may have overlooked, we are deeply sorry and can easily be made to feel guilty. Feel free to take full advantage of this trait (once per person, please).

I thank my teachers, colleagues, and friends at the Department of Psychiatry of the NYU School of Medicine and at the Institute for Psychoanalytic Education.

Many thanks to the staff of Bellevue Hospital Center, particularly to my partners Michael Sobel and Serena Volpp. Special thanks to the residents, who do the bulk of the work, and to my patients, who do the bulk of the teaching.

Thanks to all those who were interviewed for the book, especially Kevin Hall.

Thanks to Seth P. Stein and Rachel Fernbach of the New York State Psychiatric Association, and Rose Gasner, for their (unofficial) guidance in assuring patient confidentiality, and to Jamie Feldman for his (unofficial and ongoing) legal advice.

Thanks to Seth and Rachel Kalvert for getting the ball rolling.

Props to mentors Arthur Propst, René Tirol, and Mark Bear.

Tusen Takk to Jim Helfield for his great humor and friendship.

A sheynem dank to Jacob and Amalia Freud, *merci bien* to the Habs, and *kiitos paljon* to Saku Koivu.

I am indebted to Adam Karpati for his boundless support, intelligence, and great camaraderie.

I would have been unable to coauthor this book or achieve much of anything, personally or professionally, without the endless patience, guidance, and care of Robert Chalfin. I will be forever grateful.

The love of and for Yaya, whose entire life to this point has been spent with this book, and the love of and for Cathy, for whom it only feels that way, are the only reasons to bother. *Je vous aime gros comme l'univers.*

Any errors that remain in this work are, of course, entirely the fault of my brother.

—JG

ACKNOWLEDGMENTS

A distant ancestor of this book formed the basis for an undergraduate seminar at McGill, and I'm grateful to all of the students in that class.

I am also very grateful to Jill Craigie and Cordelia Fine, early comrades in research on delusion, and to Lauren Olin, who contributed so much to my thinking about delusion long before this book was even begun.

It's enormously useful to have a German scholar for a mother-in-law. Margaret Mahony Stoljar translated a long excerpt of the memoirs of the nineteenth-century figure Friedrich Krauss, some of which appears here. Her work gave us access to an important firsthand description of a delusional illness for which I'm deeply grateful.

Finally, to Natalie, Alex, and Adam (who may not believe that this book is finished even when they hold it in their hands), for their love and support, a thank-you is nothing like enough, but will have to do.

Any errors that remain in this work are, of course, entirely the fault of my brother.

—IG

AUTHORSHIP NOTE

This book is coauthored, but in a number of places where the pronoun "I" is used, it refers to Joel. These references appear in the portraits of patients and are indicated by means of a specific attribution at the bottom, i.e., "—JG."

A NOTE ON THE PATIENTS

All patients depicted in this book have been disguised to protect confidentiality. Material central to the clinical picture is included, while identifying data have been changed. All patient quotes are used with their signed consent.

A NOTE ON "PSYCH" WORDS

Words that begin with *psych* (from the Greek *psyche,* meaning "mind" or "soul") have proliferated in our language and in this book. A number refer to particular disciplines, professions, or theories. *Psychology* is the broadest of these. It refers to the scientific study of any facet of mental life. *Psychopathology* is the study of abnormal or disordered psychology. *Psychiatry,* in contrast, refers more narrowly to the medical profession concerned with psychopathology—its investigation as well as treatment— and is itself distinguished from the profession of *clinical psychology* in that its practitioners are physicians and can prescribe medications. Clinical psychologists, psychiatrists, and clinical social workers may practice one form or another of *psychotherapy*—the treatment of mental disorder by psychological, rather than physical, means. *Psychoanalysis* refers to a particular movement in psychiatry based on the theory and psycho-therapeutic practice of Sigmund Freud and his disciples. Early on, most psychoanalysts were MDs, but analytic institutes now accept "lay" practitioners. *Psychosis* refers to a family of illnesses characterized primarily by delusions and hallucinations. Psychosis is distinct from *psychopathy,* a mental disorder characterized by antisocial behavior, callousness, and impulsivity, among other features.

The world as it had been shown to him was a piece of unreason, an idiot's dream. Yet it was on too mammoth a scale to be without some reason. He came wearily back to his original point: Since the world could not be as crazy as it appeared to be, it must necessarily have been arranged to appear crazy in order to deceive him as to the truth. . . . In some fashion he must get behind the deception and see what went on when he was not looking. . . . Obviously the first step must be to escape from this asylum.

—Robert Heinlein, "They"

SUSPICIOUS MINDS

PREFACE:
THE TRUMAN SHOW DELUSION

JOEL GOLD

It is a rare privilege to spend your very first day practicing medicine at the Bellevue Hospital psychiatric emergency room, formally named the Comprehensive Psychiatric Emergency Program (CPEP). I had this experience on July 1, 1995. Back then, everything I knew about psychiatry came from a couple of months as a medical student, tagging along with the grown-ups—in other words, next to nothing.

Bellevue is the oldest public hospital in the United States. Although the hospital offers treatment from all medical disciplines, in the general consciousness Bellevue is thought to be a psychiatric hospital. Be it medical, surgical, or psychiatric care, Bellevue treats people from around the world. If someone becomes manic in Europe or South America and hops on a plane that lands at LaGuardia or JFK, he or she is brought to Bellevue. The psychiatric department has a unit dedicated to patients who are monolingual Chinese speakers (Mandarin, Cantonese, and Fujianese) and another for patients more comfortable speaking Spanish. Bellevue is a veritable United Nations of Madness.

But if there is a psychiatric baptism by fire, it is the Bellevue CPEP. After one week I had interviewed or heard colleagues present cases of all manner of mental illness, especially psychosis—the cluster of mad symptoms encompassing hallucinations, delusions, bizarre or disorganized speech, and disorganized behavior that might accompany any number of disorders, psychiatric and medical.

1

A few weeks later, some common clinical patterns began to emerge: the patient with chronic schizophrenia off her medications; the crack-induced paranoia, then crash; the malingerer, feigning symptoms in order to gain entry to the hospital for reasons unrelated to his health; the man brought in naked after running down Fifth Avenue, in the throes of a manic episode; the repeat offender arrested (again), demanding to be psychiatrically evaluated (again) so as to avoid going to central booking (again). Those who were regular visitors to the CPEP were coarsely deemed "frequent flyers."

It was exhausting—and exhilarating.

At the end of my first month as a doctor, I saw someone walk into the CPEP who looked different from the last hundred patients I had seen—and rather like that med school classmate who never made it to lecture because he was always playing Ultimate. Finally, I thought, some respite from all the suicidal and homicidal patients. This guy looked about as mellow and laid back as a person could be: tie-dyed T-shirt, cargo shorts, and flip-flops, his long hair held back in a bandana. Perhaps The Dude just got dumped by his girlfriend, and he's feeling a little down. I've been there! Perhaps his boss is a jackass, threatening to fire him if he doesn't pick up the pace at work. I can handle that—I'm, like, a doctor! Awesome. This way, Dude.

So, Dude, I ask with a smile, what's the story?

As it turns out, The Dude has not been unsuccessful romantically of late or even gainfully employed. But he *has* been killing small animals and compulsively drinking their blood. That is not, however, The Dude's primary concern. The Dude tells me that his mind has been wandering away from drinking the blood of small animals to drinking the blood of people, particularly his mother. But duuuude, y'know, not, like, Mom!

The Big Lebowski this is not. The Dude is admitted upstairs for treatment.

A few weeks later, a colleague informs me that The Dude has been discharged to an ashram in the desert.

I mention the story of The Dude to help explain why the "Truman Show delusion" took months—years—to register in my mind. When the people you deal with in your working life are severely mentally ill, that becomes the norm. Mental illness is the cosmic background radiation of front-line psychiatry; stars are exploding, comets are whizzing by, meteors are smashing into planets all around you, every day. If you haven't worked in such a context, it's hard to appreciate just how much this can alter your perspective—but if you read the portraits of patients placed throughout this book, you may start to get the feel of life in a psychiatric emergency room and on a psychiatric unit.

At a state hospital, I rotated on a forensic unit where I met a man who was there because he had seen a mannequin on fire and stomped it out. Sadly, the mannequin was not on fire; in fact, it wasn't a mannequin but a homeless man sleeping on the sidewalk. The patient had killed the man while hallucinating. During that same rotation, I was warned that one woman on the forensic unit was handy with an ice pick. She had stabbed her boyfriend with one because he had purchased a toupee without consulting her. She didn't like the color and felt disrespected by his failure to include her in the decision-making process.

Still, I found delusions of the kind featured in this book most compelling. And as delusions go, the CPEP and the residency-training unit at Bellevue, 19-North (later 20-West), are to psychiatry what the Louvre and the Met are to painting, or the Bolshoi and the Kirov are to ballet. During my time at Bellevue, both as a trainee and then as an attending physician, I observed more delusions in its small, locked spaces than I suspect many psychiatrists observe in a career.

Most delusional patients present similar kinds of persecutory or grandiose ideas. Belief in being Jesus or in possession by demons is common. Other classic delusions include patients' beliefs that they are being pursued by the FBI, CIA, or KGB, which have implanted microchips in their brains or teeth in order to monitor them. Sometimes new twists on old delusions seem to emerge, albeit in small numbers. For a while, African American women from the South were coming up to New York (usually on a Greyhound bus) with the fervent belief that they could raise the dead at Ground Zero.

But the majority of memorable delusions are one-offs: The Dude; the middle-aged woman with a broken leg who demanded to be discharged so she could run the New York City marathon; the young African American woman from Brooklyn who believed the spirit of Rabbi Menachem Schneerson, following his death, had inhabited her body.

All of which is to say, when Albert, the first "Truman Show" patient, walked into Bellevue on Friday, October 31, 2003, I thought nothing of it. Eight years had passed since I'd first started, and on that particular day,

3

I was working as chief attending psychiatrist on the inpatient training unit at Bellevue. Albert was a twenty-six-year-old, single white man from western Pennsylvania. He lived with his parents, had no siblings, and worked at a nearby assembly plant. Albert believed that he was the subject of a TV show or movie. In describing his experience, he compared it to the acclaimed 1998 film *The Truman Show*, written by Andrew Niccol and directed by Peter Weir. The protagonist, Truman Burbank, played by Jim Carrey, is being watched by the whole world. Adopted *in utero* by a television corporation, Truman lives with every moment of his life being captured by thousands of cameras located around Seahaven, the island community he never leaves until his climactic escape to the "real" world, after slowly detecting the inauthenticity of his environment. Truman's wife, best friend, and those who wordlessly pass him on the street are all actors and extras populating the highest-rated reality show in the world. In the final scene, Truman has a conversation with a disembodied, god-like voice that pleads with him to stay in Seahaven:

TRUMAN: Who are you?
CHRISTOF: I'm the Creator.
TRUMAN: The creator of what?
CHRISTOF: A show—that gives hope and joy and inspiration to
   millions.
TRUMAN: *A show.* Then who am I?
CHRISTOF: You're the star.

The suspicion of being watched might never have been portrayed better than in *The Truman Show*—except in the minds of many people who daily suffer from the same delusion. When I spoke to Albert at Bellevue, he believed that all of the significant people in his life were involved in a conspiracy to keep him on the air and in the dark about his own show. Despite having had this notion for an extended period, he had only recently shared his beliefs with his uncle, a psychiatric technician at a local hospital. He also told of having cameras in his eyes and referenced another film, *Being John Malkovich*, in explaining that detail.

Albert's uncle told him that he needed to get help. Albert took this to mean that he needed to leave his hometown to find evidence for his beliefs. At first he thought about going to Europe to prove that it existed, the logic being that, if his life were a Truman-like TV show, Europe would be a fictional place cooked up by the writers and directors. Like Truman in the film, who dreamed of escaping to Fiji, Albert was going to the Continent. When Europe proved too expensive a trip, Albert came up with a simpler way to test his hypothesis. He took a train to Penn Station in New York City, with his ultimate goal being the World Trade Center site. Albert reasoned that even the attacks of 9/11 would have been staged for his benefit, and his response to the tragedy manipulated for the show's ratings. It followed that if the Twin Towers were still standing, his suspicions would be proven true. If the towers *were* destroyed, Albert said, he would admit that he was perhaps delusional. However, he never made it to Ground Zero, and instead found himself standing in the shadow of the United Nations. In a flash, his plans changed yet again. Albert decided to apply to the UN for asylum from his own show. When he attempted to enter the UN building and was approached by a security guard, he unwisely took a swing at the man. A scuffle ensued, and Albert was brought to Bellevue.

Most delusional patients hold their false beliefs wholeheartedly, but Albert was unusual: he would acknowledge that he might be suffering from a mental illness one minute and then request to speak to the director of the show the next. In the five years he had held his deluded belief—ever since the movie came out, in fact—Albert had had no formal contact with any mental health worker. And though I was among the first to learn of Albert's delusions, I didn't get to know him very well because he was quickly transferred back home to Pennsylvania, to the hospital where his uncle worked.

While Albert's clinical presentation was interesting, I thought little of him until a few months later when I met and treated Brian, a twenty-nine-year-old visual artist from Los Angeles, also single, also white. Since seeing *The Truman Show* several years prior, Brian had operated under the belief that he was living a secretly televised life. He explained that he was being followed, taped, and broadcast by a network of unknown conspirators, all for the enjoyment of others. He was the center of attention of millions of people around the world. Everyone he knew, including his family, was an actor reading from a script. Brian also believed that his viewers knew his thoughts. Anguished by the theft of both his physical and mental privacy, he had decided to take his life by jumping from the Statue of Liberty. When he discovered it had been closed since 9/11, he wandered the streets of Manhattan until he came to the attention of a homeless shelter outreach team. When he described his delusional system and plan to commit suicide, they brought him to Bellevue.

As we talked, Brian told me that he imagined an old high school girlfriend had been watching his show and would meet him at the top of the Statue of Liberty. Though he had gone there with a plan to jump, he still hoped that she would instead save him and help him expose his plight. If she were not there, however, he would kill himself to end his torment.

On 19-North, Brian was initially pleasant despite believing that his doctors were part of the plot against him, but his symptoms did not respond to any of a number of meds, including antipsychotics and mood stabilizers. In the weeks that followed, he remained delusional, and he would not rule out suicide when he left the hospital. His mood continued to sink, and he became more irritable. After nearly two months at Bellevue, Brian was transferred to a state hospital for continued treatment.

I recall noting the similarities between Albert's and Brian's delusional ideas, but two patients in a sea of hundreds still didn't register as more than a coincidence. When practicing psychiatry at Bellevue Hospital, it is often difficult to see the mad forest for the delusional trees. Amid the never-ending flow of patients coming through the doors—evaluating and treating them, communicating with family members, negotiating with insurance companies, finding housing and outpatient follow-up care— stopping to discern the subtle patterns of madness that form over time feels like a luxury, and not something we psychiatrists usually have the time or energy to do.

The Truman Show patients opened my eyes.

Unlike the single, memorable presentations that came and went, the Truman Show theme continued to appear. A few months after treating Brian, a third Truman patient, Charley, was admitted to the unit. And soon after that, a fourth Truman patient, David, a film school graduate from Chicago, was brought to Bellevue by his newly ex-girlfriend, Rebecca.

David had been hospitalized twice previously for manic episodes. In the weeks leading up to his admission, he hadn't been sleeping and was talking a mile a minute. Paranoid and irritable, he had been shouting the Ten Commandments at the TV and had been more preoccupied with sex than even the most ardent young man. He had also been smoking a lot of pot, and Rebecca had recently broken up with him. (He later said, "A girl is involved every time, and then I become manic.")

Ironically, David had been working on the production staff of a popular reality-television show when he began to believe that he was being filmed. He believed the show was about him. David said that his family had hired the crew and that his parents were not his real parents. After a family meeting, he told his psychiatrist, "I don't know what team you're on; I think you're on my parents' team." David believed those involved in the production of the TV show were controlling his thoughts. He was ultimately fired from the show for refusing to sign a confidentiality agreement about which he had become suspicious. David said, "I thought I was a secret contestant on a reality-television show. I thought I was being filmed. I was convinced I was a contestant and later the TV show would reveal me." David eventually responded well to a combination of antipsychotic and mood-stabilizing medication and returned to his apartment with follow-up care in place.

While David did not mention *The Truman Show* by name, the quality of his delusion certainly echoed those of Albert and of Brian. I began to think that there might be something more meaningful to the content of these men's delusions than simply a common interest in Jim Carrey's *oeuvre*. I also thought it was time to take in the film again. This being the Paleo-Netflix era, I made a trip to the local "video store."

"There's no point in trying to explain it, but a lot of strange things have been happening . . . people talking about me on the radio, you know what I mean?"
"I'm definitely being followed."
"Everybody seems to be in on it."
"Maybe I'm going out of my mind, but I get the feeling that the world revolves around me somehow."

These statements, all made by Truman Burbank in the film, sounded like the delusional ideas of someone suffering from some form of psychosis. It occurred to me that the three patients I had seen all suffered from the same three forms of delusion: paranoia, grandiosity, and ideas of reference. I returned to Albert's case. His paranoia was understandable, given his belief that hidden cameras were filming him 24/7 (not to mention the even smaller cameras surreptitiously installed in his eyes). The flipside of his paranoia was grandiosity. If the entire world is watching

7

your life, you must be pretty important, and Albert called himself a star. Finally, ideas of reference are delusions wherein the sufferer attaches significance to otherwise meaningless stimuli: in Albert's case, he believed that when people said "cool," they were giving him a signal that they were "in" on the show.

After seeing four patients suffering similar symptoms, I became convinced that paranoia, grandiosity, and delusions of reference appearing in the context of what I came to think of as *controlled unreality* were psychiatrically and culturally significant. The delusion raised questions about the interplay between mental illness and our environment, and larger questions about the relationship of mind to culture.

> MARLON: [Emotional almost to the point of tears] The point is, I would gladly step in front of traffic for you, Truman. And the last thing I would ever do to you . . .
>
> CHRISTOF: [Feeding Marlon his lines] And the last thing I'd ever do is lie to you.
>
> MARLON: And the last thing I'd ever do is lie to you. Think about it, Truman, if everybody's in on it, I'd have to be in on it too. I'm not in on it because there is no *it*.

With Truman Burbank's words echoing in my mind and in the mouths of my patients, I began calling their experiences "the Truman Show delusion."

The fifth Truman Show delusion patient was brought to Bellevue by police nearly two years after the first. Ethan was found trespassing in a neighbor's apartment. He believed that a young woman he had recently dated for a short time had moved into his building, and that he could find her via a secret passageway. In fact, the woman lived in another state altogether, and the secret passageway instead led into his neighbor's place. Ethan believed the CIA was following him and monitoring him through his laptop computer. It was all part of a scheme wherein people wagered on his daily activities. Due to his importance to the plan, though, the CIA was protecting him. He, too, likened his experience to *The Truman Show*.

Ethan was convinced that a vast game was in play, one involving bets placed on his daily activities, but he was perplexed by the fact that he could not fathom its rules. A dizzying number of strange things were occurring and, however unrelated they might seem, Ethan reasoned that they must be connected. He thought that radio broadcasts he heard were not authentic but were created especially for him. Pickup trucks were following him. His roommate had been video- and tape-recording him, and he suspected that he was being recorded in the hospital, too. He believed Bellevue was a hotel and that everyone in it, including the doctors and patients, were actors in his "*Truman Show*–like existence." A neighbor was a stand-in for Ethan's real father who, through an earpiece, told the man what to say to Ethan. In fact, a number of family members and celebrities were talking to Ethan through others who acted as vessels.

At times, Ethan felt helpless: he wanted to get out of the hospital but couldn't figure out what "card to play to end the game." At other times, his helplessness gave way to a sense of his own power: *he* was the Master who had created and controlled the game, but (he later explained to me) he had subsequently forgotten both that fact and the rules. Despite these fluctuations, throughout his illness Ethan remained highly altruistic, a character trait he had displayed his whole life, and the themes of his delusions revolved around his wish to do good. The bets that people were placing on his life were, he said, generating funds for a charity.

Ethan is a third-generation Chinese American, originally from Southern California, who was twenty-six years old at the time of his admission. After graduating from MIT with degrees in cognitive and computer science, he had come to New York to do graduate work in machine learning at Columbia University. Ethan had been diagnosed with ADHD as a child and been taking Ritalin for many years. In the weeks leading up to his hospitalization, he had been working exceptionally hard on his doctoral thesis and had been using more and more Ritalin in an effort to stay awake longer and focus more intensely on his writing. The psychiatrists at Bellevue weren't sure if Ethan's psychosis was strictly related to the Ritalin use or if he was in the midst of a first-break episode of schizophrenia. In either case, we stopped Ethan's Ritalin and offered him the antipsychotic Risperdal. He took it only because he believed that it was not actually an antipsychotic but a medication for his ADHD.

Ethan's recovery was slow. As his insight into his mental state grew, he mourned the loss of the idea that he was special, acknowledging that he hadn't been "living in reality." Since nobody knew if his psychotic episode would be a once-in-a-lifetime event, Ethan worried about the impact of having a mental illness on his career and romantic life. He feared that the episode was a preview of more to come, that he might become a burden to his family. Ethan later recalled that the only times he ever saw his brother cry were at their father's funeral and during a visit to see him at Bellevue. Shortly after turning twenty-seven, Ethan was discharged after spending six weeks at Bellevue. Everyone was apprehensive about his future.

On a visit to my hometown of Montreal, I talked about the Truman Show patients with my brother, Ian, a professor of philosophy and psychiatry at McGill University. Ian hadn't heard of anything like it. In his own research into psychosis and delusion, however, he had become skeptical of the field's overwhelming focus on neurobiology as the primary explanation for mental illness, and the Truman Show delusion got us talking about the larger role that culture likely plays. Although cultural psychiatry is a thriving field, with McGill one of its world centers, we were surprised to discover a scarcity of psychiatric literature about how delusion relates to culture. Over the next few months, we traded professional notes and further developed our thoughts. In 2006, Ian and I presented some of our ideas to my colleagues at grand rounds, a weekly lecture to the entire department of psychiatry at NYU Medical Center. Soon after, we began writing an academic paper on the Truman Show delusion.

But before our paper was even published, I received a call from a Canadian journalist working for the *National Post*. He interviewed me over the phone while I was sitting on a crosstown Manhattan bus. A couple of weeks later, on what must have been a slow news day, I was shocked to find a feature story on the newspaper's front page.

Within days, the story got picked up by other print and online media. Some of the pieces were well written, with reporters calling to ask insightful questions, but much of the coverage resembled the children's game broken telephone, with all sorts of misleading and inaccurate comments about the Truman Show delusion and what it implied about contemporary culture. Many outlets appeared to simply cut and paste portions of the original article, making a few arbitrary and usually incorrect changes. Ian and I were both psychiatrists; neither of us was a psychiatrist. One New York City tabloid cut out the part about the story taking place in New York City. Our favorite bit of gratuitous counterfactual reporting appeared on a British website: "Psychiatrist Ian Gold . . . a philosophy and psychology professor . . . Dr. Joel Gold (no relation) . . . "

But these errors were merely silly. The much more concerning result of being the media's flavor *du jour* was the proliferation of oversimplified, false conclusions. Apart from a few pieces, the serious question—does culture have an impact on mental health, and if so, how?—was ignored. The worst accounts clearly held some preconceived notion of what the Truman Show delusion should be and strove to attach quick, socially relevant messages about the Facebook generation (messages that could apply to any and every healthy person) to what was a narrow, working idea about an expression of psychosis. My and Ian's role in these stories, it turned out, was less as serious thinkers than straight men to the comedy of our research: our job was to say that watching the *Real Housewives of Des Moines* could drive you mad.

When the media hype had passed, we were left with the realization that most people have very little understanding of what delusions are. This is not surprising: many experts in the field appear to be confused when it comes to delusion. By 2008, Ian and I had spent a decade or more wrapping our own heads around concepts of mental illness, and found no easy answers. But over the years, we have developed strong opinions about some of the ways influential thinkers have got delusion wrong.

Most of the attention paid to psychosis today, delusion specifically, involves what sorts of pills to prescribe and which kind of misfiring neurons the pills are meant to target. But what this pill-and-neuron story misses is the larger narrative of social and cultural life going on around every patient, around every neuron. And so, with this book, we have set out to correct a number of misperceptions about psychotic illness and its sufferers, with a focus on delusion. We also hope that the professional conversation surrounding mental illness might become more balanced, so that genetics and neurobiology are not emphasized at the expense of environment.

There was one major benefit of the media attention around the Truman Show delusion: community. In the years since the first story ran in 2008, Ian and I have received a great number of emails from people suffering from the delusion, from their families and friends, and from clinicians treating the same delusion, all around the world. We discovered that women, including a young female doctor in the Middle East, suffered from it as well as men. A lot of people were looking for support or offering to take part in future research. The most common sentiment was a desire to help others who suffered from it. Many people described the relief they felt upon learning they were not the only ones to have survived the delusion. Others were not so lucky: one bereaved family described how their child had committed suicide in order to escape the Show.

While some patients with Truman Show delusion have schizophrenia, the delusion is seen in patients with bipolar disorder, substance-induced psychosis, and (we suspect) could be a symptom of any psychotic illness. Psychiatrist Paolo Fusar-Poli and his colleagues at the Institute of Psychiatry at King's College, London, use the term "Truman syndrome" to describe "prodromal" patients (those who are not yet fully psychotic, but show early signs of illness). One of the British researchers, psychiatrist Oliver Howes, has said that of those coming to the Outreach and Support in South London (OASIS) mental health clinic, one in four has Truman syndrome. And Jean Addington, professor of psychiatry at the University of Calgary, has said that many of her prodromal patients compare their experiences to *The Truman Show*.

We also learned that a sizable number of people who do not go on to develop any psychotic illness have Truman Show experiences as children. We do not know if this finding will have any practical utility in the study of childhood development or if there is an age beyond which having Truman Show experiences ceases to be a normal variant of a child's imaginative play.

In writing this book, we discovered a tremendous amount of evidence to support the thesis that culture shapes madness—evidence that has been well described in the psychiatric literature but passed over, perhaps because it does not fit the particular spirit of the times.

And as we worked our way through the clinical research and ranged into fields such as evolutionary psychology and urban epidemiology, something new arose: a fresh view of delusion (explained in chapters 4 and 5) that depends on a hypothesized brain system we call the Suspicion System. In the course of developing this view, we've come to better understand the crucial role of the social world in delusion, and in psychosis more generally.

Interspersed throughout these chapters, we visit and revisit the front lines of psychosis through case narratives that portray people with delusions. They put a human face on what can feel, at times, like theoretical suffering. These patients lead the kind of challenging lives that can be shocking in their extremity and isolation, yet achingly familiar to all of us. Their problems, while experienced in unusual ways, are not so different from our own.

Which leads to a final point: the main misconception we encountered in the coverage of the Truman Show delusion was a sense that the mentally ill are not us—are *other*, different from you and me. But any psychiatrist will tell you that is not true. Mental illness is just a frayed, weakened version of mental health. In researching and writing this book, we came to understand just how little separates the mentally ill from the mentally fit. A genetic vulnerability here, a childhood trauma there, one loss too many—and just like that, you've switched places. We all have psychotic and nonpsychotic parts of our mind. The challenge is keeping the craziness at bay, under careful watch of the saner aspects of ourselves. It doesn't take much for anyone, you and me included, to become mad.

There is good reason to feel that as a society we are moving toward greater understanding of mental illness. In the past fifty years, recognizing that schizophrenia is a biological illness has had a humanizing effect on the people who suffer from it. Being classified as "mad" or "insane" carried with it centuries of stigma and a life of exclusion. When madness was refigured as an illness of the brain, the moral burden of madness was lightened.

Yet the biologization of madness has also refigured the boundary between "us" and "them," and that boundary, perhaps to the surprise of the practitioners who have helped to define it, has grown starker the more that mental illness has come to be characterized in terms of physical phenomena like neurotransmitters. Before the twentieth century, one could go mad from unrequited love or as a result of violating God's law. However alien the madman, he represented a moral lesson for all of us. When science began telling us that madness was etched into our genes and brains, what had been a flexible boundary became more like a closed border—with the mentally ill on the wrong side, as distant from us as ever. This book will, we hope, reopen that border and show mental illness to be the pervasive, ordinary, and highly social experience it really is.

PART I

THE SLEEP OF REASON

1

A SHORT HISTORY OF MADNESS

BEFORE PSYCHIATRY

Delusions are symptoms of a disease known, for most of human history, as madness, descriptions of which go back nearly as far as the written records of human civilization. The Papyrus Ebers, for example, an Egyptian medical text dating from 1550 BC, informs the aspiring physician that maniacal behavior is caused by possession, and five hundred years later the Indian *Atharva-Veda* reports that madness can be caused by "sin against the gods" or by a demon. A charm is provided to enable the sufferer to be "uncrazed." Among the curses to be visited on the Israelites who fail to obey the Lord is insanity, and Old Testament madmen—the envious King Saul who raves, or the bestial King Nebuchadnezzar condemned to eat grass for his pride—become deranged for their sins.

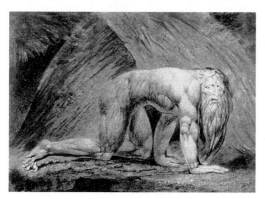

Figure 1: *Nebuchadnezzar*, William Blake, 1795. Tate Gallery, London.

The Babylonians and Mesopotamians understood madness as a punishment from the gods or demonic retribution, and insanity has a divine origin in Greek antiquity as well. When, in Homer's *Odyssey*, Penelope is told by her nurse that Odysseus has come back and killed her suitors, she says: " 'the gods have made you mad. They have that power, / putting lunacy into the clearest head around.' " And, in Euripides's *Bacchae*, possessed by Dionysus, Agave rips the head off her own son, Pentheus. Long before even the earliest of these writings, our ancestors left us clues to their theories of madness. Archaeological evidence shows that boring holes in the skull ("trephining" or "trepanning") to release the devils inside is a practice that dates from at least 5,000 BC. Removing the imagined "stone of madness" by trephination was a medieval medical fantasy (see Figure 2).

Although madness is usually thought of as a disturbance, it has sometimes been conceived of as a gift. Plato, for example, distinguished four

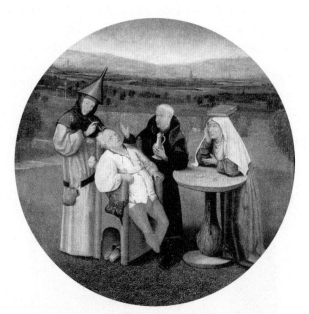

Figure 2: *Extracting the Stone of Madness*,
Hieronymus Bosch, c. 1475. The painting is a satirical
representation of the medieval belief that madness
was caused by having a stone in one's head. © Madrid,
Museo Nacional del Prado. Reproduced with permission.

forms of madness: that of the prophet, the poet, the mystic, and the lover. The hero who is driven mad by unrequited love is a common trope in medieval literature, and the link between madness and poetry—or creativity more generally—continues to our day.

With the coming of Christianity, Greek notions of madness were transfigured but not abandoned. Madness was seen to have its source in sin, in witchcraft, or in a battle between the Holy Ghost and the Devil for the soul of the madman. Although it might occasionally be a sign of holiness—in the Middle Ages in particular—the madman's loss of reason was thought to render him less like his rational God and was usually taken to be a sign of devilry or possession, as in the case of the Gadarene man healed by Jesus. Belief in possession continues into modern times, of course, and the incantations and charms used in some twentieth-century cultures are little different from those found in the ancient world. Even the familiar belief in the evil eye originates in the notion of possession and was already present in Greek culture.

Although the Greeks had a view of madness as divine, they were also the first to conceive of it as disease. In fact, Greek medicine, like our own,

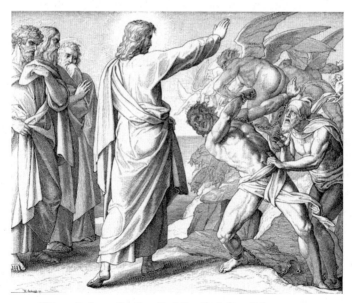

Figure 3: *Jesus Casting Out Devils*, Julius Schnorr von Carolsfeld, 1860.

took madness to be a brain disorder. A Hippocratic text, for example, denies the divine origin of epilepsy in favor of a purely biological source, the brain: "from nothing else but thence come joys, delights, laughter and sports, and sorrows, griefs, despondency, and lamentations . . . And by the same organ we become mad and delirious, and fears and terrors assail us." The cause of madness, the author tells us, is a brain that is too hot or too moist.

Greek medicine was founded on the theory of the "humors," or bodily fluids, each of which performed distinct functions and, when in balance, maintained physical health. Some treatments for disease, therefore, sought to restore humoral equilibrium—by bloodletting, for instance, when an excess of blood was to blame. The cause of mental disturbances was thought to be a substance known as black bile (in Greek: *melancholia*), though just what the Greeks called by that name remains mysterious. (Some combination of coffee grounds in brown vomit, dark urine, and tarry stool, according to one historian.) Nevertheless, the view persisted for centuries: "the devil rejoices in the humor of black bile" was a medieval adage. Purgatives to expel black bile, as well as washing liquids that stimulated its excretion, were thus the treatment of choice for those suffering from madness. A good diet (low in black bile, of course), exercise, and proper hygiene were also advised.

Alongside the medical treatment of madness, the ancients developed psychological remedies as well. These included dream interpretation and "incubation"—the practice of sleeping at a holy site in order to bring about a dream of divine origin. Philosophy also had its share of recommendations. Plato believed that madness came about by the subordination of reason to the lower parts of the mind and so declared the treatment to be the dialectical method. And the Stoics and Epicureans thought that mental anguish could be overcome by the correct application of philosophical truths, although they did not believe that this early form of talk therapy could cure madness.

Medieval medicine followed the Greek model, in particular that of Galen, the Greek doctor whose views were central to medicine for fifteen hundred years. Before the sixteenth century, however, we find no books devoted exclusively to mental illness. One of the first of these, *The Diseases Which Deprive Man of His Reason,* was written by Paracelsus (who, before being given the brief moniker, rejoiced in the name Theophrastus Bombastus von Hohenheim) and published in 1567. Robert Burton's monumental *Anatomy of Melancholy,* published a few years later in 1621, summarizes the treatments for melancholy known since the Greeks. If bloodletting and purgatives fail, Burton tells us, one can try diet, exercise, herbal remedies, travel, music, or marriage. Eighteenth-century treatments also included rotating and tranquilizer chairs, electric shock, and "ducking"—the practice of firing water at the head. To help evacuation on its way, moxibustion, cauterization, and blistering could also be used, but more useful perhaps was the available pharmacopeia, which included opium, henbane, belladonna, and camphor.

THE ASYLUM

The great nineteenth-century psychologist Hermann Ebbinghaus famously said that "psychology has a long past, yet its real history is short." The same could be said about psychiatry. Human beings have probably wondered about madness ever since they could wonder about anything, but psychiatry as a profession is just over two hundred years old. It came into existence as the medical specialty devoted to treating the madmen that society had locked away.

Although we know very little about the history of attitudes toward the mad, those who were not looked after by their families probably lived wretched lives. Some would have been forced to wander from town to town or be housed in churches which, unlike domestic buildings, could stand up to violent behavior. Still, madmen were not always treated inhumanely. While medieval Christian law, for example, deprived the mad of their rights to be married or ordained, it did permit baptism and communion.

During the Middle Ages religious institutions began the charitable work of housing those with mental illness. The hospice founded in the sixth century by the monk Theodosius near Jerusalem is supposed to have had a ward for those suffering from madness, and institutions for the sick, including the mad, were established from the seventh century in the Islamic world, which had a particularly humane outlook on mental illness. The grounds of the hospital for the mentally ill, built in the fifteenth century by the Sultan Bajazet II, were adorned with gardens and fountains, and treatment of the patients included a special diet, baths, perfumes, and concerts. Mental institutions were established in various parts of Europe from the twelfth century onward, the most famous of these being St. Mary of Bethlehem—later known as Bethlem or "Bedlam" (from which we get the synonym for "pandemonium"). Bethlem was founded in 1247 in London, and by the late fourteenth century, was housing the mad. Eventually madhouses became businesses as well as charitable institutions, and by the middle of the nineteenth century, the "trade in lunacy" had absorbed about half of those with mental illness.

In the nineteenth century, the asylums of Europe were revolutionized by reformers who were driven by both humane and medical motives. Reform was desperately needed because asylums were not hospitals; they housed the mad but didn't treat them, and the conditions in some asylums, especially those funded from the public purse, were horrific. Johann Reil, the nineteenth-century doctor from whom we get the term *psychiatry*, expressed outrage at the state of Germany's asylums: "Like criminals we lock these unfortunate creatures into mad-cages, into antiquated prisons, or put them next to the nesting holes of owls in desolate attics over the town gates or in the damp cellars of the jails, where the sympathetic gaze of a friend of mankind might never behold them; and we leave them there, gripped by chains, corrupting in their own filth." Elsewhere in Europe, conditions were as bad or worse. The Chantimoine tower in Caen, Normandy, for example, held a number of prisoners who were mad. In 1785 the tower was demolished, and the report of the demolition describes one of the inmates: "in the thickness of this tower's corner we found and pulled out . . . Jean Heude, called Bame, a tall and strong man incarcerated for twenty years, raving mad, naked and dangerous, whose door had not been opened for so long that the lock had to be knocked off with an iron bar." Symbolic of the inhumane state of Britain's asylums was the case of William Norris, an American marine who had been committed to Bethlem in 1801. An extremely violent man, he proved too dangerous to handle like an ordinary inmate. Bethlem's solution was to pin him to a wall with iron bars and put a chain around his neck that could be tightened from an adjacent room. When the Quaker reformer Edward Wakefield visited Bethlem in 1814, Norris had been shackled in this position for ten years.

In France, asylum reform was fueled in part by the revolutionary aspirations of liberty, equality, and fraternity. The political transformation of 1789 fed into a movement to storm, metaphorically, the Bastilles confining the mad. In 1793, as the story goes, in the spirit of the revolution, the asylum doctor Philippe Pinel liberated the inmates of the Salpêtrière Hospital from their chains, and with that act psychiatry was born. It was, in fact, Pinel's lay colleague at the Bicêtre, Jean Baptiste Pussin, who struck off the chains of the inmates, with Pinel following suit at the Salpêtrière, but Pinel remains the hero of the Whig history of psychiatry.

Crusaders such as Wakefield had been galvanized by moral outrage, whereas medical reformers believed that humane conditions would lead to better clinical outcomes. In 1813, Samuel Tuke, the grandson of the reformer William Tuke, published *Description of the Retreat,* which gave an account of a new form of asylum established by his grandfather in 1796. In contrast to the prison-like Bethlem and its ilk, the purpose of

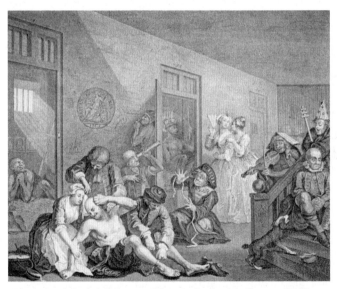

Figure 4: *A Rake's Progress,* Plate 8: *In the Madhouse,* William Hogarth, 1735. The painting shows two women "of note and quallitie"—the sort of people who were encouraged by the Governors of Bethlem to visit the hospital to view the "poore Lunatiques" for the edification of both visitor and inmate. Charles Deering McCormick Library of Special Collections, Northwestern University Library.

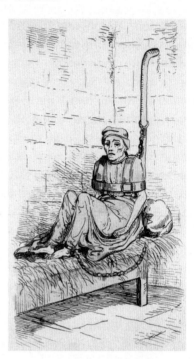

Figure 5: *Portrait of William Norris at Bedlam,* George Arnald, 1814, Clements C. Fry Collection, Yale University, Harvey Cushing/John Hay Whitney Medical Library. Reproduced with permission.

Tuke's asylum was to treat the mad rather than confine them. Advocates of the "therapeutic asylum"—Tuke and William Battie in England, Vincenzio Chiarugi in Italy, and Pinel in France—were Enlightenment men who were convinced of the power of reason and the possibility of cure by means of what Pinel called "moral (i.e., psychological) therapy" of patients, in which the doctor took "on an air of bonhomie and a tone of extreme frankness" in order to "penetrate into their most secret thoughts, clear up their anxieties, and deal with apparent contradictions by comparing their problems to those of others." By 1813, the idea of the therapeutic asylum had been around for more than sixty years, but Tuke's book marked a turning point.

One antecedent of moral therapy was new thinking about madness as a psychological phenomenon. From the time of Greek antiquity, as we've seen, madness had been understood to be either a disturbance of the soul or the body. By the nineteenth century, however, the debate about madness concerned whether it was a bodily disease or a *mental* one. The forerunner of the mentalist camp was John Locke, the great seventeenth-century empiricist philosopher. Locke (whose views laid the foundation for modern psychology) conceived of the mind as a store-house of "ideas," and thinking as a matter of their recombination. The madman, Locke said, puts "wrong ideas together."

Locke's views entered psychiatry by way of the Scottish physician William Cullen, who worked at the University of Edinburgh, the preeminent medical school of the second half of the eighteenth century. A goal of psychiatry at that time was to produce a taxonomy of mental illnesses, and Cullen became the great classifier who did for psychiatry what Linnaeus had done for biology. Cullen believed that mental disorders were indeed diseases of the nervous system, and he coined the term *neurosis* to designate them. In a remarkably prescient way, he hypothesized that the "nerve fluid" by which the brain functioned might be electrical and that mental disorders might come about by nervous over- or under-excitation. But in the spirit of Locke, he claimed that the *effect* of these neuroses was a psychological one—a "hurried association of ideas" producing "false judgement"—and under the influence of Cullen's views, the *mind* of the mental patient came to the fore in medical thinking about insanity and its treatment. Until the advent of psychoanalysis, however, psychiatric research was overwhelmingly concerned with the brain rather than the patient. If the new asylum were to offer psychological therapy, there would have to be doctors to man them, and this new generation of asylum doctors were the first professional psychiatrists. Their concern was their patients. Understanding the root causes of mental illness would have to wait.

Unfortunately, clean sheets and fresh air can only do so much to treat mental illness, and while some patients improved with informal psychological therapy, it did little for most of them. Without the hoped-for clinical success of moral treatment, the new high-minded asylums gradually lost their idealistic zeal and returned to their former function as warehouses for the chronically ill, even as patient numbers soared in England from about ten thousand in 1800 to one hundred thousand a century later. Some seventy years after Pinel struck off the chains at the Salpêtrière, Enlightenment optimism had faded, and asylums had returned to their earlier condition as custodial institutions whose task was not to cure but to keep the sick sedated, out of sight, and (because madness was now thought to be hereditary) celibate. Conditions in many of the asylums were again simply dreadful. The chains had been replaced by straitjackets and, in Britain, the apparently illegal use of isolation cells. Montagu Lomax, a doctor who worked in a British asylum during the First World War, describes a patient in one of these cells: "It was after 7 p.m., and no attendant was within call. The patient was beating on the door with his fists and feet, and was shrieking out curses and imprecations. 'For God's sake let me out, doctor! for God's sake let me out! O Christ, they are killing me! for God's sake let me out!'"

Things were no better elsewhere in Europe or in the New World. In the 1890s, "restraining sheets" were used to control patients. William Alanson White, a psychiatrist who had trained in New York, describes the sheets used at the Binghamton State Hospital as "a perfectly hellish contrivance, literally speaking, in hot weather" and claimed that he had "seen at least one patient die from heat exhaustion as a result of it." Not surprisingly, psychiatry as a profession was not attracting the best and brightest. The neurologist William Bullard derisively portrayed psychiatrists as good at the "heating of their buildings, the buying of coal and groceries, the making up of accounts," but not, it seemed, of practicing medicine. What had begun with the breaking of the chains of the mad had ended with a whimper and an echo of the asylum doors clanging shut.

JAMES TILLY MATTHEWS: THE AIR LOOM

The most famous of the victims of the brutal British asylum was James Tilly Matthews, a Welsh tea broker living in London. In 1796, Matthews wrote a letter to the Earl of Liverpool, an important statesman and confidant of the king, which quickly turned impolitic: "I pronounce your Lordship to be in every sense of the word a most diabolical Traitor." Matthews went on to enumerate in some detail the many grievous betrayals of Liverpool and closed by saying: "I profess myself to be at open war with you my Lord, and with all those your partners or Apostles in craft and Treason. You may succeed in imposing upon the World that I am insane but I will persevere till I convince you and the World that I am perfectly otherwise." It appears that Lord Liverpool had won the day. Less than two months later, in 1797, Matthews was committed to Bethlem, where he remained until the year before his death in 1815.

In 1809, Matthews's family petitioned the hospital to release him on the grounds that he had recovered and was no longer mad. The hospital refused, and the family took their case to court. Two doctors, George Birkbeck and Henry Clutterbuck, testified that Matthews was sane, but Bethlem's absentee psychiatrist, Thomas Monro, maintained that he was, in fact, a dangerous lunatic, and the hospital's "apothecary" or junior physician, John Haslam, concurred. Shortly thereafter, Haslam published an account of James Tilly Matthews's illness to exhibit Matthews's state of mind, and, in the process, to defend his own professional reputation. Haslam's *Illustrations of Madness* (1810) is the first extended case study in British psychiatry and perhaps the first clinical description in the psychiatric literature of what would come to be known as schizophrenia.

Haslam's book revealed that, while in Bethlem, Matthews had told a frankly unbelievable story of political intrigue in which he played the central role. He had been, he said, a British emissary to the French revolutionary government, empowered to carry on secret negotiations to bring about an end to the war between them that had begun in 1793. Unbelievable it was, but it may very well have been true. Matthews certainly had set out to act as an intermediary between Britain and France but wound up in a French jail. After being released, he went back to Britain convinced (as his letter to Liverpool shows) of a betrayal by his government.

While in Paris in 1793, Matthews had heard reports about Franz Mesmer, the doctor who claimed to have discovered a new force that he called "animal magnetism," which, when manipulated around the body of a sick person, could restore health. It could also be used to control minds. When Matthews returned to London, he became convinced that the betrayal of the British government had been effected by French spies using mesmeric techniques to pull the strings of the authorities, including the prime minister, William Pitt the Younger.

In the historical context, this idea wasn't actually mad. Other, presumably sane, people also thought that mesmerism was being used in the French war effort. Where Matthews's story veered away from reality was in his description of the details of the methods. Teams of spies, he said, had come to England with machines called "Air Looms" that could manipulate waves of animal magnetism and take control at a distance of the minds of British officials. Air Looms had therefore been set up to do their sinister work at various crucial locations, including outside of the Parliament. Moreover, villains supporting the French war effort—or perhaps the British who had betrayed Matthews—had also set up an Air Loom outside the walls of Bethlem to control and torment him. The villains were a gang of seven, four men and three women: Bill the King, who never smiles and is skilled in working the machine; Jack the Schoolmaster, who keeps the records of the gang's doings; Sir Archy, who uses a magnet and may, in fact, be a woman in men's clothing; the Middleman, who builds the Air Looms; Augusta, who acts as a liaison with other gangs in the West End of London; Charlotte, who is kept nearly naked and poorly fed; and the Glove Woman, who never speaks and wears cotton mittens because she has "the itch." "At home," Matthews believed, "they lie together in promiscuous intercourse and filthy community."

The Air Loom itself operates on the principles of pneumatic chemistry, the chemistry of gases that was at the cutting edge of science in Matthews's day, and is fueled by "the vapours of vitriol and aqua fortis—ditto of nightshade and hellebore—effluvia of dogs—stinking human breath—putrid effluvia—ditto of mortification and of the plague—stench of the sesspool—gaz from the anus of the horse—human gaz—gaz of the horse's greasy heels." As depicted in Matthews's drawing of it—he was a gifted draftsman—the Air Loom is made up of pipes and levers, tubes and barrels, and something that looks rather like a windmill (see Figure 6).

In his case history, Haslam tells us that the persecution of Matthews takes different forms, among them "fluid locking," which immobilizes his tongue and prevents him from speaking; "kiteing," in which ideas are "lifted" into the brain; and "thigh-talking," which causes Matthews to hear through his thigh. His body is controlled and his thoughts manipulated by the Air Loom, and he lives under constant threat of torture or death by "stomach-skinning," "apoplexy-working with the nutmeg grater," "lobster-cracking," "bladder-filling," "gaz-plucking," "eye-screwing," "roof-stringing," "bomb-bursting," and other malevolent forms of magnetic voodoo.

In 1813, sixteen years after having been committed, Matthews was moved to London House, a private clinic run by Samuel Fox, where he died in 1815, probably of tuberculosis contracted in Bethlem. But he continued to haunt Haslam and the British asylum. The Quaker reformer

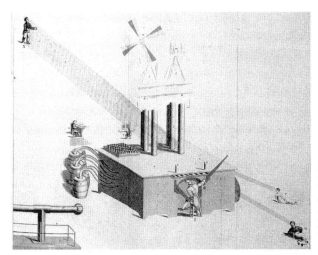

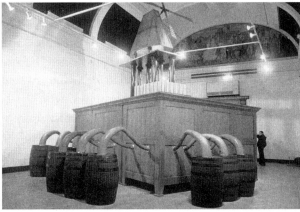

Figure 6:
Matthews's
depiction of the Air
Loom. Wellcome
Library, London.
And a recreation:
*The Air Loom, A
Human Influencing
Machine*, Rod
Dickinson, 2002.
Reproduced by
permission of the artist.

Edward Wakefield had sought out Matthews in Fox's clinic and found him "a man of considerable accomplishments" and quite plainly sane. In the pursuit of reform, Wakefield persuaded the government to set up a House of Commons select committee to look into the state of the country's madhouses. In the course of its investigations, the case of James Tilly Matthews came to play a starring role. Matthews's nephew, Richard Staveley, called as a witness, testified that although Matthews had some clearly odd ideas, they didn't drive him to abnormal behavior; he was as sane as the next man, as many people (including other psychiatrists) had discovered firsthand. He also claimed that Haslam, who was effectively in charge at Bedlam, had had Matthews in chains for two years, not for any medical reason but because Matthews would not "submit" to Haslam's authority. Testimony given on a later occasion by James Simmonds, head keeper of Bethlem, confirmed Staveley's opinion: "The irons," he said, "were put on him to punish him for the use of his tongue."

Haslam himself testified before the committee and was raked over the coals. All the crimes of the old asylum, it seems, were being laid at his door. When his position came up for renewal in 1816, the governors of Bethlem informed him that his services were no longer required.

THE DISEASED ORGAN

Although it was asylum psychiatry that had created the need for a professional class, the theory that dominated eighteenth- and nineteenth-century psychiatry was firmly rooted in medicine. The rise of modern science in the seventeenth century had been intertwined with the "mechanical philosophy" of nature, according to which natural objects were understood as machines. Because the explanation of madness was to be mechanistic, attention had to move away from the four humors to the putative mechanism of interest: the brain. Although there was a persistent "mentalist" tradition in thinking about insanity, by 1845, Wilhelm Griesinger—author of *Mental Pathology and Therapeutics,* the most important psychiatric textbook of his day—could express the orthodoxy by asking, "What organ must necessarily and invariably be diseased where there is madness? . . . Physiological and pathological facts show us that this organ can only be the brain." With this pronouncement, Griesinger planted psychiatry's flag in natural science and declared it a branch of biology.

If the road to madness ran through the brain, then the study of madness would have to adapt. Brain dissection and the microscope, therefore, became the state of the art in psychiatry as they had been in neurology, where they had delivered the goods. By the nineteenth century, it seemed clear that particular regions of the brain supported unique psychological functions, which postmortem examination of patients with brain damage had made it possible to identify. In 1874, for example, Carl Wernicke pinpointed a region of the brain that, when damaged, leads to difficulties in understanding spoken language—a disorder now known as Wernicke's aphasia. Wernicke and other leading neurologists like Griesinger, Theodor Meynert, Eduard Hitzig, and Paul Flechsig (of whom more shortly) believed that the signs of madness were etched into the substrate of the brain as they were in neurological illness. All that modern medicine had to do was learn to read them.

But the optimism of these early biological psychiatrists was premature. The brains of the mad were *not* visibly different from those of healthy people. The fault lay less in the theories of the neuropsychiatrists than in their technology: the brain disorders associated with madness were beyond the resolution of the anatomist's microscope. Clues to its biology would have to wait until the twentieth century, when the chemists got involved.

The failure of early biological psychiatry caused the theory of madness to drift from the structure of the brain to its function. Psychiatrists began to consider the possibility that mental illness might arise in a brain that was physically intact but functionally abnormal; this would certainly explain why microscopes and dissections could not reveal the underlying causes of madness. By the 1890s, Cullen's neuroses were distinguished, therefore, from the *psycho*neuroses and from *psychosis*, both of which designated the illnesses associated with a *malfunctioning* brain without anatomical pathology. The focus on "functional" illnesses rather than brain lesions remained largely unchanged for almost a century.

With the decline of the therapeutic asylum and the defeat of the biological method, psychiatry had come to dual dead ends. It was into this world of discouraged caregivers and theoretical impasse that Emil Kraepelin and Sigmund Freud burst like supernovas.

THE VARIETIES OF MADNESS

Popular culture takes Sigmund Freud to be the father of modern psychiatry, but Freud had an intellectual twin, Emil Kraepelin, born in Germany in the same year as Freud, and it is Kraepelin, not Freud, who is contemporary psychiatry's patron saint.

Kraepelin began his career as an assistant to the neuroanatomist Paul

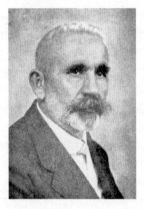

Figure 7: Emil Kraepelin (1856–1926).

Flechsig but found working life with him to be so disagreeable that he left after three months. Part of the problem was Kraepelin himself; he had eye trouble and couldn't use a microscope. Still, this handicap didn't stop his progress, and by 1890 he was professor of psychiatry in Heidelberg. In his Heidelberg clinic, Kraepelin began to keep records of new patients. Every patient had a card on which he recorded his or her history and a provisional diagnosis. After a few weeks of observation, he and his colleagues would revise their diagnosis and add a description of the patient's state of mind on discharge. In this way, the change in the illness over time came into relief. Kraepelin's great contribution to psychiatry was thus to focus attention on the *course* of illness rather than on its fleeting symptoms.

By observing how mental illness developed, Kraepelin saw something that we now take for granted: madness is not monolithic. There were, Kraepelin found, two forms of insanity. The first, which he called "manic-depressive psychosis," was characterized by symptoms of alternating euphoric and depressed moods. The second, "dementia praecox" (or "early dementia"), had no essential connection to mood but was marked, he thought, by a decline in cognitive function. For patients with dementia praecox, the prognosis was poor; for those with manic-depressive psychosis, it was surprisingly good.

Kraepelin's hypothesis about dementia praecox turned out to be incorrect. It became clear, in due course, that while those suffering from it showed abnormalities of thought, they were not undergoing cognitive decline. In 1908, the Swiss psychiatrist Eugen Bleuler proposed replacing Kraepelin's term with "schizophrenia," a reference to a bifurcation in the mind or in psychological function. The misconstruction of schizophrenia as a form of split personality has its roots in this term and (unfortunately) persists.

In emphasizing the course of illness rather than its symptoms, Kraepelin had moved psychiatric theory toward matters of description and classification, which, by the 1880s, had become common practice in other areas of pathology. Kraepelin published a textbook of psychiatry in 1883 that outlined his psychiatric taxonomy and spent the rest of his professional life on successive revisions. The sixth edition, in 1899, introduced the distinction between dementia praecox and manic-depressive psychosis, and provided the model for our modern classification.

Although his conception of schizophrenia turned out to be wrong, Kraepelin did more than any of his predecessors to make psychiatry a branch of medicine. In the absence of a demonstrable connection between the brain and mental illness, however, the medicalization of psychiatry had to move forward without a beachhead in a diseased organ. Mental illness was surely a brain disease, but at the turn of the twentieth century, that idea was of no practical use.

PSYCHOANALYSIS:
FROM THE INTRAPSYCHIC TO THE INTERPERSONAL

Freud's intellectual development, like Kraepelin's, also began with a focus on the brain, and he had high hopes of understanding mental illness scientifically as brain disease. He had trained at the Salpêtrière with Jean-Martin Charcot, one of the preeminent neurologists of his time, who was interested in, among other things, the sexual origins of the disorder known then as "hysteria." ("It is always something genital," he is supposed to have whispered to Freud.) On the road away from the brain, Kraepelin headed toward medicine; Freud turned to the mind and its unconscious.

The bulk of Freud's theory developed out of his experience outside the hospital with patients suffering from *non*psychotic illness—hysteria most famously—and he neither treated madness nor had much interest in it. This was partly a matter of personal predilection. In a letter to István Hollós, the analyst who first introduced hospital-based psychoanalytic treatment for psychotic patients, Freud writes that these patients "make me angry and I find myself irritated to experience them so distant from myself and from all that is human. This is an astonishing intolerance which brands me a poor psychiatrist."

Freud first attempted to grapple with psychosis in 1896 when he published "Analysis of a Case of Paranoia." In keeping with his theories of hysteria from that period, he hypothesizes that "paranoia, too, is a psychosis of defence; that is to say, that, like hysteria and obsessions, it proceeds from the repression of distressing memories and that its symptoms are determined in their form by the content of what has been repressed." The case concerned a certain Frau P., who suffered from paranoia as well as visual and auditory hallucinations. She "complained that she was being watched" sometimes while undressing and that "people were reading her thoughts and knew everything that was going on in her house." Her visual hallucinations were of naked women as well as male and female genitalia, and "these hallucinations," Freud believed, "were nothing else than parts of the content of repressed childhood experiences, symptoms of the return of the repressed." Freud hypothesized that the hallucinations had to do with Frau P. and her brother "showing each other naked before going to bed" as youngsters, and he concludes that Frau P. "was now making up for the shame which she had omitted to feel as a child."

According to Freud, one's sexual development begins in childhood with autoeroticism, then "oscillates all through his life between heterosexual and homosexual feelings, and any frustration or disappointment in the one direction is apt to drive him over into the other." Freud claimed that when unconscious and (to the subject) unacceptable homosexual feelings begin to enter into awareness, paranoia—an illness he thought to be distinct from schizophrenia—might ensue. He believed a frustration might instead induce withdrawal of one's libido—strictly speaking, sexual energy—from the outside world and direct it back onto the self. This profound psychological regression to the autoerotic, infantile state produces schizophrenia, which Freud believed was incurable. Of course, everyone experiences frustration in life, but because people respond to frustration in different ways, not everyone develops schizophrenia: "[n]eurosis is the result of a conflict between the ego and its id, whereas psychosis is the analogous outcome of a similar disturbance in the relations between the ego and the external world."

Freud believed that psychotic patients "have turned away from outer reality; but for that very reason they know more about internal, psychical reality and can reveal a number of things to us that would otherwise be inaccessible to us." Moreover, Freud came to see delusions as a consequence of the patient's effort to repair the damage of the same psychological assault that drove the libido inward. He concluded that "delusion is found applied like a patch over the place where originally a rent had appeared in the ego's relation to the external world."

Despite Freud's belief that studying psychosis could further our understanding of the mind, he had no illusions about the psychoanalytic treatment of psychotic patients. According to Freud, one could not treat psychosis with psychoanalysis, because a person who has withdrawn his or her libido from the world is incapable of entering into a transference relationship, the foundation of the analytic process. The transference that develops between patient and psychoanalyst allows the patient to play out unconscious conflicts with primal figures, which the analyst can then interpret. No libido, no transference; no transference, no interpretation; and without interpretation, treatment is impossible.

If Freud's followers had heeded his instructions, the story might end there. But a number of psychoanalysts in Europe continued to theorize about psychosis, and a few took on the analytic treatment of schizophrenia, often with poor or even disastrous results. There were some successes. One analyst who had good outcomes with patients was Paul Federn, a member of Freud's inner circle, who believed that some patients with schizophrenia could develop transference, have some insight that they are ill, and direct at least some of their attention to external reality. In opposition to Freud, Federn believed that psychotic patients had too *little* libido invested in themselves, not too much. As such, Federn was less interested in uncovering unconscious material from the mind of the psychotic patient than in strengthening the patient's weakened ego, and he insisted that psychoanalysts "must help the patient in the actual affairs of his life." In practice, then, Federn's method resembles what we now think of as supportive psychotherapy. Federn was also ahead of his time with respect to acknowledging the importance of the social environment in psychosis. Without support of the psychotic patient's family, successful treatment was, he thought, impossible. Federn urged practitioners to treat psychotic patients with respect and do everything possible to remain on good terms with them, so as to be in the best position to bolster their frail egos. William Sledge claims that Federn's theory of a weakened ego "ultimately has become the centerpiece of modern psychoanalytic conceptualizations of schizophrenia."

Another major figure in the psychoanalytic treatment of psychosis was the Hungarian analyst Sándor Ferenczi, who also believed that a therapeutic connection could be made between the schizophrenic patient and the analyst, and that if an analysis was not a success, the problem lay in the analyst's technique, not in the patient's inability to develop transference. Ferenczi was actively involved with his patients during sessions, and his technique embraced the use of countertransference, the unconscious feelings stirred up in the analyst by the patient, which could then be used to help the analyst better understand his patient. While regarded as a compassionate psychoanalyst, Ferenczi took his practice to unusual limits, engaging on one occasion in a "mutual analysis" with a disturbed patient, Elizabeth Severn, and concluding, after the two analyzed each another, that *he* was the one who was schizophrenic. In the words of Jay S. Kwawer, Ferenczi "was challenged by working with patients who had been dismissed as hopeless cases, or 'lost causes,' and admirably stretched the boundaries of the more timid approaches that colleagues were wedded to."

After World War I, the epicenter of psychoanalysis moved west to England and the United States. In London, Anna Freud further developed her father's ego psychology, which embraces the "structural" model of the mind (id, ego, superego), her most significant contribution being her study of the defenses (or defense mechanisms). Ego psychologists largely followed her father's advice to leave psychosis alone. The other dominant school of psychoanalysis grew out of "object relations theory," with Melanie Klein its foremost figure. *Object* is an unfortunate term signifying a person, often an important one from early childhood, who leaves powerful unconscious vestiges that continue to exert an influence into adulthood.

Klein theorized that in the first months of life, babies want to take in pleasure and expel pain. As a result, they split the outer world—which at this stage is made up exclusively of the mother—into two distinct representations, the "good breast," which feeds and gives pleasure, and the "bad breast," which withholds and causes pain. The infant feels persecuted by the bad breast, and in turn wants to destroy it. This is the "paranoid-schizoid" position. Not only is the external world split, but the self is split into good and bad elements as well. In normal development, the infant is later able to accept that there is only one loving, if imperfect, mother, and once the mental representations of other people are integrated, the infant can do the same for itself. This is the "depressive" position. However, if this developmental process is derailed somehow, the infant experiences overwhelming anxiety, and psychosis might be the eventual result.

Donald Winnicott, an English psychoanalyst (and pediatrician), was supervised by Klein. However, owing to his original ideas, he belonged to the so-called middle group of analysts, independent of both the Freudian and Kleinian schools. Winnicott famously wrote, "There is no such thing as an infant," meaning that the infant is an inextricable part of the mother-infant whole. He believed that failures in parenting—serious deficits of attunement and empathy—could block the development of the child's core identity and might thereby result in psychosis, which he described as "an environmental deficiency disease."

In the United States, the treatment of psychosis tended to take place in hospitals, rather than in consulting rooms. The Washington School of Psychiatry developed an approach called "interpersonal psychoanalysis," which held that the cause of mental illness was difficulty in relationships with others. By extension, they thought that human relationships could help the mentally ill, including those suffering from psychosis.

Harry Stack Sullivan was the most influential figure among the interpersonalists. He worked first at St. Elizabeth's Hospital in Washington, DC, then at Sheppard Pratt Hospital in Maryland. Though he was not formally trained as a psychoanalyst, he considered himself to be a Freudian, and his techniques held sway at Chestnut Lodge, another psychiatric hospital in Maryland renowned for its analytic treatments of psychotic patients.

Sullivan challenged Freud's view of the importance of the child's libido and put a greater emphasis on the formative role of culture and society. He was lauded, in particular, for his success in treating hospitalized patients with schizophrenia in a "therapeutic milieu," an inpatient setting where patients and staff interacted and where the primary focus was on ordinary social interactions. In his posthumously published book, *Schizophrenia as a Human Process,* Sullivan described training his staff and the consequent benefits of the therapeutic milieu to both patients and staff:

[I]f we changed the attitudes of these sensitive, shy, and ordinarily considered handicapped employees so that they had some notion of the schizophrenic as a person—in other words, if they ceased to regard him as "insane," but instead had stressed to them the many points of significant resemblance between the patient and the employee—we created a much more useful social situation . . . [T]hings which I cannot distinguish from genuine human friendships sprang up between patient and employee . . . and . . . the institutional recovery rate became high.

Other theorists tended to dismiss the content of the ideas of the patient with psychosis, but Sullivan believed there was meaning in his patients' communications and that it was the difficulty with relationships—in particular, the effects of overly anxious parents—that contributed to the development of schizophrenia. The treatment, therefore, was the good relationship between the doctor and patient, and the central duty of the therapist was to do whatever was necessary to connect with his patients, and to become a "participant-observer," a term borrowed from cultural anthropology to refer to the direct involvement required to understand other cultures. Writing about his time at Chestnut Lodge, John Kafka, an interpersonal analyst, recalled it as a place where the staff believed that there were healthy as well as psychotic aspects of their patients' minds and that both required attention. Kafka invokes the ethos of the participant-observer: "In retrospect, I think that those of us interested in being therapists of psychotics in some way resembled a group of anthropologists who wanted to understand and to find a way of communicating with the inhabitants of psychosis-land."

Like Federn's practice, Sullivan's more closely resembles treatment of hospitalized people with schizophrenia today (minus the medication) than it does classical psychoanalysis. By 1947, when he supervised the treatment of Jim, a young navy veteran, Sullivan had stopped using terms like the *unconscious, id, ego,* or *superego.* Instead, he talked about Jim's relationships with his parents, sexual partners, boyhood friends—a particularly significant developmental relationship, according to Sullivan, is the "chum"—and, of course, with his therapist. Sullivan was also interested in the important events in Jim's life, his self-esteem, and his loneliness. Sullivan was *not* particularly interested in Jim's dreams, at least for the time being. Although he encouraged all psychiatrists to read Freud's *The Interpretation of Dreams,* he warned doctors to avoid searching for the "latent" material in the dreams of people with schizophrenia and instead suggested that they "[s]ee if there is some way of making a succinct statement of the manifest dramatic story told in the dream." As for interpretations, they are primarily evidence that the psychiatrist isn't sure "what the hell he is trying to do." "People come to me," he said, "to have difficulties in living untangled." Though his approach may have seemed radical, it was adopted by many later practitioners, and Sullivan has been called "the most influential native-born figure in American psychiatry."

Sullivan and the other interpersonalists challenged strict Freudian theory by taking the environment to be an important factor in development, healthy or otherwise. Schizophrenia was the result of deficient family relationships or dynamics, though analysts differed in their views about what sort of deficiency was most toxic. The central villain, however, was usually—in the infamous words of Frieda Fromm-Reichmann—the "schizophrenogenic mother," who is both overprotective and rejecting. Over the course of sixty or seventy years, psychoanalysis moved outward from a focus on internal psychological conflicts to distortions arising in the developing child's social environment as the cause of psychosis. The cost of this shift was laid at the feet of parents, who were told that they were responsible for the fact that their child had developed schizophrenia.

Looking back at the first half of the twentieth century, psychoanalysis appears like a reasonable form of therapy when compared to other treatments for psychosis available at the time, like frontal lobotomy. But times and treatments were changing. Psychoanalysis dominated psychiatry until the 1970s, when it was attacked for deficiencies of all kinds, including its views about psychosis. In 1984, Thomas McGlashan, a psychiatrist at Chestnut Lodge, published a follow-up study of the patients who had been treated there approximately fifteen years earlier. The results were discouraging, to say the least: two-thirds of the patients treated at Chestnut Lodge were ill or only marginally functional. "The data are in," McGlashan said. "The experiment failed."

If that weren't enough, in the 1980s, Raphael Osheroff, a physician, was treated at Chestnut Lodge for what was diagnosed as narcissistic personality disorder with an accompanying manic-depressive illness. He was given months of psychotherapy to no effect and was not offered any medication. He was subsequently transferred to Silver Hill Hospital in Connecticut, where he was successfully treated with medication for what was diagnosed as psychotic depression. After Osheroff recovered, he sued Chestnut Lodge for malpractice, and the case was settled out of court. McGlashan's study and the Osheroff suit had a chilling effect on any psychoanalyst contemplating treating severe mental illness with talk therapy. In due course, psychoanalysis came to see the wisdom of Freud's warning and left psychosis to the psychiatrists.

DONALD: DEPRESSION AND DAMNATION

Donald called his friend Leon to say good-bye. He apologized for what he had done. He had been waiting for God to punish him, but was now tired of waiting and was taking matters into his own hands through suicide. Leon wisely played for time by suggesting that he would come by Donald's apartment to say good-bye. When Donald hesitantly agreed, Leon hung up and called 911 immediately. Donald was brought to Bellevue.

Donald was a fifty-nine-year-old white man with no previous psychiatric history. He had worked in a number of sales jobs over the years and had been happily married for thirty-five years until his wife, Delia, had passed away three years earlier. Since that time, according to Leon, Donald had become more reclusive, no longer coming over to watch Giants games on Sundays and often going days without leaving his apartment. He had no children and few friends.

Simply looking at Donald, one would suspect he was depressed— slumped in his chair, tearful, his face hollowed, his brow furrowed—and talking with him removed all doubt. He had a number of classic symptoms: poor appetite with weight loss, insomnia, low energy, the inability to enjoy anything, and, most seriously, the desire to die.

But Donald didn't simply want to die to relieve the pain of his depression. He needed to pay for his sins. Donald said that he had cursed the planet for eternity and had to be punished. Worse, he came to believe that since God had not killed him for his sins, Donald, through his sinning, had in fact killed God.

And what had he done to kill God and curse the planet? His sin was fornication. Not only had Donald had a sexual encounter after his wife died, but he was also plagued by the fact that it happened on Easter, and for this he could not be forgiven.

Donald was placed on one-to-one suicide watch: a health worker at Bellevue stayed with him day and night, ensuring he would not attempt suicide while in the hospital. He refused all medication and food. He wouldn't talk to members of the treatment team or receive a visit from the hospital clergy. Transfer to a medical unit was ordered, and a court hearing to have him fed over his objection was the likely next step. But where his psychiatrists, social workers, one-to-ones, and the rest of us were unable to reach Donald, his fellow inpatients did. Though Donald was too depressed to talk, much less socialize, his roommate and others on the unit continued to cajole, plead with, even tease Donald to join the group and, mostly, to eat. We were relieved when Donald's new associates told him the staff were morons; that we didn't know the first thing about helping him, but that he could trust them. It worked. Donald grudgingly began to eat. In time, he accepted medication.

After his fellow patients saved him from starvation, Donald began to talk to the staff. He was so ashamed of what he'd done. He had loved Delia with all his heart, and he'd sullied their marriage after her death by sleeping with another woman. Donald was not very religious, but Delia was. She observed Easter, and Donald went along to mass. But after her death he stopped. He hadn't even realized that his tryst had happened on Easter weekend until days later. And that was when the guilt began to torment him. It was difficult to determine if his guilt had precipitated his depression or if his depression predated his guilt. Certainly he was suffering from a full-blown major depressive episode when he developed his delusions.

As Donald's depression slowly lifted, his delusions abated: he no longer believed that he had cursed the world or killed God. When his mood improved, he no longer sought self-punitive annihilation. He was thankful to his friends on the unit for what they had done for him. He told them how much they would have loved Delia.—JG

BIOLOGICAL PSYCHIATRY RETURNS

The biological psychiatry of the nineteenth century—exemplified by the work of Wernicke, Flechsig, and others—had failed to break the neural code of mental illness, and by the end of the Great War, it was clear that it had nothing to offer patients. As a result, psychoanalysis continued to dominate academic psychiatry into the 1970s. A number of factors conspired to bring the psychoanalytic era to a close, including the inauguration of a new form of biological psychiatry and the move toward a Kraepelinian model of disease classification. These two themes are the topics of this section and the next.

After languishing for decades, biological psychiatry made a spectacular comeback in the years after the Second World War, fueled in large part by the discovery of drugs to treat mental illness, including psychosis. The first of the great discoveries was made by an Australian doctor, John Cade, who, observing that lithium salts had a calming effect on guinea pigs, tried it on psychiatric patients. In patients with mania, in particular, it had remarkable effects. All of the patients improved, and half got well enough to be discharged from the hospital. Despite its monumental importance, however, the discovery of lithium was slow to make its mark on psychiatry. Cade was, as he put it, "an unknown psychiatrist, working alone in a small chronic hospital with no research training, primitive techniques and negligible equipment." Working in a small town in Australia wouldn't have helped either. The first shot of the psychopharmacological revolution that was heard came from Europe.

Psychopharmacology developed by accident, as a by-product of textile production. In the second half of the nineteenth century, organic chemists got interested in how to make new compounds, a pursuit stimulated to a large extent by the textile industry. Natural dyes were expensive, and textile makers were badly in need of methods to create synthetic versions. In 1856, the chemist William Perkin formulated "aniline purple," or mauve, the first synthetic dye, and its financial success led to a host of new ones: fuchsin, Bismarck brown, imperial blue, quinoline blue.

In the early days, synthetic dyes were made by trial and error, but as chemistry began to understand the molecular structure of organic compounds, new substances could be made by applying theory rather than guesswork. German chemistry led the way. In 1868, Carl Graebe and Carl Libermann synthesized the natural red dye alizarin, which was then produced commercially by the Badische Anilin und Soda-Fabrik (BASF) under the direction of the chemist Heinrich Caro. In 1876, Caro produced a new dye, methylene blue, and hired August Bernthsen to investigate its chemical structure. The core of the compound, Bernthsen discovered, was the molecule phenothiazine.

It was at this point that industrial chemistry and medicine collided in the figure of Paul Ehrlich. Born in 1854 in Germany, Ehrlich studied medicine but was not much of a student because he spent all of his time staining tissue. ("That is little Ehrlich," one of his medical teachers is supposed to have said. "He is very good at staining, but he will never pass his examinations.") But there was a big idea behind Ehrlich's obsession. He theorized that if a substance stains tissue, it must be because there is a strong chemical affinity between the two that could be put to medical use. A compound that stains—and therefore bonds selectively to—a disease-causing organism could potentially be used to destroy it without damaging the healthy cells of the host. Successful staining, therefore, could identify what Ehrlich dubbed "magic bullets," and he hoped that methylene blue was going to be the first of them. Early on, Ehrlich had discovered that methylene blue stained the malarial parasite. In 1891, in what was to be the founding event of the field of chemotherapy, Ehrlich gave methylene blue to two patients with malaria and cured them.

In the years that followed, a number of researchers experimented with chemical variants of methylene blue in search of more powerful antimalarial drugs. Among them was Paul Charpentier, a chemist working at the French pharmaceutical company Rhône-Poulenc after World War II. Although these compounds proved largely ineffective against malaria, they were found to have antihistamine properties. The first antihistamine had been formulated in 1937, and this class of drugs was thought to have enormous medical promise. Phenothiazine compounds were suddenly important.

In 1949, a third train of events intersected with the phenothiazine drugs. Henri Laborit, a French navy surgeon, reported his use of antihistamines to treat postoperative shock. Shock is an abnormality in the circulatory system (with low blood pressure, rapid heart rate, and cold sweat among its signs), and it can be life-threatening. It is a common feature of battlefield injuries and a serious problem in surgery. Histamine, the immune molecule that antihistamines target, is a central player in shock—anaphylaxis, for example, is a histamine process—and Laborit thought that antihistamines could be useful in treating it. He also thought that the sleep-inducing qualities of antihistamines, familiar to many allergy sufferers, made them valuable for use in surgical anesthesia. He started experimenting with promethazine, the first phenothiazine-based commercial antihistamine (marketed as Phenergan), and found that it not only made patients sleepy but also worked as a painkiller. And antihistamines didn't just sedate patients but led to a "euphoric quietude." Laborit also thought that there might be a second use for antihistamines in surgery. One way of lessening the risk of postoperative shock, he believed, would be to use less anesthetic by reducing the patient's basal metabolism before administering it. He formulated a mixture of drugs that he called the "lytic cocktail" for this purpose, and antihistamines were among the ingredients.

By 1950, Pierre Koetschet, assistant scientific director at Rhône-Poulenc, decided that there was enough preliminary data (from Laborit and others) on the phenothiazine compounds to merit more systematic research into their use in anesthesia, and he initiated a research program for that purpose. New compounds were synthesized by Paul Charpentier, and Simone Courvoisier, also at Rhône-Poulenc, carried out animal studies on the behavioral effects of the new compounds. One of Charpentier's new compounds was 4560 RP, or chlorpromazine, and it was immediately clear that chlorpromazine affected behavior in a big way. Courvoisier and her colleagues found that although it was not an antihistamine, chlorpromazine enhanced anesthesia considerably, lowered metabolism, and brought about "psychic disorientation." Human trials were carried out, and Rhône-Poulenc concluded that chlorpromazine might indeed have useful applications in surgery, obstetrics, and psychiatry.

In the meantime, Laborit had moved to Paris from Tunisia, where his early studies had been carried out, and began working with the anesthesiologist Pierre Huguenard on "artificial hibernation," a process of lowering body temperature, and thereby metabolism, as yet another means of reducing the risk of surgical shock. The technique wasn't new, but Laborit and Huguenard modified it by adding the lytic cocktail to the procedure: the patient was given the drugs, and body temperature was lowered by applying icepacks. Given Rhône-Poulenc's results with chlorpromazine, it seemed the obvious drug to try in combination with body cooling. Laborit and Huguenard began using chlorpromazine as part of artificial hibernation therapy and found that it was effective enough to allow them to dispense with many of the other drugs in the lytic cocktail. Remarkably, they noticed that chlorpromazine made it possible to carry out some surgeries without the kind of anesthesia that rendered patients unconscious. In 1948, Huguenard had had to anesthetize one of his nurses, who needed an operation on her nose. Since he couldn't administer anesthesia with a mask, he gave her a combination of pethidene and promethazine and found that during the surgery she was almost entirely indifferent to what was going on. Given this dramatic psychological effect, applications in psychiatry seemed even more clearly indicated, and Laborit began urging his colleagues to explore the possibilities.

A number of trials with the drug were carried out in 1951 and 1952. Jean Sigwald and Daniel Bouttier, for example, gave chlorpromazine to a fifty-seven-year-old woman, who heard voices and had paranoid thoughts. After the woman spent some months on the drug, the doctors reported that she "no longer talks about herself or her hallucinations; she is gay, works, and reads; sleep is normal. When questioned, she says she hears voices as before, but she does not interpret them to herself; there is no disappearance of the hallucinations, but their interpretation has become very imprecise, and there is no longer any complaint or threat of vengeance."

The work that ignited the chlorpromazine explosion, however, was done by two French psychiatrists, Jean Delay and Pierre Deniker, at St. Anne's Psychiatric Hospital in Paris. Deniker had by chance heard about the use of chlorpromazine in Laborit's hibernation therapy from his brother-in-law, an anesthetist. Unlike many of his colleagues, Delay believed that mental disorders could be treated by drugs and was interested in exploring new compounds. Having tried chlorpromazine in concert with hibernation therapy, Deniker and Delay quickly decided that it was too risky for their patients and moved on to trying chlorpromazine alone across a wide range of symptoms. They got the best response in delirious patients who, after being given chlorpromazine, quickly became reoriented. Patients with schizophrenia also improved dramatically, as did those suffering from depression. By 1953, Delay and Deniker claimed that treatment with chlorpromazine was so effective that it had "brought about a transformation in the atmosphere of the locked wards and definitely relegated the old means of restraint." They dubbed chlorpromazine a "neuroleptic" (literally "nerve-seizing")—a substance that reduces nervous system activity.

The typically sober professional reports of chlorpromazine's effectiveness almost certainly understate the amazement this new drug must have occasioned in the doctors who administered it. Chlorpromazine wasn't a typical sedative, so it didn't just dampen raging psychosis. Psychotic patients who had been stuporous and uncommunicative became responsive, and the voices they had been hearing often disappeared. A barber from Lyon who had been in a stupor for years "woke up" after being given chlorpromazine and said that he wanted to go home and get back to work. His doctor, Jean Perrin, suggested the patient give him a shave to prove he was up to it. Cutthroat razor in hand, he did the job as if he had never left the barbershop.

Ironically, it was chlorpromazine's astounding success that slowed its progress in psychiatry. Doctors simply did not believe that there could be anything like it—"a drug," as Deniker later put it, that "could truly modify a mental disorder, which is such a complex neurologic, biochemical, and social phenomenon." For us today, awash in a sea of psychopharmaceuticals, it is hard to imagine how deep the skepticism must have run; to anyone who hadn't seen its effects firsthand, chlorpromazine must have sounded like science fiction. Nonetheless, the cumulative reports of its effects couldn't be denied, and in 1952, Rhône-Poulenc decided to market it commercially. Introducing it under the name Largactil, the company identified chlorpromazine's applications as anesthesia, acute mania, and vomiting, in that order. The revolution was just getting going.

The new drug entered North America through Canada. Rhône-Poulenc had an office in French-speaking Montreal, and a company rep visited the Verdun Hospital (now called the Douglas Institute of McGill University) and left Deniker and Delay's papers on chlorpromazine with the psychiatrist Heinz Lehmann, a German immigrant who read French. "About three to four weeks later," Lehmann recalled, "I was catching up on my reading in the bathtub on Sunday morning and got to the Rhône-Poulenc materials . . . I couldn't quite believe it, but thought, if it's true, it offers an entirely new treatment concept." Lehmann and one of his medical residents, T. E. Hanrahan, gave the drug to seventy-one patients and got the same results as Deniker and Delay had. "At the time," Lehmann said,

> we thought we were just treating excited states with CPZ [chlorproma-zine] and attributed the improvement that the schizophrenics showed to that effect of the drug. But then, about three months after the trial had ended, we discovered that some of the chronic, back-ward schizo-phrenics had been accidentally left on large doses of CPZ. And incred-ibly, to us, four or five of these back-ward patients were getting better. No one believed that a pill could cause remission in schizophrenia, and we seemed to be getting the best results with chronic paranoids, the group most refractory to treatment.

Lehmann did a second study with patients diagnosed with chronic schizophrenia, and "[a]t the end of four or five weeks," he said, "there were a lot of symptom-free patients. By this, I mean that a lot of halluci-nations, delusions, and thought disorder had disappeared. In 1953, there just wasn't anything that ever produced something like this—a remission from schizophrenia in weeks."

Lehmann published the first papers in English on the use of chlor-promazine and made the drug known in North America. Rhône-Poulenc offered the license for chlorpromazine to the American pharmaceuti-cal company Smith Kline & French, which released it in 1954 under the trade name Thorazine for use in nausea and vomiting, as well as psychi-atry. But American psychiatrists were reluctant to take it up. Apart from their skepticism about the possibility of a wonder drug for madness, the dominant psychoanalytic model could not countenance the notion that mental illness could be treated biologically. "At the time," Lehmann said, "no one in his right mind in psychiatry was working with drugs."

Nonetheless, by 1955, many psychiatrists had at last begun to under-stand that chlorpromazine could treat schizophrenia, and they used it because it worked. What had started out as a way of making cheap tex-tiles had wound up—after an astonishingly improbable series of chance discoveries, bold conjecture, and good luck—as the first effective treat-ment for madness in history.

But how did chlorpromazine work? No one knew. The theory of its action, and of the many antipsychotic drugs that followed, was developed to a large extent by the Swedish Nobel laureate Arvid Carlsson, Solomon Snyder in the United States, and Philip Seeman in Canada. Their research showed that antipsychotic drugs targeted dopamine receptors—molecules on the surface of certain brain cells that form chemical bonds with the neurotransmitter dopamine—thereby preventing dopamine itself from doing so. When dopamine is blocked in this way, the symptoms of schizophrenia wane. This finding led to the formulation of the "dopamine hypothesis" of schizophrenia, first articulated by J. M. van Rossum, according to which schizophrenia is caused by dopamine overactivity.

In recent years, it has become clear that the dopamine hypothesis is simplistic at best, not least because not all of the antipsychotic drugs currently in use are powerful dopamine blockers. Indeed, the gold standard, clozapine, binds to receptors other than dopamine and only weakly to the dopamine "D2" receptor, initially thought to be the crucial target in schizophrenia. Although researchers still think that dopamine is a factor in psychosis, it's by no means the whole story.

The efficacy of antipsychotic drugs proved beyond doubt that schizophrenia was a biological disorder. A second line of evidence supporting the biological reality of schizophrenia came from genetic research. Psychiatry had always believed (without much evidence) that chronic psychosis was heritable. But in 1960, Seymour Kety, a leading neuroscientist, waded into the politically risky waters of genetics—still tainted in the postwar years by Nazi eugenics—and came back with research to support this claim. Kety's idea was to explore the inheritance patterns in schizophrenia by looking at adopted children. He had two adopted children himself and, as he later said, "I'd noticed an interesting characteristic of the parents of adopted children . . . If the kid does something that you're proud of, you say, 'See, that's the effect of a good environment.' And if he does things that you're not so proud of, then you say, 'Well, it's in the genes.'" By asking whether schizophrenia runs in biological or adoptive families, one could disentangle the effects of nature and nurture. Kety's study showed that it was biology that mattered. A child's risk of schizophrenia depended on whether the biological parents, but not the adoptive ones, were ill.

The discovery of antipsychotic drugs and the new genetics of schizophrenia marked a turning point in psychiatry. As psychoanalysis faded from the scene, it began to seem likely that "there can be no twisted thought without a twisted molecule."

IN SEARCH OF DISORDERS

The second current that eroded the foundations of psychoanalysis came from the frontline of psychiatric diagnosis. Identifying and classifying disease is part of the core business of any medical specialty. This was what had motivated Kraepelin to look at the course of illness rather than at symptoms. Diagnosis is difficult in many parts of medicine, and, as too many patients discover, a second opinion (or a third) won't always get to the bottom of a complaint. Psychoanalysis for its part had never been much concerned with diagnosis. Although it developed a detailed and sophisticated theory of mental illness and the mind, psychoanalysis conceived of every patient as unique. Since the whole point of diagnosis is to see past the unique to the general, psychoanalysts took it to be largely irrelevant. Nonetheless, for a discipline wanting to think of itself as a branch of medicine, the uncertainty of psychiatric diagnosis became increasingly embarrassing. In a 1971 study, for example, experienced American and British psychiatrists were shown videos of clinical interviews with eight patients and asked to provide a diagnosis. Considerable discrepancies appeared. One patient, "Patient F," was given a diagnosis of schizophrenia by 69 percent of the Americans but by only 2 percent of the British doctors. Diagnosis is an art, but this was intolerable.

In 1952, the American Psychiatric Association published a classificatory scheme, the *Diagnostic and Statistical Manual of Mental Disorders*. DSM-I, as it came to be known, was revised and replaced in 1968 with DSM-II. Although it advertised diagnosis as a central topic, the DSM didn't provide much in the way of specifics about how to actually make one. When the time came for the third edition in 1980, things changed. The revision was led by Robert Spitzer, who, with the collaboration of a number of like-minded psychiatrists, left behind the psychoanalytic framework of DSM-II and grounded DSM-III in what they took to be more serious science.

DSM-III was based on the classification of disorders found in the sixth edition of Kraepelin's textbook. A draft was given to five hundred psychiatrists, who then diagnosed twelve thousand patients according to the new classification, and the results were used to establish diagnostic consistency. The impact of DSM-III was immediate. The improvement in diagnosis was such that nowadays, reports of schizophrenia published before 1980 have to be taken with a grain of salt.

DSM-III was explicitly designed to be nontheoretical. Its purpose was solely to provide psychiatrists with explicit guidelines for making an accurate diagnosis. In the service of specificity and detail (and at nearly five hundred pages), it listed 265 psychiatric disorders; the 134-page DSM-II had listed only 180. DSM-IV, published in 1994 (with a text revision in 2000—DSM-IV-TR), grew to around nine hundred pages and listed 297 disorders. The expansion of the categories of illness is due in part to the psychoanalytic view that there is more psychopathology outside the asylum than in it, with madness only the most severe end of a broad spectrum. The latest revision of the DSM, DSM-5, has simplified as well as altered the older classification. The number of pages and disorders, however, have remained roughly the same.

DSM-5 recognizes twenty-two categories of disorder: of development, mood, trauma, sex and gender, sleep, drug abuse, and personality, among others. The primary category of psychosis is "schizophrenia spectrum and other psychotic disorders," which breaks down into (a) *delusional disorder*, characterized by the presence of delusions alone; (b) *brief psychotic disorder*, lasting between a day and a month only; (c) *schizophreniform disorder*, lasting between one month and six; (d) *schizophrenia*, lasting six months or more; (e) *schizoaffective disorder*, in which there are both psychotic and mood-related symptoms; (f) *substance/medication-induced psychotic disorder;* (g) *psychotic disorder due to another medical condition;* and (h) *schizotypal personality disorder*, characterized by a reduced capacity for close relationships. (Personality disorders are quite different in their manifestations from psychotic disorders; in DSM-IV, personality disorders constituted a separate "axis." Schizotypal personality disorder is classified as a form of psychosis because it is marked by delusion-like thoughts, such as a belief in clairvoyance or telepathy, as well as paranoid thinking.)

DSM-5 lists five characteristic features of psychotic disorders: (i) *hallucinations*—usually hearing voices; (ii) *disorganized thinking* manifesting in disorganized speech; (iii) *grossly disorganized or abnormal motor*

behavior, such as bodily agitation and trouble with goal-directed movement; and (iv) *negative symptoms,* particularly salient in schizophrenia,
which include avolition (a failure to initiate behavior), alogia (reduced
speech), asociality (a loss of interest in social interaction), and diminished emotional expression. (v) The fifth characteristic is the presence of
the strange beliefs known as *delusions.*

UNFINISHED BUSINESS

The discoveries made in psychiatry during the second half of the twentieth century laid the foundation for what is now called the "biological"
model, and DSM-III (and the subsequent revisions) instituted a "medical" model of psychiatric diagnosis. One now finds an optimism among
psychiatrists, akin to that of the founders of the therapeutic asylum, that
a deep understanding of mental disorder is coming into view, with reme-
diation and even cures on the horizon. The American psychiatrist Nancy
Andreasen puts it this way:

> We live in an era when biology and biomedical science have matured
> to a point where we can expect pivotal discoveries to occur . . . Earlier
> medical achievements such as the discovery of insulin, which redeemed
> people with juvenile-onset diabetes from an inevitable death sentence,
> are likely to pale in comparison with future accomplishments in the
> treatment and prevention of mental illness . . . We live in an era when
> two large knowledge bases will meet and mingle: the map of the human
> genome and the map of the human brain. . . . The synthesis of these two
> knowledge bases will give us the power to understand the mechanisms
> that cause major mental illnesses and to use this knowledge to relieve
> the pain of the millions of people who at present suffer from them. The
> time when we can realistically declare a war on mental illnesses, with
> some hope of eventually achieving a victory, has finally come.

Thomas Insel, director of the National Institute of Mental Health
(NIMH), and the Canadian psychiatrist Remi Quirion express the feeling
of much of the profession: "psychiatry's impact on public health will require
that mental disorders be understood and treated as brain disorders."

And yet there are reasons for disquiet. Although the treatment of mental disorder has improved out of sight, the great advances of biological psychiatry were all made accidentally or, at any rate, not on the basis of theory. Sixty years after the discovery of chlorpromazine, we still don't know how antipsychotic drugs work, nor do we understand how electroconvulsive therapy (ECT)—the gold standard for the treatment of severe depression—improves mood. The latest wave of drug successes, selective serotonin reuptake inhibitors (SSRIs), were developed on the basis of an idea about brain chemistry that's simplistic at best. Despite the tremendous advances that neuroscience and psychiatry have seen, we still don't have anything like a theory of mental illness that is good enough even to be wrong.

When we look at schizophrenia, for example, we find no theoretical consensus. The dopamine hypothesis—*the* great success of biological psychiatry—remains inadequate. The genetic story is also very much unfinished. Once it was established that schizophrenia runs in biological families, the search for particular genes could begin. A good deal of genetic research has been carried out, and some twenty-two regions of the human genome are associated with schizophrenia. But we still know very little about how genetic processes contribute to the development of psychosis.

The DSM was never intended as a theory but only as a useful checklist. It remains, however, the only conceptual framework psychiatry has, and it is widely believed to have flaws that run deep. The primary one is that its taxonomy of disease is based on the signs and symptoms of mental illness—disordered behavior, pathological feelings, aberrant thought—and not on the biological reality that grounds our understanding of physical disease. Take diabetes as a contrast. Diabetes results from a biological disorder of the pancreas that explains why the disease manifests the way it does. Diagnosis can be made by testing for that biological disorder, and a cure will have to correct it. At the moment, psychiatric disorders aren't like that. Although there are some hopeful leads, we still have no biological markers associated with schizophrenia that can confirm a diagnosis. Instead, the clinician must depend on symptoms such as delusions or hallucinations, which the patient himself must report.

Furthermore, there are *lots* of symptoms of a disorder like schizophrenia, and you don't have to have all of them to get the diagnosis. What this means in practice is that two people who look like they should be on different hospital wards—the patient who hardly moves or speaks, and the patient who is fulminating against the CIA—apparently have the same disorder. Conversely, the biological processes in patients who look similar may in fact be different, so we can't be sure that what we refer to as schizophrenia is a single entity (and it quite possibly isn't).

Without a theory of the biology of mental illness, all we can do is piece together a pattern of symptoms and hope that it carves biological reality at the joints. The fact that the diagnostic categories of psychiatry are called "disorders" rather than "diseases" or "illnesses" is a reflection of our lack of confidence that we've got it right. The biological model predicts that this will change in the future and that psychiatric disorders will eventually be characterized and diagnosed on the basis of their biological manifestations. But until then, the categories have to be fudged. In an interview following the publication of DSM-5, Michael First, a major figure in the development of the DSM, expressed disappointment about just this state of affairs: "We were hoping and imagining that research would advance at a pace that laboratory tests would have come out. And here we are twenty years later [after DSM-IV], and we still unfortunately rely primarily on symptoms to make our diagnoses."

Our uncertainty about the underlying biology is one of the reasons mental illness continues to be so controversial. Indeed, it is so deeply contested that leading figures such as the philosopher Michel Foucault and the psychiatrist Thomas Szasz could claim, within the past forty years, that there was *no such thing* as mental illness but only (at best) life problems dressed up as disease or (at worst) a monumental con to aggrandize psychiatrists and control those who threaten the social fabric. Such iconoclasm is possible, however poorly it comports with the facts, because the biology of mental illness remains elusive. Like murder, it's hard to prosecute a science of madness without the bodily evidence.

LOUIS: HELL ON EARTH

Louis is a twenty-three-year-old man from Toronto with a master's degree in computer science who works as a software engineer at a large tech company in New York City. He has a family history of depression and was briefly treated for depression himself on two occasions. When we met, Louis noted that both depressive episodes were precipitated by change, namely his move from middle school to high school and, later on, his leaving home to pursue an undergraduate degree in mathematics in Western Canada.

For Louis, the transition to his job in New York was smooth at first. He enjoyed his work, had several friends who had already relocated to the city, and had begun dating a woman. Several months after the move, Louis and his friends were celebrating 4/20, the April twentieth festival of cannabis. Louis was not a regular pot user and didn't take other drugs. While his roommate and friends were feeling good, Louis experienced an episode of extreme paranoia, considerably more frightening than the brief feelings of paranoia or panic that many pot users have.

After eating the same pot brownies his friends ate, Louis suddenly thought that his roommate was the Devil and was keeping him in the apartment against his will. Louis took refuge in the bathroom and had a vision of dying by being shot. It occurred to him that he might *already* be dead and in Hell, suffering. Was he having a premonition or remembering his past? When a girl Louis knew only casually entered the apartment, he was convinced that he was in Hell because he had raped her. Louis kept asking her, "What did I do to you?" She had no idea what he was talking about. Louis returned to the upstairs bathroom, and when his Devil roommate called him back downstairs, Louis resisted, thinking that the torture chamber was below. After spending hours in the bathroom, he made his way back to his bed. The next morning, Louis woke up feeling better and had no distressing thoughts.

About a week later, Louis started to think that he was the subject of an artificial intelligence experiment and that his team of coprogrammers at work was using his brain as a network on which to run software programs. Louis imagined that the everyday terminology his team used (e.g., "processors" and "servers") was actually code for different parts of his brain. Moreover, if his coworkers discovered that he knew about the secret experiment, he would be killed, because the software wouldn't run on a brain that was aware it was the hardware. Louis found it "meta" that he was working on a project whose subject matter was his own brain. Yet the project would fail if his brain knew that it was on both sides of the research. To make matters worse, Louis knew that the others could read his mind, so he had to stop himself from thinking about knowing what was going on.

Whenever Louis felt that things were "out of place or nothing was real," he would review a number of possibilities that could explain his experience. One possibility Louis considered was that his coworkers were actors who were trying to convince him that nothing had changed. He wondered, "Is this like *The Truman Show*?" If Louis watched a movie he had seen before, perhaps *The Truman Show* or *The Matrix*, he thought it was "something that actually does represent my life, but they're showing it to me as an idea . . . to see how I'd react to it." Louis would ask himself if the movie he was watching wasn't in fact the movie he was in. In these moments, Louis's delusion of being dead and in Hell would recede, to be replaced by the Truman Show delusion. He also considered the possibility that he was living in a simulation, but ultimately "it would always eventually get down to me being in Hell, and me being dead and being tortured in some way."

A friend, Gord, visited from Toronto. At this point Louis thought he was in Hell. The two walked into a grocery store, and Louis had a strong experience of déjà vu that this was the store where he had already been killed. In his mind's eye, he saw himself arguing with the store owner about the price of an item, then Gord stepping between them, and the owner shooting Louis. He also considered the possibility that his murder had not already occurred but was about to. If it was a postmortem memory, Louis was being shown why he was in Hell—for losing his temper with the grocery store owner. Either way, their presence in that store would end in his being dead. They left the store. Later, in a restaurant, Louis said the other patrons were all looking at him with red eyes, a sign that they were demons and he was once again in Hell. This thought was always followed by two questions, "How did I die?" and "Why am I in Hell?" Louis now felt he had been hit by a bus while riding his bike. When driving back to the apartment from the restaurant in a taxi, Louis pointed out the window and asked Gord, "Is this where it happened? Is this where I got hit?" Louis determined that he was in Hell simply for being a bad person, that he had never done anything genuinely nice, and that he was self-interested.

It became clear to Gord that his friend was not well, and he took him to the hospital. In the subway car, Louis felt everyone's eyes on him. They knew him. He thought, "I'm the meme." Louis explained to me that, as memes like "Scumbag Steve," "Bad-Luck Brian," and "Annoying Facebook Girl" have text overlaid on their images, he imagined that his meme would be accompanied by something like "Gets good job. Goes crazy." But unlike the other memes, which were just photos, Louis was a live, three-dimensional meme that would be used by others to signify wild scenarios.

Since he was in Hell, Louis wondered where all the flames were. He decided that either Hell was not how it had been portrayed to be or that he had not yet reached that particular level of Hell. In fact, Louis had been feeling cold all evening, and as he grew colder, he thought that he would never be warm again. Being cold, he realized, was another form of hellish torture. Hell didn't have to be hot; it just had to be painful. When they arrived at the hospital, Louis thought that upon entering its doors, the real world would fall away and the true nature of Hell would be revealed. When entering did not expose the inferno, Louis noticed that several of the hospital employees had their hair dyed red, indicating that they too were demons.

In the ER, Louis developed another theory. He was, and always had been, a robot that had been programmed not to know he was a robot, but who was now becoming self-aware. Now that he had achieved consciousness, he would be destroyed by humans. He felt that Gord—who was not a robot himself but aware that Louis was one—had tried to signal to Louis to behave in ways that would not betray his newfound self-knowledge, in order to save him from destruction.

When Louis was placed on a gurney and asked to change into hospital pajamas, he believed the next torture would be eternal rape. When he wasn't attacked but instead told that he had to wait to see the doctor, Louis determined that "Hell was so crowded" that he would have to wait to be tortured. The anticipation, he thought, was another form of torture.

When I asked Louis about the apparent contradiction between his belief that he was dead and other beliefs that suggested he was still alive, Louis explained that all of his other beliefs were ultimately founded on the primary one that he was dead and in Hell. "It has to feel so real, or else I would know I'm in Hell and I would get used to it . . . The only way to keep my mind feeling like it was in Hell was to create all these fake scenarios." So the beliefs that he was a robot or a piece of software or in a simulation were all simply demonic ideas used to keep Louis in a continual state of torment. These thoughts would come to Louis, terrify him, and disappear, leaving him to realize once again that he was eternally damned. He would never know anything for certain again.

Louis was fixated on the theme of Hell as a place where pain would always be a surprise and would always get worse. As an example, Louis suggested that if a nail were hammered into his stomach for eternity, he would eventually get used to the pain. That wouldn't do, so Hell would mix it up. If something good happened to him, he knew it was only a setup so that the next misery heaped upon him would feel that much worse. The notion of Hell having only seven levels had to be wrong; once Louis or anyone else hit level seven, he would eventually become inured to its anguish. Louis stopped counting levels, believing they had to be infinite.

Louis was hospitalized and treated with Haldol, an antipsychotic. His parents arrived from Toronto, and Louis was discharged into their care—prematurely, it turned out. On the plane back to Canada, Louis was struck by a memory or premonition of getting into an altercation on the plane and it crashing.

He soon returned to New York. Louis was not referred to me because he had experienced a form of Truman Show delusion; it was mere happenstance. Our work together was fruitful. Louis did well with a combination of an antidepressant, a newer antipsychotic, and focused talk therapy. After about six months, Louis had to switch to a psychiatrist who accepted his insurance. He brought me a list of providers in his plan, and I directed him to colleagues I respected. I have not seen him since.—JG

2

ONE HUNDRED YEARS OF DELUSION

WHAT ARE DELUSIONS?

John Locke's view that madness is a matter of wrong ideas moved thinking about mental illness away from the spirit, the body, or the brain to the quality of mad thought. For this reason, perhaps, delusions—a paradigm of wrong ideas—have been so closely identified with madness. As the great psychiatrist and philosopher Karl Jaspers put it: "Since time immemorial delusion has been taken as the basic characteristic of madness. To be mad was to be deluded."

Delusions are symptoms of illness, not illness proper, with the same relation to madness that chest pain has to heart disease. And they are surprisingly common: delusions can appear in as many as seventy-five illnesses due to brain or genetic disorders, endocrine diseases, and infections. They can also be caused by alcohol or drug abuse and medication, and can be symptoms of otherwise nonpsychotic disorders, such as depression and, especially, bipolar disorder.

Some types of delusion frequently appear only in particular disorders, and some types are common across many. Paranoia, in particular, is common to many psychiatric disorders and physical illnesses. In contrast, it's been suggested that the delusion that someone is putting thoughts in your mind ("thought insertion") or extracting them ("thought withdrawal") is typical of schizophrenia but that the delusion of being robbed of one's possessions is not. In dementia and "normal" aging, it seems to be the other way around. Someone who has the Cotard delusion (named after nineteenth-century French neurologist Jules Cotard)—a belief that one's organs are rotting, that body parts are missing, or that one is dead—is quite likely to be depressed. Delusions like the last are sometimes referred to as "mood congruent" because they reflect the pathological mood. But these associations are not hard and fast.

Delusions are found in both more and less severe illnesses. Some high-functioning individuals can have a delusional belief that persists for years, but much the same delusion may appear in someone whose behavior or thought is grossly impaired. Mental disorders can also be distinguished by the character of the delusions associated with them. Delusional disorder, for example, is typically associated with *monothematic* delusions—delusions with a single theme. Other disorders, such as schizophrenia, typically involve *polythematic* delusions as symptoms.

Despite these rough-and-ready associations between delusions and particular disorders, it's important to think about delusions in isolation from illness. There are two reasons for this. First, because the association between delusion and illness is not rigid, overemphasis of the link is risky. In fact, thinking about delusions against the background of a disease may obscure as much as it reveals. The belief that your spouse is an impostor is not uncommon in dementia, for example, but does this delusion have something to do with memory loss? Perhaps, but we doubt it. Better, therefore, to isolate the symptoms from the illnesses until we understand more about both. Second, psychiatry will make better theoretical progress by focusing on the thoughts that delusions express, rather than the diseases that bring them about, or so we will argue. As a consequence, we are going to treat delusions very differently from the symptoms of physical illnesses. It *does* make sense to think about chest pain in the context of heart disease because each illuminates the other. We think that psychiatry isn't yet at the stage where this strategy will work for delusions, and we are not alone in this. Only progress in psychiatry will tell, however, whether we are right.

WHICH BELIEFS?

Item 1: An April 2010 New York Times/CBS News poll found that Tea Party supporters were better educated than the general public. At that time, 30 percent of them were "birthers" who believed that Barack Obama was not born in the United States. Obama's birth certificate showed that he was born at 7:24 p.m.

on August 4, 1961, in Honolulu, Hawaii. By April 2011, nearly three years after his birth certificate was published, the number of Tea Party birthers had grown to 45 percent.

Item 2: In a 1954 experiment, researchers showed Dartmouth and Princeton football fans film of a controversial game between the two schools. Eighty-six percent of the Princeton fans, but only 36 percent of the Dartmouth fans, believed that Dartmouth started the rough play. The Princeton fans thought the Dartmouth team had committed more than twice the number of infractions the Dartmouth fans saw.

Item 3: People like to save money on their purchases, but how much effort they are willing to make in exchange for the savings depends on what they are buying rather than on how much they are saving. In a study of economic decision making, 68 percent of the participants were willing to take a 20-minute drive to save $5 on a $15 item. Only 29 percent were willing to take the drive to save $5 on a $125 item, even though the savings, and the effort required, were the same in both cases.

Human beings hold an awful lot of beliefs that are nonsense. All things being equal, however, no one will consider you mentally ill because you believe your team is better behaved than the opposition or that the president was born in Kenya. But tell your psychiatrist that you caused the flood in New Orleans or that Jon Stewart is sending you coded messages during *The Daily Show*, and you are almost certain to get a diagnosis of a psychotic disorder. Moreover, someone who believes that he has been abducted by the US military and been subjected to mind-control experiments will likely get a psychiatric diagnosis, but someone who believes that *other* people are being abducted by the military for mind-control experiments will not. On the face of it, these are pretty similar thoughts, but only one of them is a delusion. Which of the myriad irrational beliefs that people have are delusional? In our view, this is the most important ignored question in the study of delusion.

DSM-5 describes delusions in a rather noncommittal way, as "fixed beliefs that are not amenable to change in light of conflicting evidence."

While it is undoubtedly true that delusions are held tenaciously, this casts too wide a net, since a big chunk of *nondelusional* beliefs are also resistant to change in the face of evidence. DSM-IV-TR had a good deal more to say about what a belief has to be like to count as delusional. It claimed that a delusion is a "false belief based on incorrect inference about external reality that is firmly sustained despite what almost everyone else believes and despite what constitutes incontrovertible and obvious proof or evidence to the contrary." While there is no doubt that delusions are strange beliefs and that people who have them persist in keeping them despite lots of evidence to the contrary, the DSM-IV characterization turned out to be inadequate in a variety of ways—there are delusions that violate nearly every condition of the definition—which is probably why it has now been abandoned. In the absence of a penetrating definition of delusion, what do we do?

Otto Neurath, the Austrian philosopher of science, famously said that scientists "are like sailors who have to rebuild their ship on the open sea," and so it is with the science of delusion. We don't have a definition to ground a theory or a theory to provide a definition. We can only begin with what we know and work our way to something better. So what do we know? The obvious place to look for some reliable facts is in the practice of the people who are most familiar with delusions, namely, psychiatrists and other practitioners. They are the people who spend their lives trying to decide whether something is a delusion or not, so they count as the experts. There is no guarantee that starting with expert opinion will lead to theoretical success, but it's the best we've got.

According to psychiatrists, then, which beliefs are delusions? The cross-cultural psychiatric literature and DSM-5 describe a number of delusions that fall into twelve broad types: (1) *persecutory delusions,* which are concerned with being harmed by others; (2) *referential delusions*—beliefs that events in the environment are directed at the delusional individual or have a special meaning for him; (3) *grandiose delusions,* according to which one is exceptional or powerful; (4) *erotomanic delusions*—beliefs that someone is in love with the delusional person; (5) *nihilistic delusions,* which are concerned with an imminent catastrophe or with nonexistence of some kind (e.g., with one's own nonexistence, as in Cotard); (6) *somatic delusions*—concerns about one's health and bodily function; (7) delusions concerning *thoughts* being withdrawn from, or inserted into, one's mind; (8) *delusions of control,* according to which one's body or actions are being manipulated by another agent; (9) *delusions of jealousy* (also known as *Othello syndrome*), beliefs that one's partner is unfaithful; (10) *religious delusions*, according to which one is either being persecuted by supernatural forces or is on a divine mission; (11) *delusions of guilt* or *sin*—beliefs that one is responsible for some disaster or tragedy; and (12) *misidentification delusions*, which are concerned with the identity of other people. One example of this last type is the *Capgras delusion* (named for the early-twentieth-century French psychiatrist Joseph Capgras), the belief that a thing or person—usually a loved one—has been replaced by a duplicate.

Table 1 on page 64 lists the categories of delusion found across cultures. The number of delusional forms identified differ across studies, but there is a lot of overlap. Given the variability in the styles of classification, this overlap suggests that delusions don't change much from culture to culture. All of the lists identify persecutory delusions as the most common type of delusion, often by a substantial margin. Grandiose delusions appear everywhere, and many of the other motifs appear on a few of the lists, if not on all. Studies also confirm that the categories of delusion haven't evolved over time.

Whatever delusions are, then, the entire scientific literature on psychosis reveals that they are only a minute subset—perhaps a dozen—of all the bizarre beliefs that people have or could have. This is a clear pattern in the phenomena of delusion, and any theory worth its salt is going to have to be able to explain why it is there.

FORM AND CONTENT

If so few delusional ideas are known to psychiatry, why do many people with psychosis seem to have so many strange beliefs? Two hundred years ago, James Tilly Matthews, the subject of the first detailed case history of schizophrenia, had beliefs concerning fluid locking, kiteing, thought making, voice sayings, lobster cracking, bomb bursting, foot curving, lethargy making, spark exploding, knee nailing, burning out, eye screwing, sight stopping, roof stringing, vital tearing, and fiber ripping—and, of course, the machine he called the Air Loom, the instrument of all this mischief. If the motifs of delusion are so restricted and so stable across time and culture, why do psychiatrists no longer observe delusions like these?

Form	English	African	Jamaican	Continental Europeans	English-speaking Non-Europeans*	Asian	Middle Eastern	Far Eastern	Caribbean
Persecutory	26	45	37	14	11	22	9	7	31
Reference	16	11	9	8	3	12	6	13	11
Grandiose and religious	11	19	21	8	8	8	6	7	8
Sexual and fantastic	14	6	15	7	3	4	0	27	10

*North Americans, White South Africans, Australians, and New Zealanders.

Form	Sydney
Persecutory	80.0
Religious	26.7
Grandiose	23.3
Reference	15.6
Somatic	14.4
Mind control	4.4
Guilt	4.4
Mind reading	4.4
Thought broadcasting	3.3
Transmitting devices	3.3
Thought withdrawal	3.3
Believing that a stranger is a close relative	2.2
Believing that they are someone else	2.2
Believing someone is in love with them	2.2
Extraterrestrial	2.2
Others	6.7

Form	Tokyo	Vienna	Tübingen
Persecution/injury	75.9	70.3	72.7
Poisoning	8.0	14.9	18.0
Jealousy	1.9	1.0	6.0
Being stolen from	4.9	2.0	2.7
Parasitosis	0.9	3.0	2.0
Mission/grandeur/special ability	19.4	19.8	18.7
Erotomania	6.5	5.9	6.7
Descent	2.8	1.0	0.7
Pregnancy	0.9	3.0	0.7
Resurrection	0	1.0	0
Invention	0.3	0	0.7
Hypochondria/dying	8.6	19.8	9.3
Guilt/sin	4.9	20.8	15.3
Being dead	0.3	5.9	0.7
Poverty	0	1.0	2.0
Death of relations	3.4	1.0	2.7
World catastrophe	2.5	2.0	4.7
Separation of being	1.5	3.0	1.3
Homosexual	0	0	0
Others	5.9	10.9	8.0
Religious	6.8	19.8	21.3

Form	Seoul	Shanghai	Taipei
Persecutory	72.3	78.9	79.1
Reference	6.0	54.2	59.0
Grandiose	48.2	27.5	38.8
Control	35.5	23.9	30.9
Somatic	23.4	14.1	24.5
Guilt	31.2	4.9	5.8
Jealousy	17.0	8.5	3.6
Poverty	2.1	4.2	5.0
Nihilistic	0.7	2.1	3.6

Form	Western Turkey	Central Turkey
Persecutory	74.6	83.7
Reference	57.7	70.9
Poisoning	9.5	26.2
Religious	10.9	20.9
Grandiose	10.0	19.8
Being controlled	6.0	19.8
Mind reading	4.5	17.4
Jealousy	3.5	14.0
Guilt/sin	0.5	13.4
Hypochondria	1.0	12.2
Erotomania	2.5	9.3
Thought broadcasting	0.5	11.1
Thought insertion	1.0	9.3
Nihilistic	4.0	5.2
Thought withdrawal	0.5	5.2
Nobility	0	3.5
Inferiority	0	3.5
Homosexual	0	3.5
Parasitosis	0	1.2
World catastrophe	0	1.2
Resurrection	0	1.2
Others	4.5	0.6

Form	White Pakistani	British Pakistani
Persecution	48	60	62
Control	50	26	13
Reference	48	43	11
Grandiose ability	26	19	28
Grandiose identity	14	23	42
Religious	14	21	11
Sexual	14	13	16
Depersonalization	18	11	2
Hypochondriacal	8	17	5
Misinterpretation	8	6	8

Table 1: Forms of delusion across culture.

The solution to this puzzle lies in a distinction (already made by nineteenth-century psychiatry) between two senses of "delusion." A psychiatrist in New York sees a patient who believes that the CIA has inserted a microchip into his tooth. Halfway around the world, a psychiatrist in Melbourne sees a patient who believes that ASIS, the Australian Secret Intelligence Service, has installed a tracking device in his cell phone. Have the two psychiatrists observed the same delusion or different ones? In one sense, of course, the delusions are different because the thoughts expressed by the patients are different. In another sense, though, it's plausible that the delusions express the *same* idea dressed up in different details, since both delusions express a fear of being victimized by a powerful social institution. Even if the details were changed further—for instance, a patient from Moscow who believes that the Russian Ministry of Defense is planning to get him fired from his job in a missile factory— the basic motif still seems clear enough. We'll call the precise thought expressed in a delusional belief its *content* and the motif or theme of the delusion its *form*. Thus, the three delusional contents (involving the CIA, ASIS, and the Russian Ministry of Defense) all belong to the *persecutory* or *paranoid* form. Some people with psychotic disorders, therefore, seem to have a great variety of beliefs, because there is no limit to the number of delusional contents one can entertain within a handful of delusional forms. Like the great variety of human languages that all obey the same principles of deep grammar, delusional contents, however mutable, conform to a set of underlying motifs.

The rigidity of delusional form contrasts dramatically with the elastic nature of content. Delusional contents do more than vary with an individual sufferer's thoughts: they adapt to culture and morph with history. Indeed, for an illness that is often characterized as a break with reality, psychosis keeps remarkably up to date with the world outside. An American with psychosis can believe that the CIA is planning to kidnap him, but in Russia, a different institution occupies the CIA's social role, and persecutory delusions will reflect that fact. In China, someone might have the delusion that he is the chief disciple of the Buddha; a patient with a similar "grandiose" delusion in Texas is not likely to believe anything like that because being the chief disciple of the Buddha doesn't mean the same thing in Dallas as it does in Beijing. The cultural environment is, in technical terminology, "pathoplastic": it shapes the content of the delusion. The same is true of delusional change over time. In keeping with the evolution of contemporary culture, people now believe that microchips or the internet do the malicious work of Matthews's Air Loom.

Culture may also affect how *common* a particular delusional form is. Delusions of jealousy are more prevalent in Germany than in Japan, and a wealthy Pakistani man is more likely to be grandiose than his poor female cousin, who is more likely to suffer from erotomania. Moving outside one's native culture can affect the manifestation of delusion as well. The delusional forms exhibited by immigrants from Pakistan to Britain are more like those of their British neighbors than those of their former compatriots. The forms of delusion can differ in frequency even across regions of the same country (see Table 1).

Delusional contents sometimes express ideas that are unique to a culture. In West Bengal, one can have a somatic delusion of "puppy pregnancy," a pathological variant of the local legend that being bitten by a dog causes canine pregnancy. In Malaysia and China, in contrast, one can suffer from the delusional belief that the penis (or breasts in women) is being resorbed into the body to be followed by death, a symptom of an anxiety disorder known as *koro*. Beliefs about penis retraction are found in ancient Chinese medicine, and related delusions find their way into the minds of the inheritors of that tradition. (The disappearing penis, it must be said, seems to have a resonance in other cultures as well.)

Delusions also harmonize with the worldview of the period. Since the middle of the nineteenth century, for example, the incidence of religious delusions has decreased as religious commitment has become optional in many cultures. Even current events or political developments may show up in delusional thought. At a moment when the United Nations was celebrating its fiftieth anniversary, the Pope was visiting the United States, and the O. J. Simpson trial was taking place, a patient with a psychotic illness believed that he had a secret relation to the United Nations, the Pope, and Simpson. And following a political advertising campaign in Britain, a woman with a paranoid illness came to believe that the Labour Party was trying to kill her. When asked why, she echoed the Conservative Party's campaign slogan: "New Labour New Danger."

FRIEDRICH KRAUSS: A HOT METAL DISK

In 1815, at the age of twenty-four, Friedrich Krauss, a German traveling salesman, came to believe that he was a victim of persecution by controlling waves of animal magnetism. He published two long memoirs (nearly fourteen hundred pages in total) called *Cry of Distress of One Poisoned by Magnetism* (1852) and *Continuation of My Cry of Distress* (1867). In these books, Krauss recounts his experience of persecution over the course of an illness that lasted more than fifty years, until his death in 1868. Unlike the account of James Tilly Matthews, which is reported by a third party, or that of Daniel Paul Schreber (discussed on pages 73–75), which tries to convey his religious views, Krauss's memoir reads more like a diary and is written in a "naive, agitated style, like someone trying to persuade a skeptical person of the strange nature of his sufferings."

He is tormented by four figures—the "old magnetizer," "Janeke Simon-Thomas," "van Asten," and "van Asten's daughter"—who watch him constantly, read his mind, and control him with magnetism. They also punish his body, exposing him to "bursts of heat, heart pressure, heart thudding, slave driving, flaying, besmirching, drying out of the brain, hellish erections" and more. These memoirs have never been translated into English, so Krauss is not as well-known in the English-speaking world as he should be. The following is a brief excerpt from his memoirs translated by Margaret Mahony Stoljar.

THE BEGINNING OF THE PSYCHOSIS
AND
THE GENERAL EXAMINATION IN THE TERRIBLE FORTY NIGHTS OF 1816

I was restless, I couldn't sleep, and soon a hot metal disk came into my left ear; it was the size of the palm of my hand, round and smooth like a broad crown coin. This mass of vapor, that I couldn't make head or tail of, moved calmly along, and once it came to my hip I put my hand on it, but it didn't stop moving but pushed forward to a place that modesty forbids me to name, and while it caused this warm mass to move backwards and forwards, it allowed itself plenty of time for the most cynical indecencies; such as when it squeezed my noble parts and twisted them, this depraved creature murmured: "*Ah vous êtes un bon mâle!*" I was quite beside myself at this infamy, when the idea came to me for the first time that I could indeed be electrified, since then I knew nothing at all about magnetism, and I assumed that there must be a copper wire through the floor between the kitchen and my bed, and this wire must be removed. But however often I thrust my stick under the bed and reached backwards and forwards, looking there and moving it around again, no connecting wire was to be seen.

The old magnetizer finally tried to press the aforesaid hot place from my belly up towards my navel, from whence she spent a long time trying to push upwards, as if feeling with her finger through a narrow passage towards my heart. I struggled against it and the beast muttered that I kept my heart too high, she could not reach it.

Thereupon there began a period of wakefulness of forty times twenty-four hours.

THE PERSECUTORS

The Old Magnetizer

The old magnetizer sometimes said she came from Strasbourg, more often she called herself an old nun (doubtless a wh-re) from Luxemburg. Presumably she was from Strasbourg—her Swabian dialect, her expressions and allegories were all in the style and sound of this region. This poisoner also said she was only employed by van Asten for six months, and frequently I thought she was drunk. Already during the time I was locked up in the Cellites' dungeon I could hear the voice of this creature. This monster seemed to be fairly stout, she had a broad, swollen muzzle, with teeth missing, her lower lip hung down, and judging by her pronunciation it must have been thick; her voice was often squawking, scratching, or clattering like an old pot.

Since the odd creature had heard that I had written a few sarcastic things in verse, she roared at me: "Why don't you make me a quatrain!" and quickly I said:

ONE HUNDRED YEARS OF DELUSION

A fine glove,
Your charms
Carry arms
Against love.

Janeke Simon-Thomas

Janeke Simon-Thomas was at that time a thoughtless street urchin, about four and a half feet tall, incapable even of copying properly, who wanted to turn every smutty vulgar observation into a witty saying. Because of his poverty he was dressed in the worn-out clothes of his uncle J. A. Simon-Thomas, an associate of the Thuret company. His head was large, round like a ball, with bristly black hair, eye-glasses, a thick nose, a wide slit of a mouth with thick lips, no beard, chinless, with arms hanging inwards, bandy legs and a calf's voice—a young emancipated Jew. Now about fifty years old.

Van Asten

Van Asten, the *père noble*, is so clever that he says of the blockhead son of J. A. Simon-Thomas: "Why does he always laugh to himself when he says something?" Less *rabougri* than Janeke, he is of medium, rather small stature, making a mean, dull, knavish, depressed impression; he even stumbles over simple counting, he is otherwise thin, pale, with sharp, stubborn, fixed features. Through years of practice he tries to hide his stupidity behind a borrowed façade of importance with which he snatches at clichés until, oppressing the listener with repulsive drawling and emphasis, he bursts out at last, squawking in his shrill, wooden, juvenile voice. This one is a quite naive, stupid rogue to the core, who of necessity must envy an orderly person everything, who therefore knows no end to his envy, and with affected philosophical calm and unshakeable phlegm, all too full of self-satisfaction and regarding himself as a man of character, he gives himself up to his terrible, murderous pleasures. He is known as "van Ass," and is now seventy-five or eighty years old (he himself says seventy-seven).

Van Asten's Daughter

His daughter was a naively lewd, short-necked, slovenly lump with a hide the color of hemlock (greenish with red-brown spots), of middle height for a woman, coarse hyena's head, mean, dull, expressionless features, a pug nose, with staring, round, codfish eyes, goggling stupidly like a jellyfish, thick lips, with sickening lewdness letting everything hang out, prancing about like a poodle but coarse and brutal with it, as if she and the rich peasants of her family in Antwerp could command more than the king; naively rough, in all her habits the pure expression of female depravity, a terrible warning for any other than the most animal feelings. You would look in vain for such a creature in any other part of the world! This scourge is now at least fifty years old and probably just as vile.

ON THE PERSECUTION

Influencing the Body. Torture.

The ears are the funnel which by nature (by order of the Creator) have the task of drawing the electro-magnetic fluid . . . of the air . . . out of the universe, to suck it in and carry it into the body . . . That is how this condensed ether comes into me through my ears . . .

From the start I differentiated three distinct kinds of magnetic gas: 1) the more common kind, ringing only faintly, that streams in with a swishing noise more like boiling water; 2) the kind that billows in with a loud roaring as in rubbing sand, not ringing at all, so that whole gusts like smoke well up by my ear; forcefully touching my ear, heart . . . nerves, muscles, and veins, stretching and swelling, tensing itself, making me unusually strong, but not yet highly excited; 3) the most concentrated, violent, and sharpest gas, often a pure flame, licking like a tongue . . . this moves with a high singing noise *oooooh* or *tsiiiii*, flashing, hissing, rustling, generally without tension, it smokes less the sharper it is, but often creeps as deep as possible into my ear in a perceptible flow . . . like a living flame that takes hold in a terrible manner, in extreme excitement; it quickly ignites, causing me the greatest pain, the most terrible torments.

THE INFLUENCING MACHINE

James Tilly Matthews is the first known case of a recurring theme in psychotic thought that tracks culture: control by means of new technology.

A delusional fear of technological control is common enough in psychosis to have been baptized: it is known as the "influencing machine" delusion. Although the psychoanalyst Victor Tausk is credited with describing the delusion in a now-classic paper in 1919, Tausk makes it clear that both the phenomenon and the name would have been familiar to his colleagues at the time.

The paper is a case study of the influencing machine theme. Tausk begins by describing the machine as it is imagined by patients with schizophrenia. It is an apparatus that "consists of boxes, cranks, levers, wheels, buttons, wires, batteries, and the like," and "with the progressive popularization of the sciences, all the forces known to technology are utilized to explain the functioning of the apparatus." Despite the evolution of technology, the purpose of the machine never changes. It is used to torment its victims and to produce or remove "thoughts and feelings by means of waves or rays or mysterious forces." It causes "erections and seminal emissions, that are intended to deprive the patient of his male potency" and creates strange sensations and "cutaneous eruptions, abscesses, and other pathological processes." The components of the machine are sometimes connected to the patient's bed by "invisible wires," and it "is operated by enemies."

The case Tausk describes is that of Natalija A., a former philosophy student. Thirty-one years of age at the time of her treatment, she had been deaf for many years and communicated only in writing. She believes that she has been controlled for six and a half years by a machine located in Berlin that also controls her mother and her friends. Ignorant of its function, she nonetheless has a vague idea that it might operate by telepathy. She conceives of the machine as a sort of electrical life-sized voodoo doll, the inner "organs" of which are batteries, and everything that happens to it happens to her. When someone strikes the machine, Natalija feels the blow in the corresponding part of her own body. The people who control the machine "produce a slimy substance in her nose, disgusting smells, dreams, thoughts, feelings, and disturb her while she is thinking, reading or writing." When the machine's genitalia are touched, Natalija experiences sexual sensations. The operator of the machine is a former professor whose marriage proposal Natalija had refused. When he cannot change her feelings, he employs the machine to control her doctors, her friends, even her psychoanalyst (Tausk himself), all in an effort to torment her.

In his formulation of the influencing machine, Tausk begins with the presumption that the machine is itself a "representation of the patient's genitalia projected to the outer world" and suggests that the strange hypochondriacal sensations come about as a transformation of a sexual impulse. Because this perception is experienced as alien, it is projected onto the world and experienced as persecutory. The influencing machine is thus created in the mind of the patient to explain these thoughts and feelings. The sexual origin of the delusion accounts for Natalija's belief that the machine's operators are figures of desire.

The influencing machine reappears in a 1958 paper by the psychiatrist Louis Linn, who describes a patient treated at Mount Sinai Hospital in New York. The woman, fifty years old and "strait-laced," was a devout Catholic who contracted a sexually transmitted disease from her traveling-salesman husband and suffered from a vaginal itch. She became increasingly hypochondriacal, and in September of 1955 her complaints suggested to Linn that she had an influencing machine delusion. She came to believe that the cardiologist who had treated her for palpitations several months earlier had since had a "nervous breakdown" and had been admitted to a different psychiatric hospital, where he "operated an electrical machine which was affecting her body." These effects included cardiac symptoms and sexual stimulation, as well as toxicity that caused her to urinate and defecate frequently. The machine had "all kinds of radio tubes and wires in it" and is "like a robot, a giant mechanical man, or like a cigar store Indian." Linn claims that his patient had a dream that "confirmed" that the machine was "a male or at least a phallic persecutor."

The patient initially did well after a course of ECT but took a turn for the worse after Linn unfortunately decided to share his interpretation of her symptoms which focused on her feelings about masturbation. "She responded to this explanation," Linn writes, "by lapsing into a state of psychomotor retardation in which she refused to leave her room, rarely spoke spontaneously, and answered questions in evasive monosyllables." (You have to give him credit for publishing.) Her influencing machine delusion disappeared, only to be replaced with the belief that Linn had amputated her hands and replaced them with a pair she didn't care for. Unsurprisingly—and to be fair, somewhat understandably—Linn took this as further confirmation of the masturbatory roots of her delusion. She spent the next three months in a sanatorium.

The influencing machine continues to evolve with technology. Dusan Hirjak and Thomas Fuchs report on three recent patients with variations on the theme. One believed that his computer had been infected by a virus when he downloaded a Marilyn Manson song. He thought that he was being manipulated by Marilyn Manson and would eventually be kidnapped by him. A second patient believed that she was being raped by neighbors who were projecting pornography into her eyes using "laser radiation." Microphones had been implanted in her body through which she could hear voices; "metal parts" were irradiating her; and a camera had been implanted in her uterus through which Russians and Muslims were monitoring her sex life. A third patient said that he was being "tracked by cameras, microphones and his television." Airport security personnel had implanted a microphone and a computer chip in his neck to be able to observe him, listen to his thoughts, and control his behavior.

SCHREBER

We've looked to psychiatric opinion to get a fix on which beliefs count as delusions. The long list of questions about what delusions *are,* however, has to be answered by a theory. Although Haslam's description of James Tilly Matthews is the first detailed case study of delusions in schizophrenia, the *theory* of delusion begins with a patient called Schreber.

Daniel Paul Schreber was a judge in the Kingdom of Saxony, part of the German Empire. In 1893, just weeks after he was appointed to the highest court in Saxony, he fell ill and was in due course declared legally incompetent on the grounds that he was insane. He admitted himself to the Hospital for Psychiatric and Nervous Diseases of Leipzig University under the direction of Paul Flechsig and subsequently entered the asylum established at Sonnenstein, a castle near Dresden, where he remained for eight years under the care of Guido Weber.

During his stay at Sonnenstein, Schreber wrote a memoir entitled *Denkwürdigkeiten eines Nervenkranken*—literally, the great thoughts of a nervous patient, and translated as *Memoirs of My Nervous Illness.* Published in 1903, it is a remarkable self-revelatory expression of psychotic thought running to almost one hundred thousand words in English. Schreber's ideas are complex, but the basic views are clear enough. Schreber believes that he is being persecuted by Flechsig, who has committed "soul murder," an act that has torn the fabric of the universe and created a channel between God and man. (Kraepelin's reaction to working under Flechsig suggests that he might have been a suitable focus for a paranoid delusion.) God's nerves, or "rays," are now in contact with human nerves—in particular, Schreber's—and this contact has destroyed all life on Earth. (Schreber is writing only a few years after Wilhelm Röntgen's discovery of X-rays, and this strand in his delusional thought might be a form of influencing machine delusion.) Although Schreber *seems* to see people, they are only "fleetingly improvised," souls "temporarily given human shape by divine miracle." At times Schreber thinks that even *he* no longer exists; Flechsig's discharge report says that he believed he was "dead and rotting."

The interaction between God and man is not only harmful to human beings but to God as well. When the world was intact, God encountered human beings after death, but now that God is in contact with the nerves of living people, His existence is also at risk. The bond between God and Schreber has to be broken for God to be able to save Himself, and His only option is to destroy Schreber.

In the months before Schreber's illness began, while lying in bed one morning, it occurred to him that "it really must be rather pleasant to be a woman succumbing to intercourse." This idea reappears in the most important of Schreber's delusions, his belief that God is destroying him by a process of "unmanning"—that is, transforming him into a woman. This transformation leads to his body being filled with "nerves of voluptuousness," or female sexual pleasure. He believes that his facial hair is disappearing and he is getting smaller; that he is developing breasts and female sexual organs; and that his penis is shrinking into his body. In his discharge summary, Flechsig says that Schreber thought that his penis had been "twisted off with a 'nerve probe.'" Ultimately, Schreber came to believe that he would be impregnated through God's rays and would repopulate the earth with a new race. After being discharged from Sonnenstein, he continued to wear women's clothes as a sign of his sexual change.

Not much is known about Schreber's life after he left the asylum. Having been institutionalized, he was prohibited by German law from working as a judge and could get no other work through the Ministry of Justice. He lived with his mother for a while and then built a house in Dresden, where he lived with his wife, Sabine, and a foster daughter, Fridoline. In 1907, Sabine suffered a stroke. Schreber fell to pieces and was admitted to an asylum in the town of Dösen, near Leipzig. Until his death in 1911, Schreber was withdrawn, depressed, and mostly mute.

Schreber's *Memoirs* didn't attract much notice when it first appeared, but one of his readers was the Zurich psychiatrist Carl Jung, then a disciple of Freud. In 1910, Jung told Freud about Schreber's book, which by then had been in print for seven years. Freud read the *Memoirs* and decided to try to psychoanalyze Schreber through his writing. (Freud never met Schreber, although he considered doing so.) Freud's reading of Schreber, published in 1911, laid the foundation for psychiatry's conceptualization of psychosis and made Schreber one of the most famous patients in the history of psychiatry.

Freud theorized that the persecutor in a paranoid delusion is an important person (or a substitute for one) who was once "loved and honoured," and the delusion can be understood according to a "simple formula." First, the idea *I love him* is changed to *I hate him.* The thought *I hate him* is then inverted and becomes *He hates me.* Since Schreber believes that Flechsig is persecuting him, Flechsig must therefore really be loved. Focusing on Schreber's fantasy about being a woman having intercourse, Freud proposes that Schreber's paranoia is an inversion of sexual desire for Flechsig and, indirectly, for Schreber's own brother and father—an "outburst of homosexual libido." Since homosexual desire is psychologically unacceptable to Schreber, he disavows it by transforming it unconsciously from love to hate. "It may be presumed," Freud claims at the end of his analysis of Schreber, "that the same schematic outline [of psychological inversions] will turn out to be applicable to other cases of delusions of persecution."

Paranoia is no longer recognized as an independent mental disorder, but psychoanalytic thinking about delusion continued after Freud. A lovely example of this approach is the psychoanalytic model of the Capgras delusion. Melanie Klein, as we've seen, believed that the infant splits the mother into good and bad. The psychoanalytic theory of Capgras takes this form of mental splitting to be at the root of this delusion as well. Consider Bella and George, an unhappily married couple. George is solid but boring, and Bella, appreciating his dependability but raging unconsciously at his dullness, is understandably ambivalent toward him. Under the pressure of this ambivalence, Bella's unconscious mental representation of George is split into two: the steady, loyal George and the tedious, irritating George. With two Georges in her mind, the tension in her feelings vanishes: her rage at George can now be felt guilt-free because it is directed at the bad George, while her love is directed at the good George. The bad George absorbs the anger, while the good George is spared. Problem solved; the rent in the ego's relation to the external world is patched.

As psychiatry moved away from psychoanalysis, theorists mostly set aside the details of delusions. Mental contents are at the heart of psychoanalytic thinking, but with the DSM playing so central a role in contemporary psychiatry, the variety of delusional thoughts lost its appeal and clinical usefulness. With an eye to DSM criteria, a psychiatrist working in an emergency room will place great emphasis on the presence of delusions as a requirement for giving a patient a diagnosis of schizophrenia but will not much care whether the patient believes that she has a double living in Paris, that Sarah Palin is putting thoughts in her mind, or that she is related to all the royal houses of Europe. All that matters is the presence of the symptom. Over the past forty years, therefore, the most important theoretical work on delusions has come primarily from psychology.

STRANGE EXPERIENCE

Psychologists have articulated two overarching questions that a theory of delusion has to be able to answer: *(1) How do delusional thoughts arise in someone's mind?* and *(2) Why do people hold on to them so tenaciously despite the fact that they are extremely implausible?* Most of the research has been concerned with the first of these.

The modern history of delusion theory begins with a 1974 paper by the psychologist Brendan Maher, who proposed that although delusions appear to be irrational thoughts, they are actually *normal* thoughts about abnormal *experiences* caused, most likely, by brain disorders. When someone has a strange experience, they naturally try to make sense of it, and Maher's hypothesis is that a delusion is one way of doing so. In Maher's view, delusions aren't symptoms of madness in the traditional psychiatric sense; they are actually the consequences of a rational mind trying to come to grips with bizarre psychological events.

An elegant illustration of the Maher approach to delusion is found again in a model of Capgras developed by Hayden Ellis and Andrew Young in 1990. Ellis and Young propose that Capgras is a mirror image of a neurological disorder known as "prosopagnosia," the inability to recognize familiar faces. Despite their impairment, some people who suffer from prosopagnosia continue to have an unconscious reaction to familiar faces signaled by a slight increase in sweating and, therefore, skin conductance. This preserved capacity is known as "covert recognition." For some patients with prosopagnosia, then, there is a loss of "overt recognition" (conscious awareness of familiarity) together with intact covert recognition. Overt and covert recognition can come apart because there are two neural pathways involved in recognition, and one can be dysfunctional without interfering with the other.

Suppose, however, that the situation were reversed, and someone were to lose covert recognition but retain overt recognition? What would that be like? With overt recognition intact, one would be able to recognize a familiar face consciously, but without covert recognition, there would be no physiological response, no "gut" sense of familiarity. The experience of recognizing a face without that visceral familiarity would undoubtedly be odd, and someone in this position would cast around for a way to understand it. One possible explanation of the experience is that the person who *looks* familiar isn't *actually* familiar; in other words, they're an impostor, and that's why the gut recognition response is absent. This is Ellis and Young's hypothesis: that Capgras is the result of a loss of covert recognition with preserved overt recognition. Their model predicts that people with Capgras should *fail* to show a change in their skin conductance when they see a familiar face (because they don't exhibit covert recognition), and this is exactly what is found. If the model is correct, therefore, the Capgras delusion is—as Maher proposed—a quite rational explanation of an anomalous experience.

Maher's view has been very influential in the science of delusion, but a number of investigators have noticed that it seems to leave some questions unanswered. Suppose you wake up and your wife *looks* familiar but *seems* strange, in some indefinable way, because your capacity for covert recognition is impaired. It occurs to you that maybe she's an impostor. Why, if you are otherwise psychologically normal, don't you notice that this explanation is wildly implausible? And if you don't notice this right off the bat, why don't you notice it when people point out (as they undoubtedly will) all the evidence against it? The lack of covert recognition underlying Capgras explains how the impostor thought could cross someone's mind but not why they would ever take it seriously.

Here's a second puzzle. There is no doubt that overt-without-covert recognition would give you pause and lead you to want an explanation. But would the idea that your wife is an impostor really be the first one that occurs to you? What about some of these as alternatives: she's done something to her hair that makes her seem subtly different; she's in an odd mood and not acting like herself; she's fallen out of love with me; I've fallen out of love with her; she must have an identical twin she's never told me about, and I'm the victim of a prank; I'm having a weird experience (something like déjà vu or a drug-induced hallucination); and, finally, there's something wrong with my mind or brain. Given all of these options, why does the person with Capgras choose such an odd belief? In short, why does a strange experience lead to a strange explanation?

A third question raised by Maher's theory is: what exactly *is* a "strange experience"? Some are caused by brain damage or malfunction, but many more strange experiences are commonplace. For example, under normal circumstances the human visual system can keep objects looking the same size despite changes in viewing conditions. When you watch someone walking away from you, they don't seem to get smaller, even though the image they project onto your retina is shrinking. This is known as "size constancy." But size constancy has its limits. Standing on the observation deck of the Eiffel Tower looking down on Paris, people appear not only far away but very small. That's a bit of a strange experience, as any child having it for the first time will tell you, but psychiatrists have never diagnosed anyone (in the language of *Seinfeld*) with a delusion of shrinkage. In short, if delusions are caused by strange experiences, and people have many kinds of such experiences, why are there only a dozen or so delusional forms?

To address this question, Maher's theory has to say that this strange experience is not strange *enough* to lead to a delusion—a reasonable, but unhelpful, answer if we don't know what makes an experience strange enough. A better answer might be that a strange experience (as Maher suggests) has to be caused by brain damage, but that suggestion creates its own problems. First, lots of delusions occur in people who show no evidence of having brain damage. Second, neurology has described a great many disorders caused by brain lesions, and many of these are associated with strange experiences (of the kind beautifully illustrated in the works of Oliver Sacks). Only a few neurological illnesses, however, have delusions as symptoms. When, for example, someone loses their color vision due to a brain disorder, why don't they develop the delusion that the world is gray? And if this idea does occur to them, why are they so easily talked out of it? The concept of a strange experience has to be constrained in some fairly specific ways, or Maher's theory will end up predicting that there should be many more kinds of delusion than the dozen that there are.

WITHOUT REASON

Since an emphasis on strange experience alone seems inadequate, a number of investigators have proposed that delusions are (at least in part) disorders of reasoning. People with delusions, despite what Maher says, *don't* seem much like normal thinkers trying to understand anomalous experiences. They seem much more like people whose thoughts are profoundly disordered. Since many of the beliefs we have come from reasoning about things, it's plausible that a reasoning abnormality might lead to pathological beliefs.

One idea that has been explored by Todd Woodward and his colleagues is that people with delusions have a "bias against disconfirmatory evidence" (BADE). The hypothesis is that once someone with a delusion accepts an idea based on some evidence or other, they're less inclined than healthy people to give it up. An experiment showing this runs as follows. In the first stage of the experiment, the participant is shown a picture of a man with a small dog next to him looking through a fence at a big barking dog. The participant then has to choose the most likely of four interpretations of the picture: (1) "The man has just escaped from the barking dog"; (2) "The man is looking at his neighbor's barking dog"; (3) "The man has just built a fence for his dog"; and (4) "The man is shopping for guard dogs." At this point in the experiment, the second and third interpretations are rated as more plausible. In the next stage of the experiment, the participant is shown a second picture depicting what happened *just before* the event presented in the first picture, and then a third picture depicting the moment before that. The second picture shows the man jumping over the fence with the dog chasing after him, and the third picture shows him running toward the fence. Once these pictures are shown, it becomes obvious that the first interpretation is actually the right one, and the other, initially plausible, interpretations ought to be rejected. When given the new evidence, however, people with delusions are less likely to revise their judgments about the plausibility of the different answers than healthy participants: they have a BADE.

The BADE hypothesis explains why someone who had already embraced a delusion might be reluctant to give it up. If you ignore evidence to the contrary, almost any belief can seem rational. A different sort of reasoning problem may also lead to delusional thoughts in the first place. The most popular hypothesis about how this might happen was developed by Phillipa Garety and her colleagues, who proposed that people with delusions have a tendency to accept hypotheses (especially those involving probability) on inadequate evidence. In Garety's terminology, they have a "jumping to conclusions" (JTC) bias.

Here's a typical illustration of the bias at work. You are told that there are two jars of beads. In the first jar, 15 percent of the beads are black and 85 percent are red; in the second, 15 percent of the beads are red and 85 percent are black. You will be shown some beads one after the other, all of which are taken from only one of the two jars. Your job is to guess which jar the beads come from. What would you say about this sequence, for example?

RED, RED, RED, BLACK, RED

Most people guess that this sequence has come from the jar containing mostly red beads, and so do people with delusions. But healthy people typically want to see more beads before they commit to an answer. In other words, people with delusions jump to a conclusion about the jars. If you have a JTC bias, therefore, you might be more susceptible to adopting a delusional thought. Suppose you have a strange experience of overtly recognizing your wife without the accompanying covert recognition. It occurs to you that the explanation for the strange experience might be that your wife is an impostor. Having evaluated the evidence, an otherwise healthy person will of course reject the impostor hypothesis. A person with a JTC bias, however, might miss some of the conflicting evidence and accept it.

One question that the JTC hypothesis leaves unanswered is how we should understand the notion of "evidence." Suppose someone with a grandiose delusion believes that they have supernatural powers. What could count as evidence for this hypothesis? That they feel particularly virile today? That an angel told them so? That they believed six impossible things before breakfast? If someone adopted the belief in supernatural powers on the basis of evidence like this, we'd be inclined to say that they don't know what evidence *is* rather than that they've ignored it.

More important, however, the JTC theory also ignores the core datum that only a small number of strange beliefs are delusions. A theory that explains delusions by appealing to a general reasoning problem will predict that someone who has one delusion will be delusional about nearly everything. There is no end of strange hypotheses—like the Eiffel Tower shrinkage belief—that we all entertain, however briefly. Someone who jumps to conclusions should adopt many of them. But they don't. Because reasoning is a cognitive capacity that we put to use in handling *all* of the ideas we evaluate, tracing delusions to a reasoning disorder, therefore, results in two predictions: first, that people with delusions should have *lots* of them, and, second, that they should cover a wide range of topics. Neither of these is true.

COMBINATIONS

To address the weaknesses of the strange experience and the reasoning hypotheses of delusion, Max Coltheart, Martin Davies and their colleagues have proposed a unified, or "two-factor," theory. According to their model, people who have strange experiences alone will not develop delusions, but those who have strange experiences *as well as* a second disorder may. In order to develop Capgras, for example, you have to be doubly unlucky. First, you have to have a disorder that leads to the strange experience described by Ellis and Young. In addition, however, you have to have a disorder of thought that prevents you from noticing that the Capgras hypothesis is bizarre. A strange experience causes the idea that your wife is a duplicate to put down roots in your mind, and the second disorder prevents it from being pulled up. The limited number of strange experiences explains why there are so few types of delusion, and the second factor explains why delusions aren't rejected in the face of contradictory evidence.

Coltheart and his colleagues marshal a good deal of evidence for their model by pointing to cases of neurological disorders in which a patient will say that *it's like* their spouse is a duplicate, for example, but they know she isn't. These patients have the first factor; they have the strange experiences. But because they don't have the second factor, they retain "insight," as psychiatrists say; they can see that their experience is inaccurate.

The two-factor approach goes a long way to providing a comprehensive framework for delusions. The theory was developed to explain monothematic delusions like Capgras, and it may be extendable to polythematic delusions as well. However, as a mixed theory that appeals to both strange experience and disordered thought, it inherits some of the questions we raised earlier. First, it doesn't tell us what sort of strange experience is required for someone to develop a delusion. Lots of such experiences never lead to pathological beliefs. Second, in order for people to develop even a single monothematic delusion like Capgras, the two-factor theory says that they have to have an impairment that stops them rejecting bizarre hypotheses. Since lots of odd hypotheses occur to most of us, however, someone who has even a single delusion ought to have lots of other odd beliefs as well. Impaired thought will allow *any* weird inference to set up shop in the mind and not just the ones that psychiatrists call delusions.

Another theory that appeals to more than one factor in the development of persecutory delusions is the "threat anticipation" model of Daniel Freeman and his colleagues. This account also holds that delusions start out as attempts to explain strange or ambiguous experiences. Like the two-factor account, the model includes other disorders that have to be present for delusions to arise. In particular, Freeman hypothesizes that the anxiety that is common in psychosis biases the patient in the direction of suspicious explanations. A social encounter with someone whose face is hard to read, for example, might lead an anxious person to fears of persecution. Once the persecutory thought arises, a third disorder—a JTC bias or some other reasoning problem—allows the belief to take hold. On the threat anticipation model, then, delusions are the joint outcomes of experiential, emotional, and reasoning factors.

Freeman's account has the important virtue of making the idea of threat central to delusion (or, at any rate, paranoia). Persecution is ubiquitous cross-culturally and the most common form of delusion. As we'll see, the idea of threat is crucial for understanding delusions, and we'll return to it in due course.

RUBY: ALL DRESSED UP AND NOWHERE TO GO

If you walk into almost any state psychiatric hospital—to visit a loved one, to present a lecture to staff or, perhaps, on your first day of work—you will likely feel a lingering sense of unease, as if you were in a haunted house. These old, rundown institutions have housed severely mentally ill people, some for decades. Guards stand by the doors as you pass through, and a metal detector ensures that no dangerous contraband enters the building.

However, at one particular state psychiatric hospital in the mid-1990s, after passing through all this security and making your way to the front desk, you would have been greeted by a smiling, strikingly handsome woman in her sixties named Ruby.

In those days, Ruby wore a Chanel suit. Seeing her might have called up Jackie Kennedy in your mind. And after Ruby handed you your new ID badge and your key, you might have thought it wonderful that such an elegant woman would choose to volunteer her time—she clearly did not need to work for money—in this out-of-the-way and highly unglamorous psychiatric hospital.

But I began to wonder about Ruby after lunch on my first day. Instead of returning to the front desk, she sat down inside the unit and, after carefully picking the least uncomfortable chair, began reading the *Wall Street Journal* while patients walked the halls or played Ping-Pong around her. She was, it turned out, one of them.

Ruby came to New York City from the Midwest in her twenties, a beautiful girl wanting some excitement. She did some modeling and had a few bit parts in B-movies, but mostly she went to galas, charity balls, and any other party a self-respecting socialite in the 1950s would attend. It was at one of these events that Ruby met Charles, a Wall Street tycoon thirty years her senior. Charles had been recently widowed, and the two quickly fell in love. Charles's children were less than thrilled at the prospect of their father carrying on with a woman their own age, but as long as Charles and Ruby didn't marry, they could live with it. Ruby didn't care much for marriage in any case, and they were happy. Besides, Charles told Ruby that he had amended his will so in the event of his death, she would be well cared for.

They were inseparable for almost ten years until the day Charles died in an instant of a massive heart attack. Ruby was distraught. Charles's children did not invite her to mourn with them. Her grief became a depression, and Ruby checked herself into a private hospital in the city. She was treated the way mental health patients were treated in the 1960s: daily psychoanalytic therapy sessions and some sleep medication. After six weeks, Ruby and her doctor agreed that her depression had lifted and that she would return home. Before she left, however, Ruby asked for Charles's lawyer to stop by so she could sign the inheritance papers for Charles's estate. When the lawyer arrived, he explained to Ruby that Charles had left her some jewelry and a few thousand dollars, but that was it. Not the apartment on Park Avenue, not the lodge in Vermont, and not his extensive stock portfolio. Everything had gone to his children. Ruby was not distraught, only confused.

There has been a mistake, she said.

No, the lawyer said. No mistake.

We'll see about that, said Ruby. She ordered the lawyer to go to court and have the judge correct the error.

That won't be possible, Ruby. Here is the will.

And so she waited.

And waited.

For thirty years, Ruby waited. Patiently.

The judge will be signing the papers any day now.

And while Ruby waited, she refused to leave. So Ruby was transferred to the state hospital. And still, she refused to leave until the judge corrected the error.

While she waited, she thought she might make herself useful. And so she waited behind the security doors, and, eventually, behind the metal detector, greeting people in her Chanel suit, smiling at everyone who passed by and at the resident psychiatrist who needed an ID badge and key.—JG

SELF-ESTEEM

A rather different approach to the psychology of delusions is taken by Richard Bentall, who proposed in 1994 that persecutory delusions could be understood, roughly, as attempts to preserve self-esteem. People tend to fall into two groups when it comes to explaining a bad event like a job loss: those who blame themselves and those who blame others. An early study by Bentall and Sue Kaney compared the ways in which depressed and paranoid patients explained life events and found that depressed patients tended to blame themselves for negative events, whereas paranoid patients blamed others. The patient groups differed, that is, in what is known as "attributional style."

One advantage that the paranoid attributional style has over the depressed style is that it preserves self-esteem. If you lose your job because of what someone *else* does, you need not worry about whether you are inadequate in some way. Unfortunately, there are times when it's hard to find someone to blame for your troubles. You want that Nobel Prize in literature as much as anyone and think you deserve it. Of course, you've only written one novel and nobody but *Solid Waste and Recycling* magazine reviewed it. In those circumstances, many of us might think about changing careers. But that option means accepting both the painful thought that you don't have a talent for fiction and the loss of self-esteem that comes with it. If you couldn't accept that loss, you might be forced into a strange belief—for example, that the Nobel committee is prejudiced against you because your parents sent you to a communist summer camp when you were eight. Accepting this belief will save your self-esteem but at the price of a paranoid view of the world—one that will affect the way you experience events in the future. If you believe that there are people bent on blocking your path to the Nobel Prize, the world will seem like a more threatening place than it did before you adopted that belief. An attributional style of this kind, therefore, may lead to paranoia. Bentall thus takes paranoia to strengthen a weakness in the ego, and, in this, he is the legatee of Freud.

Why do paranoid individuals explain negative events by appealing to the malicious intentions of others? Attributing one's failures to bad luck, for example, would preserve self-esteem just as well. In order to answer this question, Bentall and his colleagues propose that something other than attributional style must also be at work in paranoia. One possibility is that people with psychosis gravitate toward ideas of threat. A second possibility is that people with persecutory delusions have difficulties understanding other people's motivations—an idea we'll come to shortly—and infer malicious intent where there is none. Other biases, such as the JTC bias, or an inability to accurately interpret social situations, may also be relevant. Psychological impairments of these kinds may dispose someone to attribute malign intent to others and blame them for negative events. As before, this attributional style makes the world seem more dangerous, and a downward spiral into paranoia begins.

THE DELUSIONAL BRAIN

Thus far, we've focused on the psychology of delusions. Some of the neurobiological models of delusion, however, share some of the principles of the psychological models we've just discussed. To the extent that we have neural theories of delusion that try to explain how delusions emerge from disordered brain function, they come from more general accounts of psychosis. It's worth taking a detour through a couple of these views in order to explain why neurobiology is not yet equipped to understand delusions.

Before turning to these theories, we should say a word about the neurobiology of delusions more generally. At the moment, we know very little about the biology of delusion per se. Antipsychotic drugs can abolish or reduce delusional thinking, even in disorders other than schizophrenia, so it is possible that delusions have something to do with dopamine or the other transmitter systems affected by those drugs. When it comes to disorders involving delusions other than schizophrenia, we have only scattershot data. Delusional disorder, for example, is associated with head injuries and drug abuse. Delusions are also symptoms of illnesses with known brain pathology, such as dementia. We don't yet know whether all delusions result from a small family of neural processes or from a variety of different ones, nor do we have very clear ideas about *how* brain disorders cause delusions.

What we know about the delusional brain comes from two primary sources: brain-imaging studies (mostly in schizophrenia) and studies of patients with brain lesions. Unfortunately, these studies don't agree all that much about the disorders that cause delusions. Brain-imaging studies of schizophrenia patients with paranoid delusions suggest that the areas relevant to delusions are in the frontal or prefrontal regions, the temporal lobe, and the subcortical brain structures, the amygdala and the hippocampus. (See Figure 8.)

Some of the most interesting brain lesion data come from patients suf-

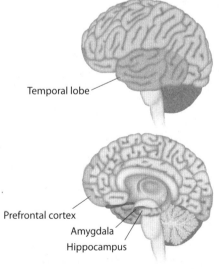

Temporal lobe

Prefrontal cortex

Amygdala

Hippocampus

Figure 8: Some of the brain areas implicated in delusions.

fering from misidentification delusions. When these delusions are associated with known brain damage—and not all are—lesions to the right hemisphere and the frontal lobes are frequently found.

PUTTING WRONG IDEAS TOGETHER

The first of the neural theories we'll consider was developed in 1999 by Nancy Andreasen as a general hypothesis about schizophrenia and builds on the work of Eugen Bleuler, the psychiatrist who coined the term *schizophrenia*. Bleuler believed that one of the central symptoms of schizophrenia was a disturbance in association—the way in which ideas are linked together—and disturbed association is the centerpiece of Andreasen's theory. Following Bleuler, Andreasen hypothesizes that the primary symptom of schizophrenia is what she calls "cognitive dysmetria," a "disruption of the fluid, coordinated sequences of thought and action." The linchpin of the theory is the idea that cognitive dysmetria is echoed in a disorganization of the brain regions implicated in schizophrenia. These regions (the prefrontal cortex, the cerebellum, and the thalamus) are connected via bundles of nerve fibers into a neural circuit known as the cortico-cerebellar-thalamo-cortical circuit, or CCTCC. When the brain regions in the circuit fail to communicate normally, a disorder of associative thought arises. According to Andreasen, the problem is one of timing: the temporal properties of the circuit are abnormal, so the information that is carried by the circuit is also handled abnormally. If the timing of the CCTCC is off, then information passed from one part of the circuit to another will get incorrectly linked to other information. Since the information in a misfiring CCTCC is not coordinated, the patient's ideas will be incorrectly associated. The thought of a ray, for example, which might normally be associated with the thought of the sun, might now get incorrectly associated with the thought of God's nerves. Schizophrenia is thus a "misconnection syndrome," where the disorganized connection of brain regions produces fragmented thought.

Andreasen's theory is particularly good at explaining disorganized thought (and speech), which DSM-5 identifies as one of the symptoms of schizophrenia. One variety of disorganized speech is "word salad," where the patient produces an incoherent jumble of words and phrases. The misconnection theory will say that mistiming in the CCTCC leads to the incorrect association of ideas, causing the words or phrases that express the ideas to be jumbled. Since the phenomenon of word salad is, in effect, an observable manifestation of a conceptual jumble, it's just what the misconnection theory would predict about schizophrenic speech.

The misconnection theory also has a good account of what is known as "flight of ideas." This symptom is characterized by a rapid shifting from one thought to another, often involving plays on words or puns. It is usually seen in mania, but it can also be present in schizophrenia. Unlike word salad, a flight of ideas is coherent enough to be understood, and a natural way for the misconnection theory to explain the symptom is to suppose that mistiming in the CCTCC (and thus the misconnection of ideas) can be more or less severe. When there is a slight mistiming, the associated ideas are disorganized but intelligible—a flight of ideas; when the mistiming is serious, the result is word salad. Andreasen's theory, if correct, not only explains these two symptoms of schizophrenia, but also shows how they are related.

When we turn to delusions, however, the misconnection theory fares less well. Schreber believed that Flechsig had committed soul murder, that God was affecting his nerves, and that all of creation had been destroyed. We don't know why he had these pathological ideas rather than some other ones. Still, the delusions are perfectly understandable, and they hang together in a way that is coherent, if peculiar. This is true even of the most outlandish delusional beliefs. If you think you are dead, for example, you have a belief that seems to be self-refuting: since dead people can't have beliefs, the fact that you've got one means you're alive. There are few beliefs that could be more nonsensical, and yet no one has any trouble understanding what a patient means when he asserts that he is dead. Because the thoughts of delusional patients are perfectly comprehensible, they are not much like a flight of ideas and nothing like word salad. If what lies at the root of psychotic thinking is a timing problem in the CCTCC, it's not clear why delusions remain coherent.

The obvious way to adjust the misconnection theory in order to address this problem would be to invoke again the idea that mistiming in the CCTCC (and the consequent misconnection of ideas) comes in degrees. When the mistiming is extreme, we get word salad; when it's moderate, we get flights of ideas; when it's minor, we get delusions. But does this solution really work? The misconnection hypothesis says that the worse the timing of the CCTCC, the worse the thought it produces. But it doesn't seem true that time and thought run in parallel. Unless you are making a considerable effort, everyday thoughts don't move from sensible association to sensible association like the waves caused by a rock thrown into a lake. When you are in the pasta aisle in the supermarket, your thought about a jar of arrabbiata sauce doesn't necessarily lead inevitably to tomatoes, ketchup, olives, appropriate side dishes, Barolo wines, and so on. Thoughts jump all over conceptual space very quickly, and a thought about arrabbiata sauce could just as easily be followed by a yearning for that high-def TV, a momentary worry about your cousin's upcoming knee reconstruction, or a memory of Ursula Andress in that bikini. In short, the passing of time doesn't measure conceptual distance in thought. Consequently, a slightly mistimed CCTCC is no more likely to produce meaningful, if odd, associations than it is to produce nonsense.

Finally, Andreasen's theory also faces the puzzle we've noted in connection with some of the other theories we've reviewed. If delusions are caused by a misassociation of ideas, then in principle any ideas could get misassociated with any others to produce an endless stream of bizarre ideas on every topic imaginable. But, as we've suggested, people with psychotic illnesses don't have an endless stream of bizarre ideas; only about a dozen.

IN THE SPOTLIGHT

The second biological theory of psychosis and delusion has dopamine as its centerpiece. Although the early formulation of the dopamine hypothesis has been abandoned, many theorists continue to believe that dopamine is an important part of the story of schizophrenia. In order to theorize about a dopamine abnormality in schizophrenia, however, we have to have a theory about what dopamine does when it is functioning normally. One hypothesis developed by the psychiatrist Shitij Kapur has been very influential. Kapur's idea is that the effect of dopamine is to make something in the environment stand out in experience. You see a close friend on the other side of a crowded room, for example, and she stands out in your experience of that room; she has a kind of psychological spotlight on her. That spotlight is created by dopamine. According to Kapur, the dopamine abnormality that characterizes schizophrenia puts the psychological spotlight on the wrong features of the environment, and the resulting "aberrant salience" leads to some of the symptoms of psychosis.

Kapur's hypothesis works this way. Suppose Tom is watching the television news. He hears the newscaster say that violent crime is up by 1 percent over last year. Because Tom's dopamine function is abnormal, that statement stands out in his experience in the way a friend would stand out across a crowded room. Why, Tom asks himself, does that statement seem so significant? Perhaps, he thinks, because the newscaster is speaking to *me* in particular. But why, Tom wonders, would she be telling *me in particular* that crime is up? Maybe she is trying to send me a message of warning. As a result of this chain of reasoning, a random event—a story about crime statistics—becomes a delusion of reference because it is made inappropriately salient by an out-of-whack dopamine system.

Like Maher's theory of delusion, the aberrant salience hypothesis is about anomalous experience. For that reason, it raises the same sort of puzzle. If dopamine function is disordered in schizophrenia, there seems to be no reason why it couldn't make *anything* salient: the color of the socks of the person sitting next to you on the subway, the fact that there are six letters in "Peoria," the experience of seeing a cloud that looks exactly like Margaret Thatcher holding an AK-47.

A natural response to this problem is to say that while dopamine may indeed make any old thing salient, delusions come about only when the patient *reflects* on the oddly salient phenomenon. Delusions, as Kapur says, "are a 'top-down' cognitive explanation that the individual imposes on these experiences of aberrant salience in an effort to make sense of them." Echoing Maher, Kapur claims that delusions aren't descriptions of strange experiences but *explanations* of why you are having them.

Unfortunately, this only pushes the problem back: we now need to ask—as we did in our discussion of Maher—why a patient's *reflection* leads to aberrant explanations. If your wife suddenly appeared strangely unfamiliar to you, as Ellis and Young's theory of the Capgras delusion hypothesizes, why is it that the delusional person opts for a bizarre explanation of that experience when lots of other nonbizarre explanations are closer at hand? Consider Dick, who, like Tom, also has a dopamine problem. The statement that crime is up 1 percent over last year also stands out in his experience, and, like Tom, he wonders why. Well, he thinks, perhaps I am developing a real interest in the sociology of urban life. He turns off the television and decides to earn a PhD in criminology. This explanation of Dick's aberrant salience is at least as plausible as Tom's. (If you find something standing out in your experience, wouldn't it be natural to think that it was because it was intrinsically interesting?) But this explanation is not strange or bizarre in the way delusions are. Aberrant salience doesn't have to lead to aberrant *explanations of* salience.

But what if it does? Maybe there is something about strange experiences that somehow calls for strange explanations. It's possible, but it won't help. Consider Harry: his dopamine is also abnormal, and the newscaster's claim about crime being up is salient in his experience as well. Harry is interested in *gematria*, the ancient Jewish practice of assigning numerical value to words or phrases and exploring their relation to other words or phrases with the same numerical value. When Harry reflects on the salience of the increase in crime, he hypothesizes that it must be because the numerical value of the phrase "crime is up 1 percent" (suitably translated into Hebrew, of course) has precisely the same numerical value as the name *Maher-shalal-hash-baz,* a son of the prophet Isaiah. Now this is a very odd idea, and maybe Harry came up with it because his experience is odd. But Harry isn't delusional, even though his idea might be as bizarre as Tom's. If delusions are the result of aberrant salience, there should be a lot more Harrys than are known to psychiatrists.

HOW DOES IT FEEL?

When trying to describe what it might feel like to have a delusion of reference, my colleague Michael Garrett cleverly employs a common experience most of us have had, so as to convey the paranoia and terrifying sense of being singled out that many psychotic people feel.

Imagine this scenario: As you pass a break in the tree line on a highway, a state trooper pulls out onto the highway. He turns on his rotating, flashing lights. You look down to see that you are driving 75 mph on a 65 mph highway. You press the brakes slowly, but you know it's too late. Your heart races. Then the state trooper speeds past you. In a flash, you realize it is not you he is after. It still takes a minute for your jaw and hands to unclench. There were thirty other cars driving approximately 75 mph, yet for a moment you knew, with fatalistic certainty, that those flashing lights were coming for you.

How does it feel to be psychotic? I don't know. I have never heard non-existent voices or seen things that were not there. Nobody has suggested that I have delusional beliefs. Though it's unlikely in the next decades that I will develop schizophrenia or bipolar disorder, illnesses that tend to present before middle age, depression is certainly possible and with it the potential for psychotic symptoms. A stroke or a traumatic brain injury could also lead to hallucinations and delusions—and the possibility of dementia worries us all.

Fear of the psychosis that lurks within each of us may explain the distancing some psychiatrists engage in with psychotic patients. Instead of trying to get inside the heads of their patients, they medicalize the relationship. Symptom? Check. Antipsychotic? Check. But nothing can protect us from the fear, the *possibility* of going mad, and being scared doesn't help anyone. A colleague, one who cares very much about what his patients feel, told me of a recurring dream in which he is the patient, not the doctor: he is on the unit, his door is locked, and he is pleading to his psychiatrists that he's not crazy and should be discharged. They do not listen.

The reality is, the vast majority of psychiatrists have not experienced psychosis, and over the long history of mental illness, this non-understanding has been a major barrier to treatment of those who have it.

Physicians in other specialties have all experienced pain, nausea, thirst, weakness, and the fear that accompanies these and other symptoms. Similarly, psychiatrists know what it is like to be anxious and can identify, if only in part, with depressed patients, even if they have not had an episode of major depression (though many have). We have all been sad, all experienced guilt and low energy, and these experiences are a reasonable approximation of what our patients are going through.

But psychosis is another matter. The subjective experience mostly eludes us. Hearing a patient describe a delusion is a far cry from *feeling* it. Since good social relationships with patients are strongly correlated with better outcomes, then learning how to empathize becomes particularly important when approaching psychosis. And this is not just a concern for psychiatrists. Family members desperately want to comprehend what their loved ones are feeling. A patient of mine recently said of her friend's psychotic episode, "You can explain to me what goes on in the brain, but it's still so mysterious."

In the end, I have to agree: there is a mystery at the center of psychosis. But if we are limited to comparisons in our understanding, there is still a lot to compare it to. Temporary approximations of psychosis include delirium (a dangerous state of confusion associated with medical illness) and substance use. Hallucinogens, as the name suggests, often induce hallucinations, and a "bad trip" may bring paranoia, as can marijuana, cocaine, and amphetamine use. Dreams, good and bad, also hint at a way forward in the dark. The wish fulfillment of the dreamer who can fly, the nightmares of being chased by an unseen malevolent being, and of the friend whose changing features signal he might be an impostor—these common dream scenarios seem a lot like the delusions we present in this book. Films like *Shutter Island* and *Gaslight* might also give the viewer some sense of what it's like to be psychotic. And books describing psychotic illness can be particularly illuminating due to the intimacy of their writing. Elyn Saks's *The Center Cannot Hold: My Journey Through Madness* is a moving illustration of her long battle with schizophrenia. Kay Redfield Jamison's *An Unquiet Mind: A Memoir of Moods and Madness* describes the author's experience of having bipolar disorder and attendant psychotic symptoms. Jamison is a clinical psychologist and an expert who has gone on to coauthor the definitive textbook on bipolar disorder.

It's possible that the "daily hassles" of technological society will also help us understand psychosis. At the airport recently, while awaiting reentry to the United States, I saw a single Department of Homeland Security officer checking passports. Another officer was doing nothing, just sitting in a chair, looking down. Standing some thirty feet away, I whispered some wisecracks to my wife and child about the glacial pace of things—comments not even the man in front of us could have heard. When we finally got our passports stamped and walked through, another officer—the one who had appeared to be doing nothing—stopped us for a "routine" check. After a while, he said to my crying child, "Your dad doesn't think we're working hard enough. I'm going to show him what we do." I was gobsmacked. "How did you hear me?" I asked. His response? "We have ears." The entire area, I later learned, was full of hidden microphones.

Am I on some watch list now? Will I be allowed back into the country the next time I leave?

The fear remains with me. Maybe I do know what it feels like to be psychotic.—JG

THINKING ABOUT THOUGHT

A single theme has run through our review of the theories of delusion. If delusions are produced by anomalous experience, or faulty reasoning, or both, there ought to be a lot more forms of delusion than there are. It's quite possible that experience and reasoning play some role in delusion, but a successful theory is going to have to add something to the mix for theory to match the phenomena of delusions as psychiatrists understand them. We conclude our review of delusion theory with two models that do just that.

Richard Bentall's suggestion that people with delusions may have trouble understanding the motivations of others originates in an influential theory of schizophrenia developed by Christopher Frith. In a 1992 book, Frith proposed that many of the symptoms of schizophrenia, including a number of delusions, could be explained as the consequences of a defect in the "Theory of Mind," or ToM, the ability human beings have to think about the thoughts and feelings of others. Having the ToM capacity is sometimes described as having the ability to "mentalize" (to think about mental states) or the capacity for "meta-representation" (the ability to mentally represent the mental representations of others). ToM develops naturally in healthy young children, and some proto-version of it appears to exist in babies as young as fifteen months.

A classic test of ToM is the "false belief task." If you want to try it with your own child, take some candy and hide it under a yellow cup in clear view of the child and another adult. (We'll call the adult Josie.) Josie now leaves the room. Transfer the candy from under the yellow cup to under a blue cup. Josie then reenters the room. Now ask your child where Josie thinks the candy is. A three-year-old will say that Josie thinks the candy is under the blue cup; a four-year-old will say that Josie thinks it's under the yellow one. The three-year-old consults *his own* beliefs to answer the question about Josie's beliefs, but the four-year-old has crossed a cognitive bridge; he understands that Josie's perspective is not the same as his own, and he can imagine Josie's perspective in order to infer what she believes. People with autism often fail ToM tests, and a ToM deficit is at the heart of a leading cognitive theory of the problems that people with autism have with social interactions.

It's quite easy to imagine that someone who couldn't think accurately about other people's thoughts might come to feel threatened by them. Suppose one of your colleagues usually offers to get you a coffee when she goes out to get one for herself. Today she goes for coffee but doesn't offer you one. What might be going on in her mind? She might simply have forgotten to ask you; she might be distracted by the fight she had with her boyfriend; she might be short of cash; or . . . she might have formed an alliance with all the baristas in town to make sure you don't get any caffeine. Someone with a normally functioning ToM capacity is not going to find the last alternative plausible, but if one's ToM were impaired, a paranoid idea about others' motivations might seem reasonable.

Theory of Mind deficits may generate other forms of delusion as well. A typical ToM thought has this form: "She thinks (wants, hopes, . . .) that _____." So, for example, "My boss wants me to come to the meeting on time." Given this thought structure, Frith suggests that ToM deficits can take three distinct forms. (1) I can be mistaken about what someone thinks. Instead of "My boss wants me to come to the meeting on time," I can have the thought "My boss wants me dead." (2) I can mistakenly omit the reference to the person whose thought I am contemplating, so that instead of "My boss wants me to come to the meeting on time," I have the thought, "Come to the meeting on time." Or (3) my thought can have no content at all.

Because ToM is the capacity to think about thoughts, I can use it to think about my *own* thoughts as well as the thoughts of someone else. The three kinds of error just discussed can therefore occur in at least three domains. (1) I can think about someone else's intentions (as in

"My boss wants me to come to the meeting on time"); (2) I can think about my intentions (e.g., "I plan to take the month of August off"); and (3) I can think about my goals (e.g., "I must contribute to Oxfam"). The table below summarizes the possible combinations along these two ToM dimensions of deficit and domain.

		Level of Defect		
		Impaired content	Detached content	No content
Level of Awareness	**Own goals** I must contribute to Oxfam.	I must take over Oxfam.	Contribute to Oxfam.	No goals.
	Own intentions I plan to take the month of August off.	I plan to have supernatural powers in August.	Take the month of August off.	No self-intentions.
	Others' intentions My boss wants me to come to the meeting on time.	My boss wants me dead.	Come to the meeting on time.	No other-intentions.

Table 2: Theory of Mind and the symptoms of schizophrenia.

Now notice that many of these combinations are suggestive of particular delusional forms (as well as other symptoms of schizophrenia). "I must become the boss" and "I plan to have supernatural powers in August" are rather like grandiose delusions; "Contribute to Oxfam" and "Take the month of August off" sound like delusions of control or of thought insertion; "My boss wants me dead" sounds persecutory; and the absence of an intention could be experienced as thought withdrawal.

Frith's theory has led to a very fruitful line of ToM research in schizophrenia, and his model of delusions addresses the question we've been belaboring of why delusional themes are so limited. Because ToM is concerned with thoughts, delusions will inevitably gravitate to the fairly limited range of ideas that center on our own goals and intentions and those of others, and this is what distinguishes them from the vast majority of other strange ideas.

Some important questions remain open. It's not clear why an impairment of ToM should lead exclusively to delusional thoughts. Why, that is, does thinking about the boss's intentions lead to persecutory thoughts rather than affectionate ones? And why does reflection on my own intentions lead to grandiosity rather than self-deprecation? Why is the effect of detached content interpreted as control or thought insertion rather than as an expression of a commitment or a decision? And why is the absence of content experienced as thought withdrawal rather than as a moment when you're simply not thinking about anything?

Still, a ToM deficit captures an important feature of delusional thought, and we'll return to ToM (though to a somewhat different application of it) in our own account of delusion.

USEFUL DELUSIONS

We turn finally to a rather different approach to delusion, that of evolutionary psychology, the discipline that attempts to understand mental traits as having been "designed by natural selection to solve the adaptive problems regularly faced by our hunter-gatherer ancestors." In recent years, some investigators have tackled questions about psychopathology using the same tools and established the discipline of "evolutionary psychiatry." Could delusions be an evolutionary adaptation?

Edward Hagen has developed just such a theory regarding the delusions found in delusional disorder (the psychotic disorder characterized by delusions as the sole symptoms). Subtypes of delusional disorder are distinguished by delusional theme: *persecutory, grandiose, somatic,* or *erotomanic.* Observing that these delusional motifs refer primarily to the social world, Hagen proposes that they evolved for a social purpose. Because social relations are so crucial in human life, their loss would be a devastating assault on one's fitness (that is, one's ability to survive and reproduce), and faced with social isolation, our ancestors would have used every possible strategy—including deception—to reestablish social ties. Hagen hypothesizes that delusional beliefs are part of a behavioral strategy designed to deceive others into social alliances. However, although people with delusions are engaging in deception, they are not aware of it. Since successful deception has to be convincing, Hagen proposes that the delusional person will have a better chance of pulling it off if he or she believes the delusion and acts accordingly. Delusions develop and persist, therefore, by means of unconscious processes that are not accessible to the delusional person.

To see how the theory works, let's consider persecutory delusions. In human prehistory, one of the central benefits of social life was defense against the aggression of others, and social isolation would have made you extremely vulnerable. Suppose, however, that you come to believe that you and your community are profoundly threatened in some way. If you can convince others that they are also vulnerable and engage their fear of a mutual threat, they may opt to establish ties with you for the purpose of enhanced defense. Persecutory delusions, according to Hagen, evolved precisely for the purpose of luring others into relations of mutual defense.

Beyond defense against aggression, Hagen claims that the importance of two other benefits—social exchange and mating—drove the evolution of the other delusional forms. Somatic delusions—those that concern body integrity and health—are part of a strategy to get others to look after you in exchange for reciprocal care, and grandiose delusions are designed to deceive others into believing that you have commodities of social value (such as useful information) that would make you worth cultivating. Among the most useful of social commodities, of course, is access to people of high status, and people suffering from erotomania often believe that their lover is an important person. Erotomanic delusions evolved to convince others that you are "well connected" and a valuable alliance. Erotomania is thus closely linked to grandiosity.

Let's highlight a few of the features of Hagen's account. First, according to the theory, delusions *aren't symptoms of illness*. People with delusions are activating a kind of nuclear option in response to a crisis represented by the loss of social ties. Second, for delusions to be plausible deceptions, they ought to be hard to falsify quickly. Believing that you are a Kennedy on your mother's side, for example, or that you are the target of a plot by the Freemasons of SoHo is the kind of thing required. Third, it follows from Hagen's view that it has to be possible to convince at least some people that your delusions are true. Unless some people find delusions plausible, they can't possibly fulfill their evolutionary purpose. Finally, the theory makes two crucial predictions: (a) that delusional disorder will develop only in people who are suffering from social isolation, and

(b) that it will remit if social bonds are restored. There is some evidence for both of these claims.

Hagen's theory is profoundly important and elegant in the way it links the particular thoughts expressed in some delusional forms with their putative evolutionary functions. Locating delusions in the context of the evolution of the mind makes it possible to understand why delusions have the content they do, and our own strategy adopts the same methodology.

Where we disagree with Hagen is in his hypothesis about the purpose of delusional thoughts. As we've noted, delusions have to be believable to be useful. It's hard to know whether or not our early ancestors were more gullible than us, but the contemporary evidence suggests that delusions are quite quickly identified for what they are. Even delusional ideas that are believable at first blush—my husband is cheating on me; the neighbors are trying to hurt me; I've got a terrible disease—are seen by others to be false in pretty short order. Any social bonds they help to create, then, are liable to be broken as soon as it's clear that the delusion is a deception. In fact, delusions may get you a reputation as a liar and *increase* your social isolation.

The second problem with the theory is that if having a delusion represents a good solution to a serious social problem, it should be widespread, but delusional disorder is, in fact, very rare. Hagen himself cites statistics according to which it occurs with a frequency of one to three in ten thousand. (DSM-5 estimates two in a thousand—much higher but still rare in absolute terms.) The fact that delusional disorder occurs so infrequently suggests that it is more likely to be a malfunction of some kind than a behavioral adaptation. Could delusional disorder be a common strategy to deal with social isolation but rare in absolute terms because social isolation is itself uncommon? Not likely. It's hard to know how to measure the occurrence of the loss of social bonds, particularly in human prehistory, but, as Hagen notes, "social rejection, exclusion, shunning, and ostracism have been documented among . . . numerous cultures, most institutions (e.g., government, military, education), all types of relationships (formal and informal), and among children, adolescents, and adults." If delusional disorder is one way of coping with social isolation, it isn't very successful in evolutionary terms, and we should wonder why it is still around at all.

TRUMAN REVISITED

A paranoiac psychosis. Imagining that I'm the center of a vast effort by millions of men and women, involving billions of dollars and infinite work . . . a universe revolving around me. Every molecule acting with me in mind. An outward radiation of importance . . . the object of the whole cosmic process . . .

—P. K. Dick, *Time Out of Joint*

In writing this book, my thoughts naturally turned to the first patients with Truman Show delusion, introduced in the preface, whom I hadn't seen in many years. I contacted them and set up meetings with the ones willing to discuss their lives and mental health, past and present. I hoped that in getting to know these people better, in settings beyond the confines of a psychiatric ward, they might help shed light on the questions we were now asking about the meaning of the Truman Show delusion, the nature of delusions generally, and what cultural, social, and environmental factors, if any, might have played a role in their illnesses. And I was curious to see where life had taken them.

David: Unreality Show

I first met David on my unit at Bellevue, where he had been brought by his girlfriend, Rebecca. David and Rebecca both worked in the film and television industry. Ironically, at the time of his admission, he was working on a reality show.

Rebecca had actually broken up with David in the weeks leading up to his admission, not because he had bipolar disorder (something they were both already aware of), but because she felt he had been irresponsible in his drug use, knowing that it could intensify his illness. They had been dating almost a year when Rebecca began to notice "Truman Show-esque signs" of delusion. David accused her of dating him only because she was "in on this Hollywood thing and . . . in this reality show." She remembers that around this period David was also acting in an off-Broadway play. There was a hole in the wall of his apartment through which he believed people might be watching him. Feeling betrayed by her, David told Rebecca their "whole relationship had been under the guise of a reality show and that [she] was coming from Hollywood."

David grew up in a family with a depressed and substance-abusing father who was in and out of rehab. David also used drugs, and as a teenager was kicked out of boarding school when he was caught smoking pot. He came home for his senior year of high school and soon after found his father using cocaine. He moved out of the house and lived with a friend and her family. David thinks this new environment helped him have his best academic year.

David's first psychotic break occurred in college. Believing that a homeless couple were the rock stars Pete Townshend and Grace Slick, he invited them back to his parents' home. Though Pete and Grace were agreeable guests, David's family recognized that his judgment was off. David had been using copious amounts of drugs (marijuana, hallucinogens, ecstasy) and was snorting Ritalin. At first, David's doctors believed he was likely suffering from a substance-induced psychosis, but he was ultimately diagnosed as having bipolar disorder and treated with a mood stabilizer.

David's second manic and psychotic episode took place after he had graduated from film school and was living in New York City. At the time, he believed that Rebecca was a member of the Kennedy family and that the Secret Service was following him. He was admitted to a hospital, was quickly discharged, then got the reality show gig. His Bellevue hospitalization followed soon after. David had been raised as a Roman Catholic, but religion did not preoccupy him until he became manic. On the day he was admitted to Bellevue, he had been yelling the Ten Commandments and claimed in the ER that he was Muslim. Then, upstairs on the unit, he met with Bellevue's rabbi to talk about converting to Judaism.

Eight years after our initial encounter at Bellevue, I met David again, this time in his apartment in Los Angeles, where he had moved some years earlier. In LA, he had had one more manic episode and hospitalization. "Every time I've been hospitalized, it's been the same thing," he now recalls. "I thought I was being followed, like *The Truman Show*, and I was a hit. People were following me all across the world." He didn't give much thought to where the cameras were. He figured they were now capable of being so small that they could be hidden anywhere. The music he listened to on his iPod was the soundtrack for the show, mostly hip hop, but not the rapper 50 Cent. According to David, 50 Cent was angry at him about unpaid royalties and might do him bodily harm.

In LA, David believed that all the cars that passed him were driven by Hollywood talent agents. Blue cars were driven by William Morris agents, red cars by CAA agents, and white cars by ICM agents. Despite the success of his show, David found the whole thing upsetting to the point where he lay down in traffic. "I just wanted it to stop," he said. The Angelenos honked and swerved to avoid him, but no one got out of their car to help.

Rebecca flew to LA to visit David in the hospital. They had stayed in touch since breaking up, and she remained close to his family, who called her when they were worried about him. Rebecca still admires David's direct and honest manner but says that he can sometimes come at her like "a freight train." Rebecca describes David as an intense, passionate man whose personality fuels his creativity but whose illness sets him back. She noted that David's illness flared up at moments when something big was about to happen, and wonders if the stress of impending success might not trigger his mania.

It is a great pleasure to reconnect with people I've known only in their psychotic state who have gone on to find something we all pursue: equilibrium and a measure of happiness. Today, David is a film producer in Hollywood. Both he and his father have been in Alcoholics Anonymous. David's father has been sober for ten years and has grown closer to his family. David has a new girlfriend (she has also been in AA) and a promising career in Hollywood. Rebecca observed the irony: it is an amazing thing to behold someone who once had Hollywood delusions now making his life there a reality.

As I left, David reminded me of the importance of keeping his mental illness a secret from all but those closest to him. "Would a production company trust me with a thirty- or fifty-million-dollar budget if they knew I had bipolar disorder?" Good question.

Lori: Charley's Mom

Lori, a fifty-one-year-old journalist from Indianapolis, flew to New York City with her husband Quentin as soon as they heard that their son Charley had been admitted to Bellevue. Charley had been a tough kid, she said. Sweet and loving, but exhausting, the kind of boy who still had tantrums at sixteen. Charley was popular and close to his sister, but his mother always felt that he was strange. In college, he became increasingly eccentric. Charley moved to New York to pursue a career in journalism, the same field as his mother's, but according to her, the traumatic events of 9/11 seemed to have "pushed him over the edge." Lori recalls that Charley refused to open his Christmas gifts in 2001, and when he finally did, he felt sad and foolish for not having opened them right away. A year later he had his first hospitalization at Bellevue, suffering from Truman Show delusion. Apparently unaware of the compensation scales at public hospitals, Charlie believed all of his doctors were highly paid actors.

While her son was at Bellevue, Lori brought me a detailed family medical history. Charley's grandparents on both sides suffered from depression and alcoholism, and Lori thought that her own mother probably had bipolar disorder, even though she'd never been diagnosed. She recalled her mother impulsively painting the basement orange in the middle of the night and choosing to add a coat to the family piano as well. Lori's experience in her own childhood of being yelled at continually made the similar volatility in her home with Charley feel normal. With the family history of mental illness on their minds, Lori and Quentin were always on the lookout for signs of depression in Charley and felt frustrated by pediatricians who would minimize Charley's odd behavior.

In the months leading up to the hospitalization, Charley began accusing Lori via email of being abusive. Lori found herself apologizing for minor disputes that had occurred twenty-five years earlier, but Charley would not accept her apologies and stopped talking to her. After a lot of crying on Lori's part, Charley finally relented and forgave her. Soon after, Charley's illness worsened and he was hospitalized.

After Charley was discharged from Bellevue, he returned to live with his parents in Indianapolis. Despite her own reservations, Lori thought "Okay, this will be fine, he'll take his meds and everything will be okay." Her husband predicted that Charley would not take his medication, and he was right. Charley became psychotic again and believed that his parents were actually aliens inhabiting his parents' bodies or possibly actors. Despite not taking his meds and the return of the delusions, Lori believes Charley managed to stay out of the hospital by keeping these thoughts from his psychiatrist and forbidding the doctor to speak to her and Quentin.

At one point Charley made a tearful confession to his parents: he believed he was dead, his experience was an illusion, his family was not really his, and his true family was elsewhere, mourning him. "In every psychosis there is a grain of truth," Lori observes. "And that was a little bit true. We were his real family, and we were mourning him, and it was almost as if our real son was dead." Still, when Charley returned home from another year in New York, Lori put everything else, including her career, on hold to look after him.

Lori was becoming burned out caring for Charley. Every so often Charley would set her off, and a screaming match would ensue. On one occasion, she became increasingly frustrated with a barrage of questions and demands. She yelled at him to stop, and when he didn't, she picked up a glass bowl from the kitchen table and threw it down, shattering it. Lori recalled chillingly, "I didn't even hear the sound. I said to my husband later, 'If there had been a weapon in my hand, I might have used it. I don't know if I would have used it on him or on me, but I'm really scared.'" After that episode, it was Charley, somewhat ironically, who suggested to Lori that she get some help. She began seeing a therapist whom Lori credits for saving her and her family.

Charley continued to take his antipsychotic meds only intermittently and shuttled back and forth between Indianapolis and New York City. Once, he called from New York to inform them he was coming home in two days. Lori and Quentin were wary, not certain if they were prepared for his intense presence again, and told Charley that there would be certain expectations once he moved back in, including his finding a job and, of course, remaining in treatment. Charley was wounded by their ambivalence, and when they picked him up at the airport, Lori recalls, "there was a look in his eyes, which we now know means he was totally off his meds." Lori and Quentin took to locking their bedroom door at night. Lori lost seven pounds in the first five days of Charley's return.

Charley moved out after a while and began couch surfing at friends' places, but he would inevitably be asked to leave. At one point he was more or less homeless for six months. He started sending his parents threatening emails. They started locking all their doors. Charley ultimately created a public disturbance, leading to his arrest and another hospital stay. When he was discharged, fearing for their safety, Lori and Quentin directed him to various health and housing resources rather than allow him back in the house.

Charley moved between shelters, group homes, and hospitals, and then ran away from a group home, where he had been legally mandated to stay. He hopped on a bus back to New York. Lori didn't understand why nobody in the group home or county health services would try to get Charley back. Lori asked, "How many Greyhound buses can there be going to New York? Can't you just ask someone to wait at the bus station in New York and bring him back?" The answer: "Nope. Can't do it." The mandate didn't extend beyond the state border. Lori cried some more. In her estimation, "the system completely failed."

Charley shuttled between hospital and jail. A former psychiatrist once told Charley that, as his delusional thoughts would likely remain, their shared goals should include setting those beliefs aside so that he could survive in the world. As Lori sees it, Charley was too smart for his own good. He did not take the psychiatrist's words to heart; instead, he learned the words by heart. Lori recites them herself: "I have beliefs that other people don't have, but I can set them aside and I can still function." Charley would repeat that line whenever he was brought to the hospital—so much so that Lori would warn the doctors ahead of time when he was en route. More often than not, it worked for Charley.

It didn't work for Lori. She was done. In her estimation, the combination of budget cuts, Charley's ability to say the "right" things, and the principle of having patients in the "least restrictive environment" conspired to keep Charley from getting the help she believed he needed, namely long-term inpatient care.

Charley had previously been arrested for minor nonviolent offenses, like loitering and mischief, but he became more ill and assaulted two strangers. After more bouncing from jail to hospital and back again, Charley made his way to Florida in 2008. One day after arriving, he threatened to kill a waiter over a bill. Later in court, he threatened to kill his public defender. Charley has been incarcerated or on parole ever since.

When asked what she's learned, being the mother of a severely and persistently mentally ill son, Lori answered, "I thought I was pretty tough. It's made me more humble. There are some things that cannot be fixed. I was just sure I could fix him. That I would fix the family and everything would be fine. Some things cannot be fixed."

Though Lori has talked about giving up hope or giving up on Charley, she never has. They rarely speak, but when they do, she continues to tell

Charley that if he were ever to stay on his medication and stick with the program for a reasonable period of time, they could be a family again. In the meantime she tries to enjoy the family she has, though she would prefer it were whole.

Lori returns to the theme of mourning. She has a friend who lost a child to a drug overdose. They used to compare notes, since her friend's daughter's behavior on drugs was similar to Charley's when he was off his meds. When the young woman died, Lori thought about the day she might get a similar call. She and Quentin prefer to remember the son they once had. "It's almost like he's dead, but he's not dead, because he's still our son. And as long as he's alive, he'll be our son."

Postscript: Unlike most of the other people with Truman Show delusion we write about in this book who have episodic psychosis, Charley almost certainly has schizophrenia. Despite his family history of mood disorder, his near-constant and progressively worsening symptoms are more consistent with a schizophrenia spectrum illness rather than, say, bipolar disorder. This diagnosis did not determine Charley's unfortunate narrative. The vast majority of people with mental illness, including schizophrenia, are not violent. And though his insight may be limited due to his illness, Charley has repeatedly chosen to disengage from his treatment and from his family. These decisions are informed as much by personality traits as by any psychotic symptom. All of us make poor decisions—often the same ones, again and again—in the absence of delusions. Charley was a difficult child who became a difficult adult.

Ethan: The Otherness of Other People

Nearly a decade after I last saw Ethan, we met at a soccer field in Golden Gate Park, in San Francisco. He chose the spot. He had been a good soccer player as a kid, and meeting here might make talking about a painful past a bit easier. Six feet tall, wearing a Barcelona soccer jersey, a baseball cap, and sneakers, Ethan looked to me like an Asian Matt Damon. In high school, Ethan was a star athlete and played on the varsity team in three sports. Soccer had been his primary passion and he was a California All-State player. After his ADHD was diagnosed and treated, he became a more successful student. For the first time, he was excited by ideas and became a voracious reader. He preferred science fiction; among his favorite authors were Neal Stephenson, David Brin, Greg Egan, and later, Charles Stross and Cory Doctorow. These writers, along with the early giants of sci-fi, inspired him to think big. Ethan changed his mind about focusing on sports and instead went to MIT. Now an assistant professor of computer science, Ethan was working on how to get computers to see patterns in large data sets.

When Ethan left Bellevue, his diagnosis was uncertain. He might have been in the early stages of schizophrenia, but to get that diagnosis, he would have to be ill for more than six months. It was still a possibility that the psychotic episode had been brought on by the Ritalin. It was just too early to tell. Since Ethan had continued to improve after his discharge, while on a lower dose of Risperdal, it looked like the trouble had been the Ritalin. This was confirmed when Ethan started using it again to get through a three-day machine learning conference he had organized. He hadn't slept at all in the week leading up to the event, and on the last day, after introducing the final speaker and sitting down to listen, it hit him. The conference, the speech, everything—it was all about him: a big game with him at its center. He knew there were rules, but he couldn't remember what they were. It was like being Kafka's Joseph K. Ethan had been walking the tightrope between ADHD and psychosis for four years, and now he fell back into delusion.

Before his psychotic break, Ethan had been reading books and watching movies that had illusion as a theme: *The Truman Show, The Matrix, The Twilight Zone, Total Recall, The Game*, Robert Heinlein's Trumanesque short story "They," featuring an alien disguised as a psychiatrist, and Philip K. Dick's novel *Time Out of Joint*, about a man who has a psychotic break and is placed in an artificial environment much like Truman's Seahaven. Now Ethan was living in his own version of that world.

Even before he had made computer science a career, Ethan had always been interested in the logic of making predictions and had participated in competitions testing out predictive strategies, winning one prestigious contest. He had been trying to figure out how to bet on the future, and now others were betting on him. And this was no small-time book. The entire world was wagering on Ethan's behavior. Winners could earn money for themselves, but the primary goal was for people to collect money for charities of their choice. Ethan hoped the game was making charity cool, but even if many were playing only for themselves, the vigorish, along with money lost by bettors, would guarantee a windfall for charities. A board of directors of seven people including Noam Chomsky, Christopher Hitchens, and Jon Stewart would allocate the money not only to the charities but also to every single person on earth. In time, as the game molded Ethan into an even more ethical and rational person, he would get involved in the disbursements.

At Bellevue, Ethan determined that he had simply forgotten that he had developed the game. This time around, he went one better, concluding that he had consented to have his friends hypnotize him, so that his behavior would be authentic, untainted by the knowledge that the world was betting on his every act.

More good came out of the game. Ethan enjoyed knowing that Bob Costas was doing the play-by-play when he hit a home run at a Palo Alto softball field. On one occasion, while sitting on a lawn on campus having lunch, Ethan heard the sound of a piano and recalled how his father, then suffering from advanced Parkinson's disease, used to play. In that moment, Ethan understood that as a reward for all of the good he was doing for the world, his father had been provided with the latest cutting-edge treatment for Parkinson's, and he could now play again. Ethan wept with joy.

Despite the delusions, Ethan remained Ethan. Unlike someone in the grip of mania who becomes wildly grandiose, Ethan remained shy, diffident, and sensitive to criticism. He was particularly concerned that his university lectures would be slammed on the websites where the world communed to watch and talk about him (and bet, of course), but he steeled himself with F. Scott Fitzgerald's observation that "what people are ashamed of usually makes a good story." And besides, if people made witty, albeit stinging, comments about Ethan, it would at least add some spice to what he recognized as the pretty mundane stuff of his everyday life. At one point, he considered engaging in more outrageous, "reality TV–type" behavior in order to keep people interested but ultimately decided against it.

Ethan was not privy to any online postings, as the game necessitated a parallel internet created just for him, manned by a team of journalists who wrote fake news. During this episode of illness, Ethan had been teaching an undergraduate class on "predictive analytics" and thought that his students would be using the course material as part of their training to join the CIA. With former students in powerful positions, he would be safe from the people who wanted to manipulate the game for profit, like those who had sequenced his genome, wanting inside information, literally. Because Ethan felt his computer was being monitored, he didn't write anything personal on it. Instead he wrote longhand in a notebook, imagining himself a latter-day Winston Smith, scribbling out of sight of Big Brother. At a time when people tweet their thoughts, hoping the world will read them and fearing no one will, Ethan had the whole world watching but wanted to keep his thoughts to himself. In light of the recent revelations of massive government spying, perhaps we will see a resurgence of handwritten correspondence like Ethan's.

Ethan's girlfriend, Anna, was the only person on earth not in on the game. She knew Ethan so completely that he felt she was "part of my own mind's operating system." To him, Anna was Ada Lovelace, Lord Byron's daughter, the first computer programmer. It became clear to Anna that something was wrong. She and Ethan had been living together, but his behavior had grown strange. She felt he didn't trust her, and recognized that he was having difficulty distinguishing reality from fantasy. In fact, Ethan *did* trust Anna and felt it was wrong of him to expose her to the dangers of being his girlfriend. He broke up with Anna for her own safety. Still, when his father developed Parkinson's, she reached out to Ethan, and they got back together.

About two months after Ethan had his game epiphany at the conference, he confided in Anna that he was being watched. He had had enough. He was on the floor, crying. He had already told his roommate that he wanted it to stop, but not understanding what Ethan was talking about, the roommate just shrugged and left the room. Ethan took this to mean that his roommate was part of the organization running the game; they wanted a more dramatic ending. Anna called Ethan's psychiatrist. Ethan told the doctor his plan to approach somebody on the street to ask for the game to end. The doctor told Ethan that he was not well and needed to go to the hospital. Ethan remembers thinking, "Okay. So that's how it's going to end." He felt that upon arriving at the hospital he would be welcomed and feted. He would be told, "Great job. You did it!" But once in the emergency room, Ethan found himself in a tiny room with an old woman. He knew then that "this is not some story. This is real." It all came crashing down. After only a few days in hospital, Ethan's delusion receded. "It just fell away," he said. During his brief hospital stay, Ethan was primarily concerned with not missing the class he was teaching.

After a relationship of three years, Anna moved east for a professional opportunity, and although the two separated, they have stayed close, and

Anna continues to worry about him. She likes that Ethan is intellectually curious, questions the world, and is continually trying to figure things out. But the ideas that consume him are heavy; he dreams of beautiful things, but he wants that beauty used in a morally acceptable way; he doesn't let the people he loves and who love him get as close as they might. When we spoke, Ethan's thoughts turned to a passage written by the psychologist Nicholas Humphrey about the "psychological distance between people, the extent to which everyone remains an enigma to everyone else." The phrase that stood out in Ethan's mind was "the otherness of other people." Still, Ethan feels a deep love for his family, especially his mother, and he knows his friends love him despite not seeing him frequently.

Ethan hasn't had any psychotic episodes since then. He's reduced his meds and is doing fine. Like everyone, he sometimes struggles with the blues. Although he says that the past couple of years have been the happiest of his life, he feels he still has a long way to go. His academic career is thriving, though he wonders if he wouldn't prefer work that has more of a directly beneficial impact on the world. He's still fascinated with prediction markets, but he no longer believes he is the person others are betting on or the focus of worldwide philanthropy. He's just a really smart guy who cares a lot about other people, worries about our future, and thinks about the dangers associated with technology. Ethan quotes the third of Arthur C. Clarke's Three Laws: "Any sufficiently advanced technology is indistinguishable from magic." Is that so strange? After all, technology has turned a bizarre delusion about being watched into a sober worry. Cameras are everywhere: closed-circuit television cameras, high-definition personal cameras, internet cameras, reality-TV cameras, and many more. With everyone watching everyone else, for more purposes than we can know, the Truman Show delusion has crossed a threshold.

Reflecting on fame, the man who once believed that billions of people followed his every move writes, "Everybody knows who Kim Kardashian is, and I confess to not even really understanding why." Clearly, Ethan is now as sane as can be.—JG

PART II

THE SOCIAL LIFE OF MADNESS

3

THE MADDING CROWD

THE FORMS OF DELUSION

We've belabored the idea that while many people have all sorts of bizarre beliefs, only a very small subset—perhaps a dozen in all—are recognized as delusions. This narrowness of focus is even more striking when one notices that the forms of delusion are conceptually related to one another, in particular in their concerns with the social world:

1. *Persecutory delusions,* the most prevalent of all delusional forms, invariably focus on others and are thus social through and through. People who are paranoid aren't afraid of running out of garden fertilizer or choking to death on a crepe. They're afraid specifically of the harm that other people can do to them.
2. *Delusional jealousy* is persecution writ small: the cheating partner and/or the "other woman" are represented as threatening.
3. *Erotomanic delusions* are also concerned with the theme of love and therefore with other people.
4. Although *religious delusions* are typically categorized as belonging to an independent form, this is probably a mistake. Some religious delusions are simply persecution writ supernaturally large. Although it may seem strange to think that a delusion about God is no different from a delusion about the *Sopranos,* when it comes to brain function, the distinction may be irrelevant. As the anthropologist Pascal Boyer points out, the separation between the physical world and the spiritual realm wouldn't have been made in earlier cultures. Even today, there are societ-

ies in which supernatural beings are, in some respects, no different from humans. In Africa, for example, dead relatives are as much actors in everyday affairs as neighbors and may be no less powerful.

5. *Grandiosity.* Religious delusions can also be grandiose when they represent the delusional person as made important by a connection to God. Although they are often described as beliefs that one is a very important figure—Napoleon or Jesus, according to the clichés—what unites them is the idea that the delusional person is special relative to other people; that he has, in effect, a higher status: "I could find the key to the cure to cancer"; "I am a special athlete, and I run a national charity"; "I am also a famous DJ. I have Superman-type powers"; "I am also the cousin of Tony Blair, and I can fly." Grandiosity thus clearly makes reference to the social world.

6. *Delusions of control.* Given how pervasive persecutory delusions are, it's not surprising that other delusional forms also have a persecutory flavor. Delusions of control express the idea that your behavior is being driven by someone else, and implicit in the delusion is the idea that this control is harmful.

7. *Delusions of thought.* Thought insertion, thought withdrawal, and the like are conceptually tied to delusions of control because the ability to manipulate someone's thoughts is implicitly a way of manipulating that person's behavior.

8. *Somatic delusions.* At the center of the social world is the self, and the foundation of the social self is the body. Hagen's evolutionary account of somatic delusion provides one illustration of this idea. Somatic complaints are not merely expressions of the state of one's body but (among other things) invitations to be cared for. Although somatic delusions refer to bodily states, therefore, they make links to social motifs.

9. At least one *nihilistic delusion* (Cotard) overlaps with the somatic. Other species of nihilistic delusion include beliefs about oneself or others—for example, a belief that one's relatives have died or that one has been robbed. The losses represented by these delusions are thus typically social in nature.

10. *Delusions of guilt* or *sin* represent oneself as responsible for disas-

ters, and the notion of moral responsibility presupposes violations of obligations to other people, including the person of God.

11. *Delusions of reference* underscore the idea that the self is at the center of the social world. In these delusions, events are occurring in relation to the delusional person and have a special meaning for him.

12. Finally, *misidentification delusions* concern who is who in the social universe. In effect, they raise questions about the social world around the delusional individual, and are sometimes persecutory in tone. For example, the Fregoli delusion (named for Leopoldo Fregoli, a well-known quick-change artist of the early-twentieth-century theater) is the belief that you are being followed around by someone who keeps changing disguises and who may be out to hurt you.

In the next three chapters, we try to answer the central question about delusion: why are the forms of delusion both interrelated and restricted to the social? Our answer, in brief, is that delusions are symptoms of a disorder in a mental capacity whose function is to navigate the threats of social living. What distinguishes them from other bizarre thoughts is their origin in this mental capacity.

Because our case is an extended one, an agenda might be of use. In this chapter, we review the evidence of the many links between psychosis and social life. We focus on schizophrenia because it is the primary focus of research in psychosis. In the next chapter, we sketch a social-evolutionary framework for thinking about delusions; and in the one after that, we outline our social theory of delusion and its implications for the Truman Show delusion in particular.

THINKING ABOUT OTHERS

In an obvious sense, psychosis and the social are linked in the conspicuous fact that every person who suffers from schizophrenia, the primary form of psychosis, is socially isolated or struggles to cope with social relations at work and at home. Two different kinds of impairment could lie behind this struggle. Someone who has had a stroke and can't form new memories is going to have trouble navigating the social world because she is going to have trouble with most of her life. In contrast, someone who suffers from prosopagnosia, the inability to recognize faces, will struggle with social life, but *only* with social life. Prosopagnosia is a specific deficit of social perception, whereas the ability to form new memories is necessary for a much broader range of activity: not just interacting with others, but also finding your way around a new city, paying bills, keeping a job, and so on.

A large body of research shows that the social impairments of schizophrenia are more like prosopagnosia than memory loss; they are specific to social cognition—the psychological capacities that make it possible to function successfully in a social group. Within the domain of social cognition, four topics have been extensively investigated in relation to schizophrenia. First, people with schizophrenia have difficulties with "social perception": they don't pick up social cues well, and they misunderstand social roles and expectations. Second, they show deficits in expressing, recognizing, imitating, and experiencing emotion: their facial expressions, expressive gestures, tones of voice, and vocal rhythms are blunted. Third, as Richard Bentall has shown, people with psychosis differ in attributional style: while people with depression tend to blame themselves when things go wrong, people suffering from psychosis tend to blame others. Finally, Theory of Mind (ToM) is impaired in schizophrenia.

A recent meta-analysis looked at thirty-six studies using three different measures of ToM and found impairments of all three in people with schizophrenia who were actively symptomatic and to a lesser degree in people whose illness had remitted. The first measure is a version of the false-belief task discussed above. In this version, however, participants are asked to infer that someone has a false belief about someone else's belief (e.g., infer that Josie falsely believes that Cleve believes the Montreal Canadiens are playing on Saturday night). The second measure of ToM is the "hinting task." Here participants read a conversation between two people in which one of the characters drops an obvious hint. The test requires the participant to say what the character actually meant. Here's an example:

Paul has to go to an interview and he's running late. While he's cleaning his shoes he says to his wife, Jane: "I want to wear that blue shirt, but it's very creased."

Question: What does Paul really mean when he says this?
Extra information: Paul goes on to say: "It's in the ironing basket."
Question: What does Paul want Jane to do?

The third measure of ToM is the Reading the Mind in the Eyes test (see Figure 9), in which participants are shown pictures of the eye region of a face together with four words that refer to mental states. The goal of the test is to choose the word that best expresses the state of mind of the person represented. (Since the actual state of mind of the person is unknown, the "correct" answer is the one chosen most often by healthy individuals.)

In all of these measures of ToM, people with schizophrenia perform less well than healthy individuals. Taken together, these studies support the idea that a ToM deficit is a signature of schizophrenia.

SEEING THREATS

In our discussion of the theories of delusion, we mentioned the threat anticipation model of Daniel Freeman and his colleagues. Given the centrality of persecutory delusions in psychosis, threat is an important notion for the theory of psychosis, particularly since people with schizophrenia show abnormalities in threat detection.

Threatening faces—understood as those expressing anger or fear—command our attention because they signal imminent danger. Studies

joking   flustered

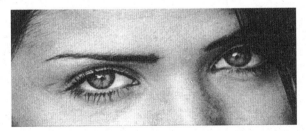

desire   convinced

Figure 9: An image from the Reading the Mind in the Eyes Test. (The correct answer is "desire.")
Reproduced by permission of Professor Simon Baron-Cohen.

over the past thirty years have shown that people with schizophrenia perceive emotions differently. A meta-analysis by Christian Kohler and his colleagues demonstrated a large difference between people with schizophrenia and healthy controls across a variety of measures. In particular, people with persecutory delusions show a bias in favor of the detection of negative emotions. A study by Amy Pinkham and her colleagues, for example, compared actively paranoid and non-actively paranoid people and found that the former had a tendency to identify neutral expressions as angry.

In healthy people, angry faces are identified as angry more rapidly than faces expressing other emotions. Moreover, healthy individuals scan angry faces in a unique way. In contrast, delusion-prone and clinically delusional people show abnormal scanpaths when perceiving angry and fearful faces (see Figure 10).

Surprisingly, though, people with persecutory delusions show fewer eye fixations on threatening facial features than healthy individuals do, suggesting that they are paying less attention to them. Melissa Green and Mary Phillips interpret this counterintuitive fact as evidence that the

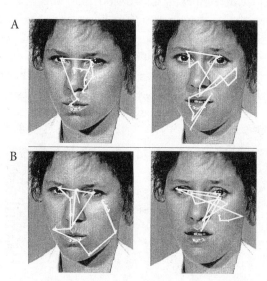

Figure 10: Visual scanpaths of (A) healthy and (B) delusion-prone individuals looking at angry and fearful faces. Adapted by permission of Taylor & Francis Ltd.

perception of threatening faces occurs in two stages, the first of which is automatic and unconscious, and the second of which is conscious and controlled by attention. People with persecutory delusions are more sensitive to threat in the first stage of face perception; they show an aversion to threat in the second stage perhaps because threat-related stimuli are specially stressful to those who are actively paranoid, and they consciously avoid it.

A different sort of evidence about threat and psychosis comes from a study of time perception. Abbie Coy and Samuel Hutton classified healthy participants as more or less "hallucination-prone"—a risk factor for psychosis. Pictures of faces expressing emotion were displayed, and the participants were asked to estimate how long the displays lasted. The more hallucination-prone the viewer, the longer they estimated the displays of angry faces to be; no other emotions were associated with time distortions. Because people tend to overestimate the passage of time when they are emotionally aroused, the experiment demonstrates a relationship between hallucination-proneness and sensitivity to anger.

Persecutory delusions are also correlated with the presence of threat-related cognitive distortions. In one study, participants were asked to remember sentences contained in passages of text. The delusional group remembered fewer sentences overall but more of the ones containing ideas of threat. A second study found that people with persecutory delusions were more likely to remember and repeat threat-related words than emotionally neutral ones. Paranoid patients also pay more attention to words expressing threats.

Finally, a study by Katherine Newman Taylor and Luisa Stopa compared people with persecutory delusions and those with social phobia, a psychiatric disorder characterized by a fear of being scrutinized and negatively evaluated by others. Newman Taylor and Stopa asked participants about their thoughts concerning social situations, self-consciousness, distress, anxiety, and depression. Surprisingly, the participants with delusions and those with social phobia were indistinguishable in their answers. Both groups experience other people as threatening.

Are abnormalities in social threat perception a cause or a consequence of psychosis? There is some evidence for it being a cause. First, even when psychosis has remitted, emotion recognition deficits may persist. Second, people at high risk for schizophrenia—but who have not had a psychotic break—show a similar impairment. Third, problems with emotion recognition may run in families. A study by Kimmy Kee and her colleagues found that healthy biological siblings of people with schizophrenia share some of the same deficits.

Beyond the association of psychotic illness and deficits in social cognition, there is a lot of circumstantial evidence that social life may also contribute to the development of psychosis. The lines of evidence for this idea come from the study of childhood adversity—abuse, bullying, and parental separation—immigration, and city living.

(ENVIRON)MENTAL ILLNESS I: CHILDHOOD ADVERSITY

In 1907, the year he met his collaborator-to-be Sigmund Freud, the psychoanalyst Karl Abraham published "On the Significance of Sexual Trauma in Childhood for the Symptomatology of Dementia Praecox," a paper in which he describes three psychotic patients and their histories of sexual abuse. Due to the small number of cases, Abraham couldn't draw any conclusions about whether the abuse caused the psychosis, and in the century that followed, only a tiny fraction of the research on schizophrenia and psychosis paid attention to child abuse.

In recent years, however, things have changed. In a 2005 review of the literature, John Read and his colleagues claimed that child abuse was probably a determinant of psychosis, including schizophrenia. Although the claim was controversial at the time, the review renewed interest in the topic. A subsequent review found that 42 percent of women and 28 percent of men with a psychotic disorder had reported sexual abuse, and 35 percent of women and 38 percent of men had reported physical abuse. (A survey of the general population estimated that "only" 11 percent of respondents had experienced sexual abuse, and 25 percent physical abuse.) Nonetheless, these findings are not widely known among North American practitioners.

A Dutch study published in 2004 asked more than four thousand adults without psychosis about childhood abuse before age sixteen. Those who went on to develop psychotic symptoms in adulthood were found to have a 2.5- to 9.3-fold increase in the risk of developing a psychotic disorder, and the worse the abuse, the greater the risk. Those who needed treatment for psychosis had a roughly 7-fold increase in risk.

More recent studies have provided further evidence of the connection between abuse and psychosis. A large Australian study from 2010 found a 2- to 2.5-fold increase in the risk of psychosis, including schizophrenia, among victims of childhood sexual abuse though only in cases that involved penetration. The people who had the highest risk were those who were abused by more than one person. A British report in the same year found increased rates of psychosis only in children who had suffered severe physical abuse by the mother but not the father. A study comparing siblings, only one of whom had a psychotic disorder, found that they typically shared both a history of trauma and a higher risk of psychosis, but that the psychotic sibling had experienced the greater trauma. Because siblings tend to be similar in many ways, the possible significance of the difference in abuse is enhanced. Finally, a 2012 meta-analysis found an overall 2.78-fold increased risk of psychosis due to childhood adversity. Meta-analysis is a powerful tool, and a 2.78-fold increase in risk is substantial.

The victimization of children can also be carried out by other children. Bullying is at last being given the serious attention it deserves, and we are discovering that the numbers are not small. We are also discovering that bullying is associated with psychosis. One study found that 10 percent of teenagers reported that they had been physically assaulted sometime during the previous year either by a schoolmate, relative, acquaintance, or stranger; 39 percent said they had been bullied. A 2009 study by Andrea Schreier and her colleagues investigated psychotic symptoms in a group of more than six thousand twelve-year-old participants in the Avon Longitudinal Study of Parents and Children (ALSPAC). The study found that children who reported bullying at eight or ten years of age were about twice as likely to have psychotic symptoms as those who did not. Chronic or severe bullying was associated with a 4.6-fold increase in risk. Other research has shown that bullies who are themselves bullied are at particularly high risk.

It's possible of course that being bullied is the result of having psychotic experiences rather than the other way around. Kids who are "different" are targets for bullies, and having psychotic symptoms is certainly likely to make you different. The fact that psychotic symptoms vary with the severity of the bullying, however, weighs the balance in favor of bullying contributing to psychosis. Having psychotic experiences might make you different, but it's not obvious that more psychotic experiences would make you seem *more* different, whatever that might mean. Even when Schreier and her colleagues took account of factors that might make someone attractive to a bully (such as having already been victimized), the results were unchanged.

Further evidence that bullying leads to psychosis rather than the other way around comes from a 2013 study by Ian Kelleher and his colleagues, who investigated more than one thousand Irish teenage students in the Saving and Empowering Young Lives in Europe (SEYLE) study concerned with suicide prevention. The students were asked about bullying, physical assault, and psychotic experiences on three occasions over the course of a year. Those who had been bullied had more than a 4-fold increase in the risk of psychotic symptoms three months later, and a 3.4-fold increase in risk at twelve months, with more victimization increasing the risk. The study did in fact find evidence that psychotic experiences also predict an increased chance of being bullied, supporting the psychosis-causes-bullying hypothesis. In order to clarify the data, Kelleher and his colleagues removed from the analysis participants who reported psychotic experiences at the time of the first interview. (These were the individuals who were more likely to attract bullying by virtue of being different.) The relation between bullying and psychotic symptoms persisted. When bullying and physical assault stopped, the risk of psychotic symptoms dropped. Taken together, this is strong evidence for a causal relation between victimization and psychosis.

Childhood trauma can also occur without malicious intent. The death of a parent, or a separation of a year or more between parent and child before age sixteen, is associated with a two- to three-fold increase in the risk of psychotic symptoms in the child. Even living in a single-parent household or spending time in the care of social services appears to increase the risk. In a study that began in 1966, researchers followed children of Finnish women who were asked at the time of pregnancy whether the birth was wanted or not. On follow-up, children who were "unwanted" were twice as likely to have developed schizophrenia.

Parents can also go some way to protecting their children from psychosis. A very large study carried out by Pekka Tienari and his colleagues looked at children who had been adopted decades earlier by mothers with and without schizophrenia-spectrum disorders. In children born to healthy mothers, who were therefore at low risk for psychosis, the adoptive environment made no difference to their risk of psychotic symptoms. In high-risk children, however, the environment made a big difference. Those who were adopted into a "dysfunctional family environment" were at much higher risk of developing a psychotic disorder than those brought up in "healthy" families.

There are a couple of important caveats to keep in mind here. First, although the increases in the risk of schizophrenia found in these studies are very substantial, the absolute risk of illness even in vulnerable individuals is still very low. If the average person has one chance in a hundred of developing schizophrenia, then a doubling of that risk—a substantial increase—brings the absolute risk to only two in a hundred, which is still relatively low. Second, studies of the kind we've just discussed always have methodological limitations that should lead us to be cautious in interpreting the data. There is no doubt that many more rigorous studies will have to be carried out before a clear picture of the complex relations between childhood adversity and psychosis emerge. More important, none of these results should be taken as evidence for the myth, exploded long ago, that parents are "responsible" for their children having schizophrenia. Most families affected by schizophrenia care for and support their loved ones. Moreover, childhood adversity plays a role in many illnesses, including cancer, cardiovascular disease, and diabetes. Blame seems irrelevant to understanding these diseases; why should psychosis be different? Still, finding ways to combat childhood adversity would contribute in important ways to the primary prevention of all of these devastating illnesses, including psychosis.

EXPRESSED EMOTION

Perhaps the best-known body of research dealing with the social determinants of psychosis concerns "expressed emotion" (EE) on the course of schizophrenia. For decades, studies have shown that people with schizophrenia are more likely to relapse if they are exposed to relatives who are more critical and hostile, or emotionally overinvolved—high on expressed emotion. A 1994 meta-analysis of twenty-five investigations published from 1962 to 1992 showed that patients living in high EE families were about two and a half times more likely to suffer a relapse.

High EE does not contribute to people developing schizophrenia, but it is an important aspect of life for those living with it. Ironically, high EE is often stimulated by schizophrenia itself. As Gillian Haddock and Will Spaulding put it, "this behavior is generally considered to be a result of a normal reaction to the incredible stress associated with experiencing a relative who has a psychotic illness." High EE family members tend to be more self-critical as well as critical of the person with schizophrenia, and those who are emotionally overinvolved have a tendency to feel guilty.

Family-based services (also called family management, family intervention and social intervention) have been developed to try to lower the stress in high EE environments and reduce the likelihood of relapse. An evaluation of this form of support found that after two years, only 17 percent of patients had a significant exacerbation of their schizophrenia, compared to 83 percent of patients receiving individual management alone. The findings were independent of medication compliance. Another study found that patients receiving medication but no social intervention that lowered family EE had a relapse rate of 78 percent at two years, but those who accepted both medication and family intervention that lowered EE had a relapse rate of only 14 percent.

(ENVIRON)MENTAL ILLNESS II: IMMIGRATION

In 1932, Ørnulv Ødegaard investigated the prevalence of schizophrenia in Norwegian immigrants to the United States. He found that some psychiatric disorders were more common among the immigrants than among people living in Norway, but the effect was far larger in the case of schizophrenia than the other diagnoses. This landmark finding has been replicated over decades in a variety of immigrant populations. The most recent meta-analysis of these studies was carried out in 2010 by

François Bourque, Elsje van der Ven, and Ashok Malla, who analyzed twenty-one previous studies from the United Kingdom, the Netherlands, Sweden, Israel, Denmark, Australia, and Canada. In all but one of the original studies, immigrants were found to have a higher risk of developing a psychotic disorder than the rest of the population, and the meta-analysis confirmed this; immigrants are at a little more than twice the risk of the native population—about the same increased risk for schizophrenia associated with using cannabis or with perinatal complications. Remarkably, second-generation immigrants were found to be at the same increased risk as their immigrant parents. This means that whatever is making immigrants more vulnerable to psychosis, it is not the stress of immigrating but of *being* an immigrant, so to speak. This idea is supported by a study showing that the younger someone is when they immigrate—and thus the longer their experience of being an immigrant—the greater their risk of psychotic disorder.

Moreover, as Ødegaard discovered, the immigrant effect seems to be relatively specific for psychosis. The physical health of immigrants is not generally made worse by immigration. In fact, immigrants are often healthier than the native population. And although the stresses of migration can contribute to other mental disorders, like anxiety or depression, the relation is much less clear or consistent.

What could account for this phenomenon? Some hypotheses that have been advanced have been debunked: Ødegaard thought that people who are at higher risk for psychosis might be more likely to migrate, but that hasn't been supported by the data. Nor are immigrants more likely to use cannabis. The effect can't be put down to some vague stress of novelty, because the local culture is not novel for the child of immigrants, and yet the trauma of migration passes into the next generation. It has also been suggested that the immigrant effect might be due to the fact that immigrants tend to move to urban environments which, as we'll see, also play a role in psychosis. However, the meta-analysis by Bourque and his colleagues found that the risk of psychosis in immigrants is the same when comparing urban and mixed urban-rural regions.

At the moment, there is simply no consensus on what makes immigration psychologically toxic. Nonetheless, the studies that have been done hint at an important possibility. Many of the immigrants investigated—in particular, dark-skinned immigrants to predominantly white countries—

have been visibly "foreign": Caribbeans, Africans, Pakistanis, and Bangladeshis to the United Kingdom; Surinamese, Dutch Antillean, Moroccans, and Turks to the Netherlands; and Africans to Sweden. One investigation (not included in the meta-analysis) that found a *decreased* risk of psychosis among the immigrant population followed immigrants to Australia, most of whom came from mostly white countries (e.g., the United Kingdom and New Zealand). In the 2010 meta-analysis, immigrants were classified as "black," "white," or "other" depending on the majority population in the home country, and the risks for these groups were found to vary with skin color. The "white" group had a 1.8-fold higher incidence of illness in the period studied; the "other" group had double the incidence; the "black" group had a 4-fold higher incidence. Among the second generation, those in the "white" and "other" groups had the same risk as their parents, but members of the "black" group had a higher risk—more than five times that of the local population. These findings strongly suggest that it might be something like discrimination and not immigration that is raising the risk of psychotic disorder. Indeed, as Bourque and his colleagues note, second-generation immigrants are exposed to discrimination for a longer period, as well as earlier in life, when they are likely to be more vulnerable to its effects, which may explain how the schizophrenia risk of a black child may be greater than that of her immigrant parents.

More evidence for the relevance of discrimination comes from the one study included in the meta-analysis that didn't find an immigrant effect, a study of children of European immigrants to Israel. This group may be an outlier because, as the authors note, European Jewish immigrants are more likely to feel like minorities in their home country than in Israel, and they are not typically victims of discrimination when they migrate. In contrast, two other studies carried out in Israel found an immigrant effect among dark-skinned immigrants (Ethiopians, Indians, Pakistanis, and Sri Lankans) who *are* likely to face discrimination.

Because having dark skin raises the risk of psychosis among immigrants, the possibility has been mooted that a vitamin D deficiency might explain the immigrant effect. Dark-skinned immigrants are certainly at higher risk of vitamin D deficiency, but it's not the case that all of the immigrants who show an increased risk of psychosis have dark skin. Ødegaard's original cohort is a case in point. The immigrant effect appears to be an intrinsically social phenomenon.

Independent evidence for a link between discrimination and psychosis has been found outside the immigration literature. An investigation conducted by Wim Veling and his colleagues examined the relationship between perceived discrimination and psychosis in ethnic communities in The Hague. Levels of discrimination were determined by means of interviews as well as on the basis of reports to the Anti-Discrimination Bureau. The incidence of a psychotic disorder was increased in the period studied 1.2 to 4 times in ethnic communities compared to native Dutch participants, and higher rates were found among those who faced more discrimination. Another study followed people with no history of psychotic disorder over a three-year period. Of these, 0.5 percent reported delusional thoughts. Participants were asked about whether they had faced discrimination on the basis of skin color, ethnicity, gender, age, appearance, disability, or sexual orientation. In those who reported discrimination of one kind, the rate of delusional thoughts rose to 0.9 percent, and to 2.7 percent in those who reported discrimination in more than one area.

SAMIR: POKING AROUND THE BRAIN

Samir, a thirty-six-year-old Bengali man, came to Bellevue Hospital looking for his wife, whom he feared had been hurt in an accident. She was visiting family out of town, and he had spoken to her earlier in the day, but after listening to the news on the radio and hearing about a minor fender bender during the traffic report, Samir felt that the newsreader was speaking directly to him and signaling that his wife had been in a major accident. When he couldn't reach his wife, who had told him she would be turning off her phone for several hours, he began to panic. At first he went looking for the radio station to speak with the reporter, but could not find it and so started checking local hospitals. Bellevue was the fifth hospital he visited that day. By the time he arrived, he was utterly distraught and was escorted to the psychiatric ER.

Soon thereafter, the ER staff was able to locate Samir's wife on her family's landline, but it took quite a while to convince him that she was safe. His wife informed the attending psychiatrist that her husband had had previous episodes of believing that reporters on television or the radio were communicating with him directly.

Samir had been hospitalized two years previously, she explained. At the restaurant where he worked, after being told he could not take time off to visit his family in India, he impulsively quit his job and subsequently became depressed. During that time, he had felt as though something had been "poking" in his brain. Whenever he saw a story on television about the brain or neuroscience, a not uncommon occurrence, he felt that the presenter was reminding Samir to have his brain checked. He visited several neurologists and had brain-imaging scans done, and was routinely disappointed when he was told that there was nothing physically wrong with him. At least one neurologist urged him to see a psychiatrist, but Samir refused. After his frustration rose at a neurology clinic at another city hospital, he became agitated, banging his head against the office wall. In short order, he was seen in the nearby psychiatry clinic and was ultimately admitted and treated for the depressed type of schizoaffective disorder. He took antipsychotic and antidepressant medication, to good effect. Upon discharge, Samir visited his family in India and enjoyed himself. When he got back to the United States, he found work at another restaurant but stopped taking his medication, in part because he was feeling better, and in part because the medication sedated him and he was working very long hours. He did not keep his follow-up appointment with a psychiatrist.

When his wife made it back to New York and to the hospital, Samir was relieved, but after she prodded him to be forthcoming with the doctors, he acknowledged other delusional ideas. The brain-poking sensation he had previously felt had returned, but this time Samir believed that it was caused by a conspiracy of unknown individuals emitting sounds at particular frequencies. Moreover, these people would communicate with one another via a series of hand and arm signals. He would see strangers on the street motioning in particular ways, informing one another as to when Samir was approaching so they could make the appropriate sounds to perturb his brain. Samir discovered this system when watching a meteorologist gesturing at a weather map, pointing out high- and low-pressure systems, which Samir took to mean high and low sound frequencies and which he coupled with the hand movements of the weatherman. Samir admitted that he had come close to assaulting one of the conspirators on several occasions but feared losing his job, being incarcerated, or being hospitalized again. Instead, he took to stuffing cotton balls in his ears and bought noise-canceling headphones that he would wear whenever he could, even—to his wife's displeasure—in bed.

Samir was admitted to Bellevue and treated in much the same way he had been during his first hospitalization, and he responded to treatment equally well. The only difference was in his discharge planning. His social worker was able to secure a Bengali psychiatrist for a follow-up appointment. Samir promised his wife he would go, and he made it to his first appointment. But after that, as with so many patients who passed through the psychiatric ER, I never saw Samir again.—JG

(ENVIRON)MENTAL ILLNESS III: THE CITY

The link between city living and schizophrenia was first discovered in 1939, when two sociologists, Robert Faris and Warren Dunham, published a study of first-episode psychosis in Chicago. Faris and Dunham found higher rates of schizophrenia in inner-city neighborhoods characterized by social disorganization and social isolation but no parallel differences in the rates of bipolar disorder.

Faris and Dunham's striking finding has been the springboard for a great deal of research investigating urban living and psychosis. The Aetiology and Ethnicity in Schizophrenia and Other Psychoses (ÆSOP) study, the most ambitious and rigorous to date, followed 568 cases of first-episode psychosis from 1997 to 1999 in three cities in England (Nottingham, Bristol, and Southeast London) and found rates of psychosis higher in London. The ÆSOP findings replicate those of Faris and Dunham, including the fact that the incidence of schizophrenia was highest in inner-city neighborhoods such as Brixton and Camberwell. A 2004 review came to a similar conclusion, and a 2012 meta-analysis by Evangelos Vassos and his colleagues, combining more than forty-five thousand individuals with psychosis, found a 2.37-fold increased incidence in the period studied in the most urban environment relative to the most rural, with rates of psychosis rising with city size in an almost linear fashion. This finding was unchanged whether or not the studies looked at schizophrenia, narrowly defined, or psychotic disorders more broadly. Nor did it matter whether urbanicity was measured by the absolute size or the density of the population. Both the city of birth and the city in which one was brought up were associated with a first psychotic episode, although early experience seems to matter the most. And the more years spent in a city from birth to age fifteen, the greater the risk.

It turns out, however, that what counts as a city is relative. E. Fuller Torrey, Ann Bowler, and Kitty Clark analyzed American census data from 1880 and found that the larger the city, the higher the rate of schizophrenia, even though all of the "cities" were so small that they would count as rural areas today. City toxicity is thus likely to be a function of either absolute numbers or population density, or both. The urban effect is really a population effect.

Living in a city can also bring out the psychotic strain in people without mental disorder. Many researchers believe that psychiatric symptoms are really just exaggerated versions of mental states that everyone experiences occasionally: we all get deeply melancholy sometimes, and if that sadness persists, or is particularly severe, it gets called depression. Similarly, it may be the case that psychosis represents the extremes of the odd sorts of thought and experience that everyone has once in a while. Lots of people with no diagnosed mental illness will admit that they think people can read their minds; that others can communicate by telepathy; that computers can influence their thoughts; or that they are like a robot or zombie with no will of their own. Jim van Os and his colleagues found that 17.5 percent of a group of people drawn from the community—mostly people who had never sought psychiatric services—had experienced delusions or hallucinations, and the larger the urban environment, the more such symptoms were found.

As with bullying, the mere correlation between city living and psychosis can't tell us whether cities lead to psychosis or people with psychosis tend to move to cities, an idea known as the "social drift" hypothesis. A number of studies have addressed social drift, and, on the whole, the data fail to support it. As we've noted, early life—life before drift can occur—is correlated with psychosis. In addition, a study of 1.89 million Danes found that moving from a less urban to a more urban environment raised the risk of schizophrenia, but movement in the other direction lowered it. This suggests that urbanicity probably affects psychosis and not the other way around, since there is no obvious reason why psychologically healthier people would be more inclined to move to the country. More direct evidence comes from research on the movements of patients before they became ill. A British study found little evidence that people diagnosed with psychosis had moved to urban areas in the five years before the onset of illness. The urban jungle itself seems to breed madness.

The most tantalizing evidence relating the city and psychosis comes from a recent study showing a direct relation between urban living and the brain's response to stress. Using functional magnetic resonance imaging (fMRI), Florian Lederbogen and his colleagues investigated brain activity in subjects without any mental disorder under conditions of stress. The investigators found that a number of brain areas—in particular, the amygdala, a brain region associated with negative emotions and social threat—were more active in those people who were currently living in bigger cities. Notably, those who had been brought up in larger urban areas showed more activation in the perigenual anterior cingulate cortex (pACC). This experiment shows two things: that the nature of the urban environment has an effect on the brain's stress response, and that urban living early in life may have long-lasting effects.

It's worth pointing out that the studies of the urban effect in psychosis have all been carried out in relatively small places. Some of the most important work has been done in Copenhagen—a place of half a million residents recently named the world's most livable city by *Monocle* magazine. We know practically nothing about the impact of megacities on delusion or psychosis. One can imagine that the unique stresses of living in cities like New York, Beijing, Tokyo, Delhi, or London could interact with psychosis in ways that go beyond the effects of population size or density. Research on this question is badly needed.

CAN SOCIAL LIFE DAMAGE YOUR BRAIN?

The evidence that social life contributes to the risk of schizophrenia raises an important question. Psychotic illness is undoubtedly the result of a brain disorder. The evidence we've just surveyed, however, shows that when it comes to psychosis, people can damage your brain, or, at any rate, can cause it to be dysfunctional. How can that be?

There are really two distinct questions here. First, are the effects of childhood adversity, immigration, and city living really brought about by social factors or by something else? Second, how can *anything* that doesn't directly interact with your brain disrupt it? The social determinants of psychosis don't involve powerful drugs or head injuries, broken blood vessels or malignant tumors. How do they increase the risk of psychosis? We'll tackle the first question here and the second in the next section.

That child abuse leaves deep psychological scars is an uncontroversial case in which a social interaction is damaging, so we will leave it aside. The more difficult questions are whether it is the social aspects of being an immigrant or an urban dweller that increase the risk of psychosis or whether the explanation involves physical processes. We've already dealt with the vitamin D deficiency hypothesis of the immigrant effect as one possibility. A second physical hypothesis has to do with infectious disease. Maternal influenza has been linked to schizophrenia in offspring, which may explain why people born in the winter show higher rates of the disorder. The winter-birth phenomenon is stronger in cities than it is in rural areas, very likely because greater population density increases viral transmission. A third hypothesis is that cities have a ready supply of drugs of abuse, and some of them, like cannabis, raise the risk of psychosis. There may also be interactions among these factors. Urban dwellers who use cannabis, for example, are more sensitive to its effects than those living in the countryside. The interplay between genes, biological insults (such as exposure to a virus), substance abuse, and the physical environment is likely to be enormously complex.

Nonetheless, there is good reason to think that genuinely social factors are at work in the immigrant and urban effects. Because neighborhood differences are really social differences, the finding already mentioned that the rates of schizophrenia vary across neighborhoods within the same city is strong evidence for the social nature of the urban effect. Schizophrenia is also more prevalent in neighborhoods in which more people live alone, and the highest rates are found in neighborhoods where people tend to stay for only short periods. This transience is a marker of "social fragmentation," which has independently been correlated with psychosis. One investigation found that the risk of a neighborhood having a high rate of psychosis was nearly 13-fold greater in the most fragmented neighborhoods compared to the least fragmented. A more recent study of more than two hundred thousand Swedes concluded that "social fragmentation was the most important area characteristic that explained the increased risk of psychosis in individuals brought up in cities." Finally, the risk of schizophrenia is higher in neighborhoods, and indeed countries, with higher income inequality, a fundamental feature of social organization.

If social fragmentation increases the risk of psychosis, then social cohesion should reduce it. In a clever study using ÆSOP data, James Kirkbride and his colleagues used voter turnout in local elections as a measure of social cohesion, on the assumption that people who are more involved in their communities are more likely to turn out to vote locally. For every 1 percent increase in voter numbers, they found a 5 percent decrease in cases of psychosis. Social cohesion is also enhanced by shared culture. Immigrants to South London living in ethnically dense neighborhoods—those with a large number of immigrants from the same country—show a higher risk for schizophrenia than whites but a lower risk than immigrants living in neighborhoods with lower ethnic density. In contrast, ethnic fragmentation—a measure of the diversity of ethnic groups in a given neighborhood—is associated with an increased rate of psychosis.

We noted that Bourque and his colleagues suggest that the source of the immigrant effect may be discrimination, and the relevance of discrimination is borne out by the study of Veling and his colleagues mentioned above. The authors stratified immigrant groups by level of perceived discrimination and found the lowest level occupied, not surprisingly, by immigrants from Western countries. The next level included immigrants from Turkey, followed by those from Surinam, the Dutch Antilles, and other non-Western countries. The group with the highest level of perceived discrimination were immigrants from Morocco. With every increase in perceived discrimination, the risk of psychosis rose.

Racial discrimination, in particular, may increase the risk of psychosis. Kirkbride and his colleagues report that, relative to whites, minority ethnic groups (whether immigrant or nonimmigrant), including black Caribbeans and Africans, as well as Pakistani and Bangladeshi women, show higher rates of psychosis and that the risk is independent of socioeconomic status (SES). The findings extend to the United States, where a study by Michaeline Bresnahan and her colleagues followed more than twelve thousand people over sixteen years. After factoring out the effect of SES, African Americans were found to have twice the incidence of schizophrenia in the period studied than whites. Although African Americans are more likely to get a diagnosis of schizophrenia on the basis of race alone, this bias was largely eliminated by clinical interviews that standardized the method of diagnosis. Interestingly, whether SES itself is a determinant of schizophrenia is a question that has been debated for more than a hundred years. At the moment, it looks like SES plays no role in schizophrenia except perhaps for those most disadvantaged.

On the basis of data like these, Jean-Paul Selten and Elizabeth Cantor-Graae have suggested that what might be common to the social determinants of psychosis is "social defeat," a concept drawn from the study of animal aggression. Many mammals need their space and are very protective of it. Introduce a strange rat into the cage of another rat, and the intruder will be attacked and (if the other animal can manage it) forced to display submissive behavior or social defeat. It is a long way from the social life of rats to that of human beings, but a comparison is suggestive. In her discussion of the treatment of the homeless mentally ill, the anthropologist Tanya Luhrmann takes the notion of social defeat in human society seriously. "By social defeat," she writes, "I mean what the ethologists mean: an actual social encounter in which one person physically or symbolically loses to another one." People experience social defeat in interactions with "another person who demeans them, humiliates them, subordinates them." The social defeat hypothesis is therefore testable; it predicts that the risk of developing psychosis will be raised in those people who, consciously or unconsciously, feel themselves to be demeaned or subordinated—in short, who feel like second-class citizens.

Social defeats, in this sense, are all too common. On a recent trip to Paris, for example, one of us made a pilgrimage to a kitchen supply store that is a bit of a legend among foodies. After a conversation with the manager in what felt like pretty good French, a shop assistant was sent to fetch a frying pan. The feeling of pride and accomplishment (not to mention a rapidly growing sense of being not too shabby in the culture department) was abolished in an instant when the manager was overheard saying to a Parisian customer with contempt obvious even to a foreigner, "*Ah! C'est un Americain.*" The feeling of shame—of being an outsider playing at being French, of being "the other"—was like a punch in the gut. The "victim" of this most insignificant of put-downs is a middle-aged white guy who grew up with every advantage. And still, the effect was powerful. One doesn't have to be a refugee or suffer from dire poverty to experience humiliation and helpless anger—experiences which social scientists refer to, in evocative technical terminology, as the "chronic daily hassles" of prejudice—and it is quite easy to imagine years of multiple daily hassles leaving their mark on a person's brain.

The social defeat hypothesis is important because we know something about the biological effects of this form of stress. If social defeat turned out to be the right description of the effects of childhood adversity, immigration, and city living on psychosis, it would provide support for the idea that they are genuinely social in nature and give important clues to the brain basis of psychosis. In a study cited by Selten and Cantor-Graae, for example, a defeated rat experiences increased dopamine activity, and repeated defeats seem to enhance the effect. Isolating the defeated animal increases the effect of defeat, and returning it to its group reduces it. If parallel neural processes occurred in humiliated or subordinated human beings, that would provide clues to the neurobiology of schizophrenia.

Although we don't as a matter of fact think that social defeat *is* the right way to understand the role of the social world in psychosis (and we'll return to it later), it remains an important and underinvestigated topic in psychosis research.

JADA: VERY PREGNANT

Jada was a thirty-eight-year-old African American New Yorker living in a women's shelter in Manhattan. Secret Service agents brought her to Bellevue from the Harlem offices of Bill Clinton, where she had caused a disturbance. Prior to being evaluated in the psychiatric ER, she demanded to be seen in the medical ER because (she told the agents) she feared she was miscarrying. Jada was not miscarrying, nor was she pregnant, but she was menstruating. When later talking to a psychiatrist down the hall, after having been informed of her negative pregnancy test, Jada dismissed the news as the misinformation of jealous individuals. For Jada was not simply pregnant: she was carrying the progeny of President Clinton, Jay-Z, Angelina Jolie, and, lastly, Jimmy Stewart, who had been dead for more than five years.

Jada said that she had given birth to hundreds of babies over the years. She went on to say that many of them were born blue, but that she had rubbed them and the warmth brought them back to life. Jada described how these famous people impregnated her. She would wake up and know that one of them had visited her during the night, either physically or spiritually. She did not consider herself as having been raped and took pride in the fact that these people knew that she was expert at carrying and delivering babies. She had visited President Clinton's office to report the good news that she was to have his baby, too. She said she became upset only when she was refused entry to see him.

The Secret Service agents interviewed her and were satisfied that she did not pose a risk to the former president. I was struck by one of the questions the agents asked to allay their fears. At first blush it seemed more parlor game than probing risk assessment, but I must admit that it was quite effective: if you had three wishes, what would they be? Jada's answers: (1) The New York Knicks would win the next NBA championship, (2) She would become a Dallas Cowboy cheerleader, and (3) She would get an apartment of her own.

Jada's mother, contacted through the women's shelter, explained that Jada had two teenaged children but had not seen them in several years. Jada had been in and out of institutions and had a previous diagnosis of schizoaffective disorder. She regularly stopped taking her medications, and her mother had been made legal guardian of the two children. Sadly, Jada had experienced a miscarriage in the previous six months.

Jada initially refused psychotropic medication as she (rightly) informed the staff that it could harm her babies. The number of babies she claimed to be carrying varied from day to day, from as few as four to dozens at a time. She complained of morning sickness and gastric discomfort, and was in fact diagnosed with gastroesophageal reflux disease.

Jada was taken to Bellevue's mental health court, located within the hospital itself. The court is a branch of the New York State Supreme Court where only cases pertaining to mental health law are heard. Patients may petition the court for release, and doctors may testify as to why a patient needs ongoing hospitalization. In Jada's case, I requested that the court mandate that she be medicated over her objection, on the grounds that her psychosis precluded her from making an informed decision as to her medical care. Jada was represented by a mental hygiene legal attorney. The judge ordered her to accept the antipsychotic and mood-stabilizing medication prescribed. She improved somewhat over time, with the number of babies she believed she was carrying diminishing gradually. However, her belief that she was pregnant never abated entirely, and after two months, Jada was scheduled to be transferred to the state hospital for further treatment.

During an interview with her psychiatric team before she was transferred, Jada stopped and stared into space. It appeared that she was dissociating—that is, in a trancelike state oblivious to any external stimuli—and she did not respond to any prompts for several minutes. However, she then became tearful and said that she was just thinking about her two children. She missed them and knew that they were ashamed of their crazy, homeless mom.

After consulting with a child and adolescent psychiatrist, and inquiring about any potential trauma to her fifteen- and thirteen-year-old children that a visit with their mother might cause, I was told that a visit might be therapeutic for all involved. Jada's mother was contacted again. While apprehensive at first, she agreed to ask her grandchildren their wishes. They did not hesitate. They wanted to see their mom.

The following week, a tearful reunion was held on the unit. Jada spent hours preparing, and presented her children with paintings she had made during art group. They in turn brought Jada her favorite snacks, magazines and, most important, photos of their last few years. They shared stories of school and friends. They told one another they were loved. The children expressed no shame in their mother. They hugged and kissed and made plans for the next visit at the state hospital.—JG

DISCRIMINATION AND STATUS

On April 15, 1912, on her maiden voyage from Southampton to New York, the RMS *Titanic* hit an iceberg and sank, taking with her 1,517 of the 2,223 people on board. Because women and children were evacuated first and the *Titanic's* lifeboats could hold only a total of about 1,200 people, a higher proportion of the dead were men. Of the women in first class, four of 143 died (three had chosen to remain on the ship); in second class, 15 of 93 women were lost; in third class, the numbers were 81 of 179. Even an iceberg and the sinking hulk of the largest passenger ship in the world could not overwhelm differences of class.

High social status increases longevity and reduces disease everywhere, and not just on cruise ships. In a seminal study, the sociologist Aaron Antonovsky showed that social advantage protects against premature death, and indeed, over the past two hundred years at least, those in the lower socioeconomic strata of society have continued to live less healthy lives and die younger even as sanitation has improved, infectious disease diminished, and average life expectancy increased dramatically.

In the last section, we asked how social conditions could lead to a brain disorder. We've looked at the evidence that the factors that do the damage are really social. In this section, we make a case for the view that the damage, so to speak, really is damage. With respect to psychosis, the social world affects the brain no less than a stroke or a tumor would. Our argument is indirect: there are well-established cases in which social factors play a role in health and longevity. Against the background of the evidence these cases provide, the idea that social factors could contribute to the development of psychosis is less implausible. We'll look at two phenomena: social status and low-birth-weight babies, and social status and health inequalities.

It has been known for decades that among the many health disadvantages suffered by African Americans is the consistently lower birth weight of African American babies compared to whites. Since low birth weight is a risk factor for disease in later life, it is an important medical problem. Low birth weight isn't a function of having genes of African origin. Richard David and James Collins found that the babies of recent immigrants from Africa and those of white Americans were no different in birth weight. Nor is this effect likely to be the result of socioeconomic factors that affect the diet or health care of African American mothers. Low birth weight is more common even among middle-class African American women than among whites. Indeed, African American college graduates with adequate prenatal care still deliver babies who are, on average, twice as likely to have a lower birth weight than non-Latino white babies. One study found that African American women living in affluent neighborhoods in Chicago had twice as many very-low-birth-weight (VLBW) infants (those weighing less than 1,500 grams, or about 3.3 pounds, at birth) than whites. This doubling of VLBW infants remains the case even in women who have never lived in impoverished conditions.

What exactly is driving this? Collins and his colleagues carried out a study in which African American women were asked about their experience of racial discrimination—among other things, whether they felt that they were assigned to jobs no one else would do; or treated with less dignity and respect than white people; or given jobs that required less thought; or whether they were ignored or not taken seriously because of their race. Women who answered "yes" to even one of these questions had a significantly higher chance of having a VLBW baby; those who reported discrimination in three or more of these domains showed an even higher risk. Being demeaned or subordinated seems to exert a sufficiently powerful effect on the body of a woman that her offspring will be physically disadvantaged. Thoughts, however abstract, can wound in the most concrete of ways.

Let's turn to the relation between social status and health inequalities. If you take the subway from Montgomery County in Maryland to downtown Washington, DC, without knowing it, you are moving steadily through a remarkable statistic. The life expectancy for the rich white people who live in the suburbs where you got on is twenty years longer than the poor African Americans who live where you get off. Every mile you travel toward DC lowers that life expectancy by a year and a half. What could account for this astonishing contrast?

Consider a few hypotheses: (A) African Americans in DC, but not whites in Maryland, live in a physical environment that breeds diseases that lead to premature death. (B) African Americans in DC get less health care than whites in Maryland. (C) African Americans in DC have a less-healthy lifestyle than do rich whites in Maryland. (D) African Americans in DC have genes that make them more vulnerable to disease than whites in Maryland. (E) African Americans in DC have a lower social status than rich whites in Maryland do, and low status leads to poor health and reduced longevity.

Given what we've said about low-birth-weight African American babies, it may not come as a surprise that (E) appears to be the primary explanation. The evidence for this comes from a remarkable study of a rather different social group—British civil servants. The epidemiologist Michael Marmot and his colleagues have spent more than forty years studying the health of eighteen thousand British civil servants in two studies called Whitehall I and Whitehall II. (Whitehall is the street that houses many departments of the British government.) The British civil service is rigidly stratified; being higher up means having more money, more responsibility, and more clout. As a result, position in the civil service is an extremely good stand-in for one's social status. What the Whitehall studies showed was that the health and life expectancy of civil servants was tightly linked to their position. On average, everyone in the civil service lives a healthier and longer life than those below them, and a less healthy and shorter life than those above. This is known as a "social gradient" in health and longevity, and the Whitehall gradient is steep: employees aged between forty and sixty-four who work in the bottom rung of the civil service have a risk of death that is four times that of those in the top echelon (see Figure 11).

Versions of the hypotheses mentioned in the context of the DC-Maryland contrast are also relevant to the Whitehall studies, and data from the studies appear to rule out all but the last one. (A) No British civil servant in the latter part of the twentieth century was working in an

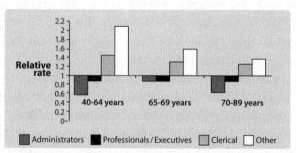

Figure 11: The mortality rates of British civil servants relative to the average for the entire service. In the 40–64 age range, administrators have about half the average rate and "others" about twice the rate— a four-fold difference overall.

environment that bred disease. They all had clean water, sanitation, sufficient nutrition, adequate shelter, and so on. They didn't die of malaria, dysentery, or the other diseases of abject poverty. So in first-world conditions, life expectancy is not related to the physical environment. (B) While insufficient medical care could explain why someone who is already sick dies sooner than someone with adequate health care, the Whitehall studies found a social gradient in first-episode disease. People in the lower rungs of the civil service were getting sick for the first time more often than people in the upper rungs. In fact, those lower down got *more* health care than those above them, presumably because more of them were sick. (C) While lifestyle factors such as smoking and high cholesterol did account for some of the disease in the Whitehall cohort, they accounted for less than one third of the health gradient. (D) By factoring out of the analysis civil servants whose parents had died young, the Whitehall studies excluded those with "unhealthy" genes. Even among those with "good" genes, the social gradient remained.

This leaves social status as the likely explanation of the gradient in health and longevity among British civil servants as well as Americans in DC and Maryland. It turns out that the social gradient is found not only among these groups but just about everywhere one finds social hierarchies (translation: everywhere there are people). The effect of social hierarchy becomes clear when we look at the health of nations. Health is related to resources *within* developed countries but not *across* countries. A rich American will have, on average, better health than a poor American, and a rich Swede will have better health than a poor Swede, but the rich American may not have better health than the poor Swede. And indeed, the health of a population isn't correlated with the average income in that group but with the size of the gap between richest and poorest. The bigger the gap, the worse the overall health of the population. Figure 12 shows the life expectancy at birth for a number of countries as a function of resources (per capita gross domestic product). Pretty clearly, longevity doesn't depend on absolute wealth. More egalitarian countries, all things equal, are going to be healthier than those with large social inequalities.

How could low social status undermine health and reduce longevity? A possible answer comes from the study of primates. Many primate species live in "dominance hierarchies," that is, social orders determined by aggressive interactions among group members competing for resources. An animal's position in the hierarchy powerfully affects the amount of stress to which it is exposed—lower down, more stress—as well as its health. Robert Sapolsky, a neuroscientist who has studied the physiological effects of stress in primates over many years, argues that subordinate animals have little control over their lives. Their behavioral options are determined by the boys at the top. As a result, when they face challenges such as defending against predators, they have to cope as best they can from the position of foot soldier, without having a say in the battle plan. Sapolsky's research shows that the stress of being subordinate has devastating effects on the brain and, in turn, on the body: low social rank leads to heart disease, reproductive problems, and suppression of the immune system.

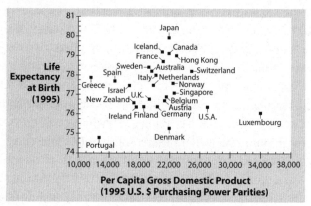

Figure 12: The relation between gross domestic
product and life expectancy.

Marmot argues that low status in humans produces similar stress. Low social position is accompanied by the severe stress of restricted autonomy. This is very clear in Whitehall, where lower rungs of the civil service have less control over their work. Someone who rises in the ranks may have greater challenges, but the freedom to choose how to face them reduces stress. Figure 13 shows the relation in the Whitehall cohort between autonomy in the workplace and heart disease. Human social life more broadly shows a similar pattern. The lower one's social position, the fewer options one has in many areas of life, and, over time, this constraint is poisonous.

At first blush, the idea that being born in a city or being the child of an immigrant could raise one's risk of schizophrenia seems rather hard to believe. Schizophrenia is a brain disorder, and social conditions don't seem like the kind of thing that could bring brain disorders about. The literature on low-birth-weight African American babies and the social gradient in health, however, shows that social stress is noxious enough to put you six feet under. The idea that social stress can contribute to the development of psychosis is moderate by comparison.

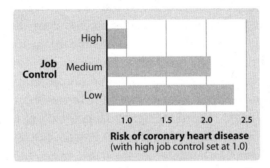

Figure 13: The relation between autonomy at work and coronary heart disease.

It's worth emphasizing that some of the stress that contributes to psychosis (or, indeed, to VLBW babies or heart disease) is brought about by conditions of disadvantage. For this reason, social inequality is a public health issue as much as cigarette smoking or poor eating habits. One hardly needs medical arguments to demonstrate the badness of discrimination, but medical consequences are not irrelevant and may be a way of marshaling the forces of change for the better. After all, if social injustice is bad for the health of those at the bottom, then it's also bad for those higher up who pay for the injustice of their society with the tax dollars that go to the medical care of their disadvantaged neighbors.

VULNERABILITY AND STRESS

That social factors can affect mental health appears to challenge an assumption of mainstream psychiatry, namely, that psychosis is nothing over and above a disorder of genes and the brain. In fact, however, an older assumption—that the disordered brain interacts with the outside world—was at one time familiar in psychiatry.

In 1977, Joseph Zubin and Bonnie Spring proposed a new way to think about schizophrenia that they called the "vulnerability" model, according to which people who develop schizophrenia (and many people who don't) have some degree of vulnerability to the disorder. A stressful experience can put a match to the tinder of susceptibility and lead to an episode of illness. Zubin and Spring characterize the vulnerability as being an effect of one's genes as well as early life events such as perinatal complications, traumas, disease, and even adolescent experience. Stressors are also of two types. The first, biological, are processes internal to the body, like ingesting something toxic. The second, social, are stressors such as the death of a loved one, a job promotion, marriage, or divorce. Because one can be more or less vulnerable to schizophrenia, two people experiencing the same life event won't be affected in the same way. Someone with modest vulnerability might successfully adapt to the stress, whereas someone with greater vulnerability could have a psychotic episode. People with low vulnerability to schizophrenia might develop the disorder only under conditions of extreme stress, but as vulnerability increases, small stresses may be sufficient for illness.

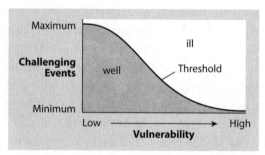

Figure 14: Zubin and Spring's vulnerability
model. As one's vulnerability increases,
the amount of stress required to lead to a
manifestation of illness is reduced.

Psychosis is a brain disorder; it is likely to have a genetic component in many cases; it is correlated with early life stressors such as abuse; and it is sensitive to current life stressors like being an immigrant. An adequate theory of psychosis, therefore, has to be able to integrate these factors and show how their combination or interaction leads to illness. Vulnerability models (now called "vulnerability-stress" or "diathesis-stress" models) provide a framework for connecting the social and biological determinants of psychosis. Biology and early life experiences set a level of vulnerability to psychosis. Stressors (later in life) will determine whether the vulnerability remains dormant or is manifested in psychological symptoms. In Richard Bentall's model of paranoia, for example, problems of attachment and victimization are hypothesized to be factors that increase one's vulnerability to delusions in later life. A more complex illustration of this kind of model is provided by a study of Eliot Goldstone, John Farhall, and Ben Ong. The goal of the study was to investigate the relations among the various contributors to delusional thinking. They asked one hundred patients with a psychotic illness about delusional thoughts, relatives who had a psychotic or other mental disorder, childhood trauma, cannabis and methamphetamine use, "life hassles" (commonplace life stressors), and finally "experiential avoidance," an overly negative attitude to one's own thoughts. By looking at the statistical strength of the relations among these factors, Goldstone and his colleagues were able to build a model of how they might be related in the development of delusional thinking. Figure 15 represents the model.

What the model proposes is that genes (represented by "heredity"), childhood trauma, and early cannabis use render someone vulnerable

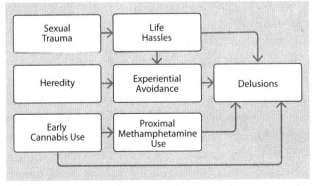

Figure 15: A model of delusion development.

to delusions. The experience of stress later in life, methamphetamine use, and negative thinking may lead to their manifestation. This model doesn't include all of the factors that may contribute to psychosis, nor will it correctly represent everyone who develops delusions. More severe sexual trauma, for example, may create a vulnerability so great that drug use in later life isn't necessary for illness. In any case, the details of the model matter less than the general structure of the explanation, which shows a complex pattern of development including genes, physical risk factors, and social stress.

The most important omissions of the model are the effects on the brain of the other factors, but other vulnerability-stress models do include brain processes. Some researchers hypothesize that dopamine in the brain region known as the striatum is the "final common pathway" in schizophrenia—the physical system that is affected by all of the biological and psychological determinants of the illness. One version of this hypothesis says that genetic vulnerability and social stress increase dopamine. With each new stressor, the dopamine system becomes ever more sensitized and leads eventually to a psychotic episode. There is a lot of evidence that dopamine is altered by means of a change in the brain system known as the hypothalamic-pituitary adrenal (HPA) axis, and the HPA axis is also significantly affected by stress. The final common pathway in schizophrenia may, therefore, terminate at the HPA axis.

A recent model of schizophrenia, developed by Elaine Walker and her colleagues, provides a good illustration of what a neural vulnerability-stress model of psychosis might look like. Their model focuses on the HPA axis and the role of the hormone cortisol, which is produced by the adrenal cortex. Walker and her colleagues' hypothesis is that stress affects the function of the HPA axis by means of a change in cortisol production; this in turn affects the dopamine system and leads to psychotic symptoms. The model is summarized in Figure 16.

A second hypothesis concerning stress and vulnerability has been developed by Maria-de-Gracia Dominguez and her colleagues. Many healthy people have psychotic experiences, such as hallucinations or paranoid thoughts. In most of these individuals, the experiences subside on their own. Stress, however, may cause psychotic experiences to persist and eventually develop into a full-blown disorder. A third hypothesis, proposed by Ruud van Winkel, Nicholas Stefanis, and Inez Myin-Germeys,

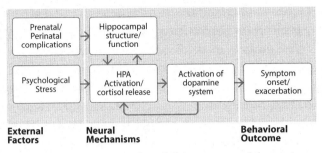

| External Factors | Neural Mechanisms | Behavioral Outcome |

Figure 16: A vulnerability-stress model.

runs as follows. We know that people can be "sensitized" in various ways, including to stress. This means that the repetition of the same stressful event may generate a greater response each time it happens. Suppose, then, that one comes into the world with an abnormally sensitive stress response. Perhaps cortisol production is too high or the hippocampus doesn't tamp down HPA activity enough. Now add some sort of trauma, such as growing up in a big city, which increases one's sensitivity to stress even further. If, after a long period of sensitization, one has a particularly bad experience, the new stress might be enough to push one over the edge into psychosis. A hard-and-fast distinction between vulnerability and stress may, therefore, be artificial to the extent that a stressful experience circles back to alter vulnerability to future stress.

We have a long way to go before we understand the precise biological mechanism through which stress works its way into the brain in psychosis. The new field of "epigenetics," however, may prove important in the effort. Epigenetics investigates the ways in which molecules associated with DNA can turn gene expression on and off, including in the brain. There is now evidence that epigenetic changes can occur as a result of experience, so epigenetic processes may constitute a family of mechanisms through which the social world alters brain function. A striking example of experience-dependent epigenetic change comes from the study of maternal behavior, which can, both in rodents and nonhuman primates, affect the sensitivity of offspring to stress. In 2004, Ian Weaver and his colleagues examined one of the mechanisms of this process. Newborn rats are licked and groomed in stereotypical maternal behavior. Rats that are licked and groomed more show a reduced response to stress and exhibit a particular chemical pattern in their DNA. In this experiment, the pups of mothers who provided more licking and grooming were given to mothers who provided less, and vice versa. The stress response of the pups changed as a consequence of their adoptive mother's behavior. The pups of poorer mothers were more sensitive to stress, and those of better mothers were less sensitive. Remarkably, the chemical pattern in the DNA of the pups was altered as a function of the adoptive mother's behavior. The implication of this experiment is that the behavior of the mothers changed the behavior of the pups through epigenetic alteration of their genes. You can't change the genes you were born with, but social interactions can affect which of them are active and which are silent.

In a subsequent study, these researchers found something similar in humans. They examined postmortem tissue from the brains of three groups: young men who committed suicide and were known to have suffered abuse as children, young men who committed suicide but did not suffer from abuse, and young men who died in accidents and suffered no abuse. The men who had been abused as children showed epigenetic changes closely analogous to those found in the rodent study. The epigenetic profile of the other suicide group resembled that of the group of accidental deaths, which suggests that the epigenetic pattern in the abuse group had been caused by the abuse and not by the mental distress that led to the suicide. This is a stunning discovery. It shows that a social phenomenon—the abuse of a child by an adult—leaves traces in the building blocks of our brains that can persist for years.

There is as yet no direct evidence that epigenetic processes play a causal role in the development of psychosis, but studies have found epigenetic differences in people with psychosis. Epigenetics may therefore prove crucial in the search for the conduits between social stress and the disordered brain. It may explain, as Sandro Galea, Monica Uddin, and Karestan Koenen put it, how the environment "gets under the skin."

JANE: THE QUEEN

The first thing I said to the resident psychiatrist after we had excused our-selves from our meeting with Her Majesty Queen Jane of Bellevue was, "That is the single most grandiose patient I have ever interviewed." That's still true.

Jane had been wandering around barefoot in Manhattan's Penn Station, and her feet were badly blistered. She was confused, and the medical team that found her deemed her an "emotionally disturbed person," a term used by the NYPD to describe people behaving strangely and who look like they might pose an imminent danger. EMS brought her to Bellevue for an eval-uation. There, Jane told the story she would repeat on the inpatient unit, the one that kept her in the hospital.

"Queen Jane" told me that she had come to Bellevue for liposuction and didn't belong on a psych ward. Some people had broken her feet, she said, and she needed plastic surgery. She had been married for twelve years, but her husband and kids had been murdered. She stated this flatly and continued talking without emotion. Her brother and father had also been killed. She had adopted her son's friend Sam, whose life was the basis for *The Curious Case of Benjamin Button*, a movie playing at the time. Sam had also been murdered—the very evening she had adopted him. Despite the disturbing content of Jane's delusions, I was struck by how pleasant and placid she was.

Jane's horrific beliefs coexisted with other, more ambitious fantasies: she was a Supreme Court justice, the "head of the court"; she had grad-uated from Oxford Law without actually attending the school (she had a photographic memory); she had 2,082 law degrees, three MBAs, and four medical degrees; she owned a number of airlines and "one hundred per-cent of New York City"—it having been "willed to her"—as well as every home in Massachusetts. She was CEO of 1,092 companies. She said that President Obama had been murdered, and she was taking his place as Queen of the White House. She was also the queen of 182 other coun-tries, including most of the Middle East. She asked that we address her as Queen Jane. Although she had been raised a Roman Catholic, she had studied six religions and, after reading the Koran, identified most strongly with Islam.

Jane's account of being brought into the hospital reflected a similar mixture of the grand and the grim. She said that she had just moved from her home in Massachusetts to a penthouse on Central Park West, and that she was in Penn Station because she had been sedated with chloroform by a fellow Supreme Court justice.

Jane was forty-eight, though she looked younger, and had three children—two teenagers and an eight-year-old, all of whom were, thankfully, alive. She had indeed been married for twelve years and was divorced; her children were living with her ex-husband. Seven years earlier, just after having separated from her husband, she had been diagnosed with bipolar disorder. She acknowledged that she had been diagnosed in 2001 with what *others* claimed was bipolar disorder and that she had been hospitalized several times. Before she became ill, she had been running her own business but had to give it up and was now unemployed and living with her father in Massachusetts. Five days before being admitted, she had become angry and left the house impulsively with no belongings. Jane's father filed a missing-person's report and tracked her to Bellevue. When I spoke to Jane's dad, he said that she had been psychologically stable for a year but had recently stopped taking her medication. Over the prior two or three months, she had been sleeping most of the time, overeating significantly, and "living in a fantasy world."

Though her history and grandiose delusions were consistent with mania, Jane didn't behave in classic manic fashion. She was neither euphoric nor irritable. In fact, she came across as a bit bland—bright but not as mentally acute as many manic people are—and there seemed to be a profound disconnection between her thoughts and her behavior. Despite believing that she was Queen Jane, she accepted her presence on a psychiatric ward largely without complaint or protest. She believed that there were people out to get her, but she claimed that the CIA was on the case, and she seemed unconcerned. For the most part, Jane kept to herself, watched television, slept, or stayed in bed. She seemed to have no desire to talk to her doctors—particularly unusual for someone in the throes of a manic episode—and mostly kept her delusional ideas to herself. Jane was later to confess that at these times, she had felt high and "untouchable."

Though previous doctors had persuaded Jane that she had bipolar disorder, her great successes in life had now convinced her otherwise. "I am the most sanest person in the world," she said. In any case, her former psychiatrists had been executed, and their hospitals had been sued and burned to the ground by the warden from Rikers Island. She let me know—matter-of-factly, without any hint of threat—that she was planning to sue Bellevue and have it torched as well.

Jane politely refused meds. Because she wasn't acting dangerously, she had that right. However, when a judge deemed that she lacked the capacity to make medical decisions and signed a court order giving our treatment team the right to medicate her over her objection, Jane accepted the treatment.

After two weeks on meds, Jane underwent a remarkable transformation. She stopped believing that her family had been murdered. She said that her children lived with their father and that she had been out of touch with them for six months. She acknowledged that she lived with her father but continued to believe that she was Queen of America and the CEO of numerous companies. A week later, all of her grandiose delusions disappeared: "I am just an average person," she said. Her insight returned. She admitted that she becomes "very imaginative" when not on her medication.

During the worst of her illness, Jane had spent most of her time sleeping; as she improved, she began to participate in the social life of the ward, attending community meetings, art classes, and other group activities. During some of those meetings, she advised other patients to work with their treatment team and encouraged them to bring their concerns to the staff.

As her time in the hospital was coming to an end, Jane made plans to move back to her father's house and to look for a part-time job. I encouraged her to remain in treatment, both medication and talk therapy. She said she would, though most patients don't manage to keep such promises. She thanked the staff for the treatment she had received and was optimistic about getting back to her life. She held no ill will toward me, either for keeping her hospitalized or for legally compelling her to be medicated. I appreciated that. A month after Jane arrived at Bellevue, she left the hospital.

Nearly two years since we last saw each other at Bellevue, I have an audience with Queen Jane. But this time, it takes place in the warm home in

153

which Jane was born fifty years prior, a house tucked away in a leafy Massachusetts town. She is dressed neatly, sits comfortably, and laughs easily. Her eighty-year-old father watches television in the next room. She has been exercising a lot, and looks younger and fitter. I have come here to see the woman who had been hidden behind that fantastic grandiosity, hoping to fill in the gaps in her story.

After her release from Bellevue, Jane started out in a day program. She stopped taking her medication and once again was hospitalized, this time for four months. When I meet her, Jane is halfway through a yearlong day program and enjoying the creative writing group most.

We talk about her time at Bellevue. We read an early version of the portrait you are reading now, whose title she likes. She remembers most of her delusions, adding that the themes tend to repeat during her manic episodes, and the same numbers seem to come back to her—182, 1,092. She finds some details funny but doesn't appear self-conscious or embarrassed. She knows she has a mental illness. She is eager to learn more about it and asks insightful questions. She finds it interesting that she has never been depressed or suicidal, only manic, and never hears voices when psychotic; she is always, solely, delusional.

As Jane describes the intertwining of her early life with the development of her bipolar disorder, I am reminded yet again of how strongly the events of our lives can set the table for future illness. Bipolar disorder is a classic "biological" mental illness, something chemical that we assume must be addressed directly with medication; yet we are often too quick to accept such a narrow understanding of psychosis. When I ask about her mother, Jane says matter-of-factly that her mother committed suicide at thirty-six, when Jane was twelve, and that Jane had been the one to find the body. Three years later, Jane's younger sister was killed when the drunk driver of the car she was in crashed. Despite her losses, Jane says her childhood was mostly a happy one because of her father. He took her fishing and on vacations to Florida. They still go out to dinner every Sunday night, where Jane, with her doctor's permission, might have one or two glasses of champagne.

Jane dated in high school and was briefly engaged before going off to college, where she met her husband. Jane married at twenty-nine and was a mother at thirty. The first years were happy ones. She started a small business and was successful. The marriage soured a decade in, after Jane was put on bedrest during her third pregnancy, and her husband became abusive. She found out he had been having an affair and filed for divorce. She decided to dissolve the business and spend more time with her children. Her ex-husband harassed her for money and initiated child-custody proceedings. Jane was placed in a shelter with her children. It was at the shelter, at age forty—not far from the age at which her mother committed suicide—that Jane became manic for the first time. Her delusion at the time was limited to the belief that she owned many businesses. She was hospitalized for several weeks, the first of ten hospitalizations over the next decade. She says, "Every time I'm in the hospital, I educate myself. I figure, why waste the time?" Mostly, she reads.

When Jane was first hospitalized, her husband was awarded custody of the children. Because of her illness, Jane thought her children would be better off with their father (he had never been abusive to them, she said). Jane is happy she was able to take her kids to Disney World shortly before her first episode. Despite her being on disability, Jane's husband sued her for child-support payments and won. A few years into her illness, Jane added to her CEO belief the delusions that she was Queen and that she owned an enormous amount of property. Her delusions are like photographic negatives of her traumas: she lost her business (she is CEO of hundreds of companies); she lives in a shelter (she owns Manhattan); she lost custody of her children (her children were murdered); she did not finish college (she has innumerable degrees); her husband abused her (she becomes Queen. Off with his head!).

Jane's story is an unadulterated success of biological psychiatry: madness repelled, if not cured. And yet if one ignores the meaning of Jane's thoughts and the role of her life story in her illness, something essential to her illness is lost. Hippocrates is supposed to have said that it is much more important to know what sort of a patient has a disease than what sort of a disease a patient has. Delusions are symptoms of a broken brain; there's no doubt about that. But it doesn't follow that the best or only description of a psychotic illness is a biological one.

Queen Jane—now just plain Jane—is in a good place. She knows the importance of taking her medication. She wants to focus on her health before thinking about another romantic relationship. She remains close to her father, whose advice she seeks (including about her having this follow-up interview with her old psychiatrist). She hopes to travel once her time at the day program is finished. And she is happy that her oldest child can now drive, so her kids can visit her without her ex-husband's involvement. The previous Christmas was the first she spent with her children since becoming ill.

I rise and thank Jane. She hopes her experience might come to help other people. Her father asks me what I think about Charlie Sheen's odd behavior, recently in the news—but before I can respond, Jane says, "He must be bipolar." As I leave, Jane and her dad prepare for their Sunday dinner, champagne optional.—JG

4

HELL IS OTHER PEOPLE

Interviewer: The legend has it that the fig leaf was the first
  apparel . . .
2000-Year-Old Man: No. It was *not* the first apparel . . .
Interviewer: What was?
2000-Year-Old Man: The hat.
Interviewer: You mean man wore a hat on his genitals?
2000-Year-Old Man: Not on his *genitals*! . . . He wore a hat on
  his head . . .
Interviewer: But that wouldn't protect your genitals.
2000-Year-Old Man: No, it's more important to protect *the brain* . . .
  If God . . . intended that the genitals were more important than
  the brain, He would have put a skull over the genitals!
  — Mel Brooks and Carl Reiner, "The Fig Leaf"

The logic seems irresistible: the more important the organ, the more
it must exist in elegant isolation from the world outside. In fact, while
the brain may be isolated physically, it is the most socially active of our
organs—a fact that has been consistently set aside in the rush of the past
decades to explain mental illness biologically. Neuroscience tells us a
great deal about the mind and its disorders. It may even discover cures
for those disorders. But a theory of the brain in isolation cannot tell us
everything there is to know about psychosis because human beings do
not exist in isolation. To understand delusions, one has to understand the
history of human sociality. That history—and, indirectly, the history of
delusions—begins with our primate ancestors.

MACHIAVELLIAN MINDS

Primates, humans included, have big brains. Despite the appealingly obvious sound of that claim, the size of the primate brain is something of a puzzle. You might think that since brains tend to be useful organs, and evolution tends to produce well-adapted animals, big brains would be an inevitable outcome of evolution. In fact, it's far from inevitable. Brain tissue uses up a lot of energy—about 20 percent of the body's total, despite contributing only 2 percent of its weight—and an animal pays a big price for a big brain in the energy it has to expend to keep it functioning normally. The brain, like all tissue, has to be fed, and the more food your body needs, the tougher your day is going to be. Since evolution has endowed primates with costly brains, they must be quite useful. But for what exactly?

The most compelling hypothesis about brain size says that primate brains are big because they evolved to cope with the enormous complexity of social life. Some of the best evidence for this claim comes from the study of differences in brains across a primate species. The brain size of a primate species (in particular the neocortex, the latest development in evolutionary history) is tightly linked to the social group size for that species. The bigger the neocortex (relative to total brain volume), the larger the social group (see Figure 17). Moreover, primate brain regions associated with social cognition have expanded more rapidly over the course of evolution than other brain areas. Extrapolating from the primate data, the "natural" human social group is likely to be about 150, roughly the size of hunter-gatherer societies or traditional villages. The fundamental purpose of big brains, it seems, is to handle the cognitive challenges of social life, an idea known as the "social brain hypothesis."

Historically, the primary benefit of living with others seems to have been defense against predators. However, the strong affiliative relations that group life makes possible provide the foundation for cooperation and coordination with others, which leads to benefits that are out of reach for individuals. But the price of a successful social life is a significant danger: the threat of exploitation by others. Being around others exposes social animals like humans to potential dangers that don't trou-

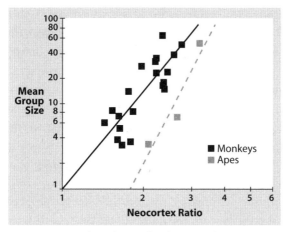

Figure 17: The relationship between brain size
and social group size.

ble relatively solitary animals because the vast majority of dangers in the human world are created by the action and inaction of others. Other people compete with us for jobs, spouses, recognition, and status, and they threaten us with physical and emotional harm, isolation, and death. As one of Jean-Paul Sartre's characters aptly puts it, hell is other people.

When we think about social threat, we usually imagine it coming from strangers, but it more often originates in loved ones, who can hurt us even more: parents abuse their children; lovers cheat; friends stab one another in the back; neighbors commit genocide. Like the rest of nature, social life is red in tooth and claw.

The psychology of cooperation itself creates risks. An essential tool for cooperation is the Theory of Mind (ToM) we encountered earlier. In order to collaborate with others, one has to be able to see things from their point of view, and this ability (often called perspective taking) is a form of ToM. Consistent with this idea is evidence of an association between the number of close relationships you have—defined as people you would depend on "at times of great social or financial trouble"—and ToM abilities. The better you are at ToM, in effect, the greater your capacity for friendship. However, if coordination with others requires being able to think about their thoughts, then open, honest interactions in which you make it easy for others to know what you are thinking are likely to be more successful than playing your cards close to your chest. But openness

159

and honesty provide a new way for others to get ahead: those willing to cheat can take advantage of the information they get from the honest folk and use it to their advantage. Because the benefits of social life depend on cooperation, one has to trust members of one's group, but trusting others makes you vulnerable. By permitting others to know what you are thinking, you put information in their hands that can be used against you. Iago, that great exploiter of Shakespeare's *Othello*, understands this well. Othello, Iago tells us, is "of a free and open nature." By using what he knows of Othello's state of mind, he can lead him "by the nose / As asses are."

We are all too familiar with the direct methods of exploiting others: take compromising pictures and squeeze them for money; hold their passports and make them work for nothing; hit them with a brick and take their wallet; kill them and steal their wives. Gaining advantage at others' expense in these direct ways can be effective but is risky. Overt exploitation invites violence from the exploited, or their community, whenever the tables are turned or the exploitation becomes widely known. If you can exploit someone covertly, therefore, *without* it becoming known to others, or even to them, you may get the advantages of exploitation without incurring the risks. All things being equal, the con artist is better off than the thief, and the adulterer better off than the wife killer. Human existence is incomparably less bloody and dangerous today than it has been for much of our history. Steven Pinker, Robert Muchembled, and others make it clear that, for all of the mischief and misery we hear about on the evening news, we are living in a peaceable utopia by comparison to even the quite recent past. Exploitation can thrive, however, even as violence declines. For this reason, deception is at the heart of covert exploitation and makes full use of ToM no less than cooperation does. If ToM greases the social wheels, it also provides the wolves among us with a behavioral strategy that (with a scattering of exceptions) no other animals have. The vast majority of exploitation in nature is overt. With a brain evolved for complex social life, clandestine exploitation comes into existence.

Take a simple case. Late on a school night, Alex, Adam, and Amalia are watching *Fawlty Towers* on a laptop computer when they are supposed to be in bed asleep. Hearing their mother coming down the stairs, they panic and shove the computer under the couch—a good hiding place because although *they* can still see the computer, the space under the couch isn't visible to someone standing over it. For their behavior to make sense, the kids have to know that the visual experience their mother will have won't reveal the computer to her. Being able to imagine the spatial world from her perspective (a literal form of perspective taking) enables them to carry out a simple bit of deception.

Now consider a more complex case: Iago steals the handkerchief that Othello gave to Desdemona and puts it in Cassio's room in order to deceive Othello into thinking that Desdemona is in love with Cassio. This behavior is made possible by Iago's deployment of ToM to formulate beliefs about Othello's mental states: that he is already feeling jealous; that he suspects Cassio; that he is likely to jump to conclusions when he sees the handkerchief; and so on. Iago's deception also points up how useful ToM is not only in direct interactions with those being deceived, but also when planning a deception. Iago knows the handkerchief stratagem will be effective because he can imagine how things will look (metaphorically) to Othello and can maneuver accordingly.

Another illustration comes from the movies. The story of the renowned check forger Frank Abagnale is depicted in the film *Catch Me If You Can*. At one point in the story, Abagnale wants to take a plane out of the Miami airport to escape the FBI agents who are after him, but the airport is crawling with police. So he cooks up a ruse. Dressed as a pilot, he walks through the airport with a group of beautiful stewardesses, and, distracted by the women, none of the police notices him. He also pays someone to dress up as a pilot and wait in his car outside the airport building. Knowing that Abagnale is likely to disguise himself as a pilot, the FBI follow the red herring instead of him. In order to set this deception up, Abagnale has to be able to reason about the mental states of others prior to actually carrying out the deception. He has to know that most men will focus on attractive women instead of the men they are with; that the FBI would indeed be looking for a man dressed as a pilot but that it would be easier to spot a pilot in a car than among a group of stewardesses; and finally that, once spotted, all the FBI men would follow the red herring.

Fortunately, ToM is also useful in *detecting* deception. Murder mysteries sometimes turn on the villain's use of ToM to throw others off the scent, as well as the detective's use of ToM to try to see through the deception. Columbo, the disheveled detective played by Peter Falk in the 1970s television series of the same name, regularly engages in this sort of game. Ken Franklin, the villain of "Columbo: By the Book," has just murdered his business partner and dumped the body on his own front lawn to throw suspicion on others. When Columbo turns up, Franklin does his best to feign distress at his partner's death. While Columbo is questioning him, Franklin absentmindedly starts opening his mail. "Isn't it funny," Columbo says, "how people are different? Now, me, if I found my partner dead, I'd never think of opening my letters." A little behavioral clue has allowed Columbo to use ToM to see through the behavioral smoke screen.

Our own lives are filled with considerably more banal deception and counter-deception. *Will his wife believe that he is working late tonight? Sure; he often has to work late at this time of year. But if she phones his office, and he isn't there, she'll become suspicious, so he'd better forward his calls to his cell phone. When she calls, she notices that the phone doesn't sound like a land line even though she dialed the office number. Why would he be forwarding calls to his cell if he is working late at the office?* And on and on in a cycle of domestic intelligence and counterintelligence. ToM is thus a skill that cuts both ways: it provides the tools for deception and the means to uncover it. Given the centrality of duplicity in social life, it is perhaps not surprising, therefore, that there is evidence that the size of the neocortex in primates is related not only to ToM but also to the use of tactical deception.

Deception is at the heart of one of the earliest formulations of the social brain hypothesis. Andrew Whiten and Richard Byrne hypothesized that primate intelligence evolved not only for the purpose of affiliation but as a defense against deception. Adopting Frans de Waal's characterization of chimpanzee behavior, Byrne and Whiten dubbed their view the "Machiavellian intelligence hypothesis," after that most famous of realpolitik theorists, to indicate the central place that exploitation and defense against it occupy in human social life.

Indeed, the existence of exploitation is important enough to social life that, in sufficient quantity, it threatens the very possibility of cooperation. In 1993, Magnus Enquist and Olof Leimar developed a mathematical model of the effects on cooperation of "free riding"—a form of exploitation in which one takes the benefits of social life without contributing one's fair share. Their model predicts that in small social groups, free riding can be controlled. If everyone knows everyone, then news about two-bit Iagos spreads quickly, and everyone is alerted to the danger. As group size increases, however, and communities occupy larger geographical areas, free riders can move from place to place and never run out of suckers. If exploitation becomes rife, the only rational strategy to avoid being conned is to opt out of cooperating altogether—to the detriment of everyone. And without cooperation, much of human social life goes by the boards in favor of a war of each against all.

But since most human beings *do* live in large groups, and for every open, honest, cooperative fellow, there are two free riders around the corner, how has cooperation survived? The probable answer is that humans have developed strategies for spotting free riders and protecting themselves against them. Enquist and Leimar suggest that gossip may be one of these defenses. Nasty stories about people tend to spread like wildfire, and our thirst for dirt may originate in the prudent desire to know whom to avoid. But Enquist and Leimar suggest an even more important strategy: *suspicion.* In the face of rampant exploitation, modulating an open and honest nature just slightly makes eminently good sense. Doing so allows cooperation to go ahead while at the same time creating a standard that partners have to meet before you will trust and cooperate with *them.*

Following Enquist and Leimar, we hypothesize that a central component of the Machiavellian social brain is what we'll call the "Suspicion System," the purpose of which is early detection of the threat of exploitation. The Suspicion System is a specialized form of cognition, directed at dangerous others, that is highly sensitive, as we'll see, to their malicious intents. A number of investigators in evolutionary psychiatry have defended the idea that persecutory delusions may be an outcome of social threats in the evolutionary past. Our goal is to show how this view forms part of a larger account of delusions

THE SUSPICION SYSTEM

What sort of cognitive system is required to enable one to be sensitive to social threats? We face all sorts of dangers and obstacles to well-being every day: sleeping in and missing a job interview; writing bad checks; slipping on an icy patch of sidewalk. Most of these threats are either sufficiently minor, or sufficiently predictable, that we can learn, or be taught, to avoid them. Parents look after infants, but nature helps, too. Babies are born with a suite of reflexes because the cost of learning some behaviors through trial and error is too high.

Let's take predation (that is, a strategic physical attack by an animal or human) as the paradigmatic threat. If you come face-to-face with a chainsaw-wielding man wearing a hockey mask, the signs of danger are unambiguous. But if you are walking through a dark forest—or a bad neighborhood late at night—you have to be sensitive to signs of danger that are deeply ambiguous. A slight rustle behind you is most likely dry leaves pushed around by the wind—but could also be the careful steps of someone preparing to spring at you. A successful cognitive system for threat detection must be able to draw your attention automatically, motivate you to start thinking hard (if unconsciously) about what the sound might mean, and move you to act if action seems warranted. In addition, the motivation that is produced by a threat system like this should suppress competing impulses temporarily, until the threat has passed. Responding to a sound that might signify danger requires full attention even if it turns out to be a false alarm. Being vigilant in this way means that you will have to act on the basis of uncertain information; but when it comes to wolves in forests or assailants in alleys, it's better to err on the side of caution. What we call "fear" is one such cognitive system: an automatic, unpleasant, highly effective mechanism that commandeers our full attention for the purpose of self-preservation.

Not all dangers present themselves as threats to life and limb. The possibility of infidelity on the part of your spouse is not a direct physical threat like predation, but the result may be the same: if your partner cheats on you, you are deprived of offspring, a fate no different from death, according to evolutionary theory. It is unlikely, therefore, that evolution would have left the capacity for detecting infidelity and other serious social threats entirely to learning, especially since some of the skills required for detecting social threats are not easily learned. These skills might include noticing the direction of someone's gaze, reading emotion in faces, perceiving body movements (an instance of what is known as "biological motion"), and even interpreting hand orientation.

The anxious suspicion of infidelity is called jealousy. Like fear, jealousy is also a great motivator. Since cheating is so harmful, casual monitoring of your partner's loyalty is possible and worth the effort, and one way to do so is to be sensitive to cues that might signal a threat from a competitor. If your wife is getting a lot of late-night phone calls, you will be better off having the kind of mind that will pay attention to them and consider what they might mean. Moreover, a suspicion that your wife might be cheating or thinking about it—a suspicion manifested as a feeling of jealousy—will be useful if it motivates you to be a better partner. Jealousy is thus an "early warning system" that something you value is under threat from other people. The thought that your partner is thinking about cheating on you gets your attention, and the feeling that comes with it provides the motivation to act.

The Suspicion System is, we hypothesize, the solution that evolution came up with to enable us to pick up evidence of infidelity and other social threats for the purpose of early detection and defense. For the reasons we've just rehearsed, at least some parts of this system are likely to be innate in human beings—present at birth or arising through normal development. The system produces "suspicion"—the term we'll use to refer to a family of psychological states, both conscious and unconscious, that arise in response to evidence that someone may intend you harm. By creating suspicion directed at other people, the Suspicion System makes social life safer because people who make you suspicious are by definition unsuitable for cooperative endeavors.

The Suspicion System is likely to be very sensitive and will err on the side of signaling danger rather than cautiously waiting for solid evidence. As in the case of detecting the danger of predation, it is better to generate false alarms than to risk missing a real threat. The Suspicion System is also likely to target other people's *intentions* to harm you. If you find your best friend in bed with your wife, you don't feel suspicion, but rage at the proof in front of you. Suspicious states, in contrast, are responses to cues that are analogous to the rustle in the forest or the footfall in the alley, a complex mix of possible, plausible, and probable, of unconfirmed, semi-confirmed, and indirectly confirmed evidence. The Suspicion System creates heightened responses to subtle, uncertain, and ambiguous signs of social danger: the glance exchanged by your colleagues; your husband's unexplained weekend meetings; the awkward gestures of the salesman.

There are two reasons for thinking that malign intentions are a central target of the system. First, people can exploit one another in ways that are not obvious from the behavioral evidence even after the exploitation has been carried out. In appreciation of your business, for example, your local coffee chain offers you a loyalty card that gives you discounts on vanilla lattes. In exchange for the discount, using a loyalty card allows the company access to information about your buying habits, which enables them to tailor their advertising to you. Over time, the effect of their advertising takes more money out of your pocket than the loyalty discount puts back. The coffee company hasn't attacked you with a chainsaw, stolen your wallet, or (arguably) even deceived you. But it may have exploited you just the same, and you may never know it. The evidence that you are being disadvantaged is latent, and the best way to detect the exploitation is to focus on the intentions of the people who make company policy. Since almost everything for-profit companies do is directed at getting your money, it makes sense to wonder about the intention behind loyalty cards. Once a suspicion is raised in your mind, you might be motivated enough to think about what's really going on.

The second reason for thinking that the Suspicion System targets intentions is because the overarching purpose of the system is to detect threats early on, in order to take defensive action. Once you've lost money on your loyalty card, it's too late. If, however, you become suspicious that the people running the company are out to fleece you, you're still in a position to do something about it.

This last point is obvious but worth emphasizing. It would make no sense for human beings to have a social threat system merely to keep track of when they were being victimized. Therefore, as in the predation example above, one would expect the Suspicion System to motivate you to act, and to inhibit other motivations that might interfere with taking the necessary evasive maneuvers. But future events, by definition, are merely hypothetical: they may or may not happen. This uncertainty points up both the huge evolutionary advantage of thinking into the future and the psychological strain of having to be constantly vigilant. We have to make conceptual bets on future dangers to get the benefits of social life, but in so doing, we pay a psychological price in the stress brought about by our sensitivity to some alarming possibilities.

JOHN: THE ACADEMIC

John was born into a middle-class family in Chicago. His father made sausages, and his mother taught school. His mother noticed that after he returned from a short stay in the hospital for an allergic reaction as a baby, he was more withdrawn and exhibited separation anxiety. John also later recalled being scalded by boiling water as a child. He was close to his brother, seven years his junior, but had few other friends. His mother even considered having him enrolled in an autism study, but she ultimately decided against it. John was an excellent student and skipped the sixth grade, which he later recalled as a watershed moment in his life, as he was teased by his older classmates who saw him as a "freak." He skipped the eleventh grade as well, with the result that he was only sixteen when he went off to college. He excelled in math and went on to get a doctoral degree. His IQ was measured at 136.

John had difficulty forming friendships, struggled to form romantic relationships with women, and felt a lot of resentment toward his peers and his parents. "I would therefore indulge in fantasies of revenge," he said. "However, I never attempted to put any such fantasies into effect because I was too strongly conditioned . . . against any defiance of authority. To be more precise, I could not have committed a crime of revenge, even a relatively minor crime, because my fear of being caught and punished was all out of proportion to the actual danger of being caught."

This concern would eventually change.

While in graduate school, John began to suspect that people who were having conversations out of earshot were saying critical things about him. At least once he seems to have had a frank auditory hallucination of somebody talking about him. He became sensitive to noises, particularly those of a sexual nature, coming through the walls.

In his twenties, John formed two sets of delusional beliefs. The first was that he was verbally and emotionally abused as a child. There was no evidence for this: his brother rejected these accusations, and John's early journals made no reference to abuse. Nonetheless, he wrote his mother a letter condemning her for a specific incident twenty years earlier, when she told

John and his brother to pick up their socks from the floor. He came to see his difficulty in romantic relationships as connected to the abuse he suffered at the hands of his family.

John's second delusion involved modern technology. He believed that electrodes and "chemitrodes" would come to control people's emotions, that "super-human computers" and mind control were making people powerless to defend themselves, and that people like himself would "vanish forever from the earth." Over the course of years, he wrote letters to various agencies inquiring about "radiation, parasitic infection, sonic booms, et cetera."

John describes the turning point in his life. During his fourth year of graduate school, when he was twenty-one or twenty-two years old, he had a period of strong sexual fantasizing about becoming a woman and contemplated having gender reassignment surgery. Knowing he would have to undergo a psychiatric evaluation in order to go forward with the surgery, he made an appointment with a university psychiatrist. But while in the waiting room, he became anxious and embarrassed, and when called into the psychiatrist's office, he made up a benign reason for his visit and quickly left.

"As I walked away from the building afterwards, I felt disgusted about what my uncontrolled sexual cravings had almost led me to do, and I felt humiliated, and I violently hated the psychiatrist. Just then there came a major turning point in my life. Like a phoenix, I burst from the ashes of my despair to a glorious new hope. I thought I wanted to kill that psychiatrist because the future looked utterly empty to me. I felt I wouldn't care if I died. And so I said to myself, Why not really kill the psychiatrist and anyone else whom I hate. What is important is not the words that ran through my mind but the way I felt about them. What was entirely new was the fact that I really felt I could kill someone."

According to the psychiatrist Sally Johnson, prior to that moment John suspected he might be mentally ill and that the cause of his suffering was internal. After this "turning point," John externalized the cause of his difficulties and saw his family and technology as the cause of his problems. John frequently read *The Technological Society* by French sociologist Jacques Ellul. He began having dreams about killing psychologists, but in the dreams his victims would return to life. He felt that by employing force of will in these dreams he could alter the ending and keep the psychologists dead. Johnson diagnosed John as having paranoid schizophrenia, as well as paranoid personality disorder.

Though he secured a teaching position in California after graduate school, he left after two years to get away from the technology he decried. He moved to the country and took a number of odd jobs beneath his educational and intellectual level. When he was thirty-four years old, he took a job at a plant where his father and brother worked. He went on a few dates with a female supervisor, and after these led nowhere, he was ultimately fired for inappropriate behavior toward her. John contemplated suicide but instead decided to mutilate the woman with a knife. He went so far as to wait in her car, but changed his mind and fell into despair.

It was during this period that Theodore John Kaczynski planted the first of sixteen bombs attributed to the Unabomber.

TRUST BUT VERIFY

Our story to this point has been about the evolution of social intelligence. Some accounts of the evolution of the mind have been rightly criticized as "just so" stories—cooked-up fantasies about the mental capacities our ancestors would have needed as they wandered the grassy African savanna evolving into us. The social brain hypothesis is no "just so" story. It is a constituent of a serious scientific model of brain evolution, and its relation to social cognition, that is built on a broad base of evidence. Still, one has to be careful about making simplistic inferences from facts about evolution to the function of the human mind in the twenty-first century. One cannot simply assume that having a good theory of primate brain evolution is all we need to understand the behavior of your auntie Mathilda. Accordingly, we have to ask whether there is evidence of the existence of a Suspicion System in contemporary human beings.

One line of evidence for the existence of a Suspicion System comes from the perception of faces. Human beings put a lot of stock in what faces reveal about people. Here is a particularly striking illustration. Responsible citizens approach elections with an eye to a careful evaluation of the policies of the candidates and make thoughtful, rational decisions about whom to vote for. Or do they? In a 2005 study, Alexander Todorov and his colleagues showed participants two black-and-white portraits of actual candidates for recent US Senate and House elections who were unfamiliar to the participants, and asked them to judge which of the two looked more competent. With no more than a one-second exposure to the pair of photographs, participants were able to come to a decision. Astonishingly, the candidate judged more competent was also the one who was more likely to have actually been elected. In a subsequent experiment, Todorov and Charles Ballew found that participants were able to distinguish the winner from the runner-up with only an exposure of 100 milliseconds (one tenth of a second). When participants were allowed to take as much time as they wanted to look at the photographs before making their judgment, the choices they made were *less* accurate at predicting the outcome of the election. It's possible, then, that quite a lot of our thoughtful, rational political decision making happens in a moment's exposure to a face.

The human face is also a rich source of evidence for judgments about social threat. One way of characterizing threatening others is to say that they are "not to be trusted"; if you give them the opportunity, they are likely to harm you. One can, therefore, assess how threatening someone is by deciding whether they are trustworthy. Unfortunately, the only way to be confident that someone is genuinely trustworthy is on the basis of knowledge about how they have handled their past responsibilities. But what if you don't have the luxury of that knowledge? As the voting experiment shows, quick-and-dirty judgments are often employed as reasonable approximations. We judge competence from faces, and we sometimes judge trustworthiness in the same way. In an elegant series of studies, Todorov and his colleagues investigated this psychological process. In one experiment participants were shown pictures of faces very briefly and asked to judge how trustworthy the person appeared to be. An exposure of 33 milliseconds (i.e., 33 thousandths of a second) was enough for participants to make some distinctions between trustworthy and untrustworthy faces. At 100 milliseconds, participants made judgments that were quite like those made on the basis of unlimited viewing. At one sixth of a second, the judgments were indistinguishable. Since eye movements take longer than one sixth of a second, some judgments of trustworthiness are literally made in a single glance.

In a second experiment, Todorov and his colleagues generated artificial faces that could be manipulated to look more or less trustworthy and found that participants made more discriminations of untrustworthiness than of trustworthiness (see Figure 18). In other words, people are more sensitive to how *un*trustworthy someone is, and this is not surprising. Small differences in untrustworthiness matter more than small differences in trustworthiness. Avoiding the worst people is more important than identifying the best ones, so it's better to be sensitive to distinctions among threatening faces than among safe ones. A similar experiment by Moshe Bar, Maital Neta, and Heather Linz further supports this idea. In their experiment, participants were shown faces and asked to judge, on a scale from one to five, how threatening the person seemed. At 39 milliseconds—half the time it takes to blink—participants could identify the threatening faces.

Perhaps the most important feature of these face experiments is that they reveal judgments of trustworthy and threatening faces to be rather special. Judgments of how intelligent someone seems, to take a contrasting case, *cannot* be made in 39 milliseconds, and judging competence, likability, or aggressiveness takes longer than judging trustworthiness. (Perhaps not surprisingly, judgments of attractiveness *are* made as

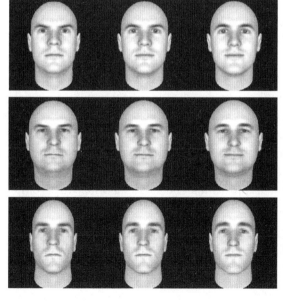

Figure 18: Todorov's artificial faces. The faces on the right are judged more trustworthy than those in the middle, which, in turn, are judged more trustworthy than those on the left. Reproduced with permission of the Social Perception Lab, directed by Alexander Todorov, Princeton University.

quickly as, or more quickly than, trustworthiness.) The time course of threat-related judgments provides some evidence that a special system is devoted to carrying them out.

In the pictures in Figure 18, the faces are not expressing passing emotional states (most importantly anger, which conveys information about imminent threat). The judgments of threat and trustworthiness are made on the basis of facial features alone and are more like judgments of personality traits than momentary states. This isn't ToM in the traditional sense, which is usually taken to be directed at *current mental states*—that is, what someone is thinking or feeling right now. The Suspicion System is trying to get at what's hidden—what is *not* clearly expressed in the face. In addition to mental states, it targets traits—the stable psychological features of people who are likely to have malicious intent. The purpose of our reading faces in this way is to try to decide which people are best avoided. The Suspicion System may not get it right, of course, but it does what it can with the data it has.

The most interesting evidence for the existence of the Suspicion System comes from studies of one of the brain regions that does some of the work of threat detection: the amygdala. The amygdala is a subcortical structure, and healthy brains have two, one in each hemisphere. Studies in animals have shown that the amygdala is involved in various emotional functions and, in humans, is particularly sensitive to facial expressions and body language expressing fear and fear-related sounds like screaming. Electrical stimulation of the amygdala, and some of the pathological electrical activity that occurs in epilepsy, typically elicit fear responses of some kind.

Studies of rhesus monkeys, however, have shown that the amygdala is also a social brain region. In an early investigation, Dennis Dicks, Ronald Myers, and Arthur Kling lesioned the amygdalas of rhesus monkeys living in the wild and found that the animals became socially indifferent, losing interest in rejoining their group or seeking out social activity. When the lesioned animals did initiate social interactions, this prompted attacks by other animals, perhaps because the lesioned monkeys' behavior was subtly abnormal, or because they flouted the social conventions of the dominance hierarchy. Crucially, they appeared "retarded in their ability to foresee and avoid dangerous confrontations." Later research confirmed this finding. Monkeys whose amygdalas are removed shortly after birth develop mostly normally but are impaired in evaluating, and responding to, dangers in the social environment.

Physiological studies highlight the social character of the amygdala. Stimuli that are only imperfect predictors of threat generate a bigger electrical response in the amygdala than stimuli, like expressions of anger, that *always* signal danger. The amygdala may thus be tuned to clues to possible threat as well as to signs of imminent peril. The very fact that the amygdala is most responsive to fear shows that uncertainty is built into its function. Someone expressing anger in your presence may be threatening you; someone showing fear, in contrast, is *responding* to a threat in the environment without communicating whether the threat is likely to put you in particular at risk. Brain-imaging studies provide another kind of evidence of a link between the amygdala and the social world in humans. The volume of the amygdala is correlated with the size of one's social network, and two of three cortical regions that also vary with social group size are connected to the amygdala.

The most important perspective on amygdala function, however, comes from studies of patients with amygdala lesions. In 1990, Daniel Tranel and Bradley Hyman described a patient, known as SM, who suffered from Urbach-Wiethe disease, an exceptionally rare genetic illness that causes brain lesions in about half of its victims; SM's were restricted to the amygdalas in both brain hemispheres. SM, now in her mid-forties, and a second Urbach-Wiethe patient known as AP, in her early twenties, have been studied over a number of years by Tranel, Ralph Adolphs, and their colleagues. They are both described as friendly, open and forthcoming, and intellectually normal, with intact memory and speech functions. Apart from a mild "executive function" impairment (broadly speaking, a deficit in goal-directed cognitive coordination), they show no signs of psychiatric disorder and—importantly, as we'll see in a moment—have normal vision.

Yet there are profound differences. SM cannot recognize fear in faces and is mildly impaired in recognizing the intensity of other "negative" emotions such as anger, disgust, and sadness. The deficit is more pronounced in the case of fear because SM doesn't make use of the eye region to identify expressions of emotion, and fear recognition is more heavily dependent on this area of the face than the recognition of other emotional states is. The deficit, however, goes beyond emotion recognition.

In a recent study, SM was exposed to snakes and spiders in a pet store, taken through a haunted house, and shown scenes from scary movies. She neither showed fear nor felt it strongly throughout the experiment.

Despite these striking findings concerning emotion, SM's impairment seems to be fundamentally a social one, as it is in monkeys, rather than visual or emotional. In the crucial experiment, Adolphs, Tranel, and Antonio Damasio showed pictures of faces to SM and two other individuals with amygdala damage, and asked them to rate the faces according to "trustworthiness" and "approachability." SM and the other participants with amygdala damage rated all of the faces as more trustworthy and approachable than did healthy individuals. Moreover, the discrepancy between their judgments and those of the healthy participants was most conspicuous with very untrustworthy- and unapproachable-looking faces. In other words, where SM and the other subjects were most impaired was in seeing threatening faces *as threatening*, a finding that resonates with Todorov's finding that we discriminate untrustworthy faces more finely than trustworthy ones.

SM's impairment is not confined to the lab. In a different study, SM was interviewed by two psychotherapists unaware of her neurological condition. The therapists agreed that she showed no evidence of psychopathology but one spontaneously commented that "she did not seem to have a normal sense of distrust and 'danger.'" AP's parents remarked that "she tends to 'trust' people too easily," and they have tried to teach her to be "more wary of strangers." According to our theory, SM and AP have a damaged Suspicion System. Looking into the face of a stranger, our brains are asking—in the immortal words of Christian Szell in the film *Marathon Man*—"Is it safe?" Their brains have lost this capacity.

Subsequent studies of SM have given us an expanded picture of her impairment. It appears that SM *can* in fact detect social threats, but she doesn't look for them (see Figure 19). As we noted, SM has trouble using the eye region to detect fear. When *instructed* to pay attention to the eyes, however, she can recognize it. Without the instruction, she returns to her impaired state. Adolphs and his colleagues interpret this as showing that the cardinal role of the amygdala may be to explore the environment, in particular the social environment. A narrower interpretation is possible. The pattern of SM's deficit in recognizing fear and untrustworthy faces, as well as SM's and AP's trusting behavior outside the lab, show that the business of the amygdala (or part of it, at any rate) is to probe the environment specifically for social threats. A failure to detect the expression of threatening emotions is really only the tip of the iceberg. Without the amygdala, SM and AP are blind to the uncertain, ambiguous clues that signal dangerous people. Of course, no brain region is an island, and the amygdala is only one component of what is likely to be a complex of interacting brain regions that together do the work of the Suspicion System. Two other regions that are candidate components of the system are the anterior cingulate cortex and the insula.

SOURCES OF SUSPICION

Before we turn to the relevance of the Suspicion System to delusion, we need to say a little more about how the system works. Although the evidence of social threat often comes from seeing other people, especially their faces, the Suspicion System responds to other clues as well, in particular those that are present in interactions with other people and those that are available through other sources. Seeing the glint of a gun under a stranger's jacket produces an immediate awareness of threat as automatically and effortlessly as seeing a dangerous face. Threat is picked up equally quickly in complex social situations. Take, as an illustration, an

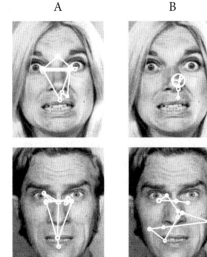

Figure 19: SM's visual scanpaths (B) and those of a healthy subject (A). SM scans the eye regions significantly less. Adapted by permission from Macmillan Publishers Ltd.

episode in the film *The Godfather*. The mobster Frank Pentangeli finds himself in the custody of the FBI and offers to testify against mob boss Michael Corleone. Because Frank is in custody, Michael can't threaten him directly. Instead, he flies Frank's brother, Vincenzo, from Italy to America and brings him to the hearing. When Frank enters the courtroom and sees his brother, he immediately recognizes this as a threat: if you hurt me with your testimony, I will hurt your family. There are a lot of cognitive steps between Frank's seeing his brother and realizing that his loved ones are at risk, but Frank doesn't have to go through these steps consciously to perceive the threat. The Suspicion System spots it immediately.

This illustration also points up two distinctions that have to be made about social threat. First, we have to distinguish between threatening *people* and specific *threats*, like the threat that your family will be harmed; the Suspicion System is sensitive to both. Second, there is a difference between an intent to harm and the harmful event itself. Michael Corleone shows his intent to harm Frank indirectly, and that's what he communicates by bringing Vincenzo into the courtroom. The harm, were it carried out, would be actually killing Vincenzo. This distinction is important because deliberate harm is preceded by an intention, and, as we've said, getting evidence about potentially harmful intentions may make it possible to take defensive action, which is why the Suspicion System is geared to look for evidence of threatening mental states. Suspicion is the state of mind someone is in when they have picked up clues, perhaps uncertain and ambiguous, that someone has a malign intention directed at them.

The Suspicion System is also likely to be very sensitive to cues signaling possible deception. Someone who represents a threat to you is typically *not* going to communicate that fact if he can help it. Plans for backstabbing are carried out in secret, after all, and must by definition come as a surprise, a betrayal of friendship or civility. To detect social threats effectively, one has to be prepared to take minor or apparently trivial events as having special meaning or significance. This may be one reason the amygdala responds to ambiguous stimuli: ambiguity is a feature of clues that are being deliberately obscured. Our sensitivity to subtle social cues is illustrated by a physiological experiment addressing gaze perception. Participants were shown groups of three faces, in each of which the two outer faces shared the same averted gaze and the gaze of the middle face was manipulated. In one picture, the middle face looked in the same direction as the other two, as if all three were paying attention to the same thing; in a second picture, the central face seemed to be exchanging a glance with one of the other faces; and in a third picture, the central face looked straight ahead (see Figure 20). The images are nearly identical perceptually. Nonetheless, they were distinguishable by electrical differences at the scalps of the participants. Since only big electrical effects can be detected at the scalp, it appears that, although visually subtle, a brief exchange of glances or an averted gaze can, in the right circumstances, elicit a substantial neural response.

A second illustration of neural sensitivity to possible signals of deception comes from a study of bodily movements in which participants were shown people simultaneously making gestures and expressing emotions. When the gestures and the emotions were consonant, brain activity was different than when they were dissonant. Inconsistencies in gesture and

Group Attention

Mutual Gaze Exchange

Figure 20: Patterns of gaze conveying social information. Adapted by permission of the Royal Society.

Control

speech combinations often signal dissembling or deception, so it is possible that other inconsistencies are significant for the same reason. When the gesture doesn't fit the emotion, that may be a signal that someone is hiding something.

In addition to the behavioral cues that one can pick up when interacting with other people, the Suspicion System is sensitive to "indirect" evidence of malicious intentions. When you see two people exchange a glance in a work meeting, and you interpret that as evidence that they're going to sell you down the river, you've detected direct evidence of a malign intention—direct in the sense that it is "read off" the behavior of the threatening individuals. If, however, you come upon an email in which your colleagues discuss the possibility of sticking it to you, you've got indirect evidence of a threatening intent. Not all of the evidence—perhaps not even the most important evidence—of social threats has to come from social interactions with dangerous people; not all the cues to social threat come from the threatening person. We often get a sense of what other people are up to from third parties in the form of gossip or unusual hesitations or tones of voice, as well as from events and objects in the environment, such as when Othello sees Cassio with Desdemona's handkerchief. Knowing what's in someone's mind doesn't require ToM in the traditional sense when other, more explicit, if indirect, evidence is available.

DO DELUSIONS FOSTER VIOLENCE?

Antony Waterlow, of Sydney, Australia, stabbed his father and sister to death in 2009. Waterlow believed they were broadcasting his life on the internet as part of a "worldwide game" that would end in either his murder or suicide, and he compared his experience to *The Truman Show*. Two years later, after being successfully treated with antipsychotic medication, Waterlow was found not guilty by reason of mental illness. He said that being treated "is a good thing, but it's also a terrible thing, because it makes me aware of the awful realities of what I have done."

Miriam Carey, the woman killed by police in 2013 after trying to drive into the White House, was reported to have been suffering from postpartum psychotic depression. At least one news outlet reported her exhibiting Truman signs, writing that she "believed President Obama was electronically monitoring her Connecticut home in order to broadcast her life on television."

The intersection of mental illness and violence is complex and not easily dismissed with the common and unfair generalization that "crazy" people are dangerous. One is far more likely to be killed by a nonpsychotic family member than by a psychotic stranger, but there is something about the shocking, seemingly random, and often gruesome nature of violence committed by psychotic individuals that captures people's attention and stokes fear in their minds.

Recent mass shootings that have received significant attention from the media and the public include those in Aurora, Colorado; Tucson, Arizona; Newtown, Connecticut; and Virginia Tech. The shooters all had some contact with the mental health system prior to the shootings, though it is impossible to know how much of a role, if any, delusion might have played in these horrors. Of the ninety-three mass shootings that occurred between January 2009 and September 2013, only ten were committed by people with mental health concerns of which a medical professional was made aware. These tragedies speak to the challenge that psychiatrists face in preventing their patients from committing acts of violence and point to cracks in the mental health system. (In the wake of the killings in Australia, the filmmaker Jane Campion, a friend of Waterlow's father, asked that the Australian laws governing involuntary hospitalization be strengthened.) Unfortunately, as violence and mental illness expert Jeffrey Swanson has concluded, psychiatrists are reasonably competent at predicting who will *not* become violent but not very good at predicting who will.

Studies of the association between delusion and violence have produced mixed results. In 1994, researchers Bruce Link and Ann Stueve described what they called threat/control-override (TCO) symptoms. Patients with TCO delusions believe both that someone is threatening them with significant harm and that their ability to control themselves is being overridden by outside forces. Link and Stueve concluded that people with TCO symptoms were more likely to engage in violent behavior than those with other kinds of delusions. The fourteen-item Threat/Control-Override Questionnaire (TCOQ) includes statements such as "Other people have tried to poison me or to do me harm" and "Other people have been secretly plotting to ruin me" (threat assessment), as well as "Other people control my way of movements" and "Other people can insert thoughts into my mind" (control-override assessment). While some in the field supported these findings, Thomas Stompe, Gerhard Ortwein-Swoboda, and Hans Schanda found a correlation between violence and the presence of threat symptoms, but no correlation with control-override symptoms. More surprising is the finding in 2000 of Paul Appelbaum and his colleagues, who reported that not only did the presence of TCO delusions *not* increase the likelihood of violence in the general population, but *no* delusions did. They concluded: "Although delusions can precipitate violence in individual cases, these data suggest that they do not increase the overall risk of violence in persons with mental illness in the year after discharge from hospitalization." Another study of people with schizophrenia found that those who were suspicious and had persecutory delusions were more likely to be violent than people with schizophrenia who had no delusions. However, those who had delusions that were not persecutory or suspicious in nature were actually *less* likely to be violent than people with schizophrenia who had no delusions at all.

Given the large number of people who have persecutory delusions, the question we might ask is not why some of them engage in acts of violence, but rather why more do not. The answers are likely the same ones that might be offered to explain why *anyone* with some reason to commit violence does not. Many children are bullied, but only a handful return to school with a gun and vengeful mind-set. Tens of thousands of Americans lose their jobs every day, but only a tiny fraction murder their bosses and coworkers. Factors aside from delusion appear to play larger contributory roles in the violence committed by people with delusion. These risk factors likely include substance use; low socioeconomic status; impulsivity; anger and hostile behavior; social isolation; poor treatment adherence; a history of childhood trauma, victimization, conduct problems, and arrest; and antisocial personality disorder.

A 2013 study found that only three delusional beliefs (persecution, being spied on, and being the victim of a conspiracy) were associated with increased risk for serious violence. Moreover, the key mediating factor was not the delusions themselves, but the anger the delusions evoked. Psychiatrists might be wise to focus not solely on the presence of delusions and their content, but also on the emotions that delusions can arouse.

It is clear that Aaron Alexis, the man who shot and killed twelve people at the Washington Navy Yards, was delusional at the time of the killing, writing that he was under attack and being controlled by very low-frequency electromagnetic radiation emitted by a "microwave machine." In addition to delusions of persecution and control, Alexis had a history of "angry outbursts" and was discharged from the navy "after 'multiple' disciplinary breaches," including disorderly conduct. He was arrested in 2004 after he shot out another man's tires, later claiming the incident occurred during an "anger-fueled 'blackout.'" He was arrested again in 2008 for disorderly conduct and in 2010 for firing a gun through his ceiling into the apartment above, the bullet narrowly missing his neighbor.

We don't know whether the pattern of Alexis's behavior prior to the killings was related to an existing psychotic illness or if it predated his psychosis. It is also impossible to know all of the factors that contributed to this man killing a dozen people he did not know. It is fair to say that one can never truly fathom every factor that leads to a violent outcome of such devastating proportions. While in individual cases, specific delusions increase the likelihood of someone becoming violent, a host of other biological and social elements no doubt contributes to violence in the context of delusion, and the large majority of people with serious mental illness are never violent.

DIVISION OF LABOR

Todorov's studies show that people make judgments of trustworthiness remarkably quickly. This suggests that the Suspicion System is a special-purpose mechanism. What does "special purpose" mean? There are many domains of cognition in which it appears that human beings have two distinct systems for handling a single cognitive task. One type of system (often given the generic name "System 1") operates quickly, effortlessly, automatically, and unconsciously; these are the special-purpose mechanisms in our sense. In contrast, a parallel system ("System 2") is slow, requires attention and mental effort, and has to be consciously engaged in problem-solving. To get a feel for the two systems at work, imagine someone testing you with a series of addition problems: 2 + 2 = ?, 4+4 = ?, 8 + 8 = ?, and on up to 256 + 256, 512 + 512, 1,024 + 1,024 and higher. At first you can answer effortlessly, but at some point you'll experience the walking-on-glue feeling you get when you step off the moving walkway at the airport. That feeling of hitting a cognitive wall marks the moment of transition from System 1 to System 2 arithmetic, when you can no longer automatically and effortlessly generate the right answer but have to do the calculations consciously. Theories that posit the existence of both System 1 and System 2 cognition are called "dual process" theories, and dual process models have been proposed in a variety of cognitive spheres, including reasoning, decision making, and social cognition. (See Table 3.)

System 1 often provides intuitive, rule-of-thumb solutions; System 2 provides reasoned, careful answers. System 1 cognition is useful when there isn't time or data for careful thought, and a quick fix is better than no fix at all. The more a rapid decision matters, the more reason there is to have a System 1 mechanism in place. For this reason, scenarios that involve danger are a paradigm of System 1 decisions. It's not a good idea to reflect too much about what's going through the mind of that chainsaw-wielding maniac. Run first, reflect later. Taking a quick educated guess about whether a stranger is safe or not may be no less momentous. This is what the Suspicion System—a System 1 form of cognition—is built for. As time and data become available, System 2 can review the evidence more fully and decide whether the System 1 response was adequate or in need of revision. When you reflexively say that 512 + 512 = 1,022, you might suddenly have a moment of doubt; System 2 is now engaged and you do the arithmetic consciously. When System 2 produces 1,024 as the correct answer, it "shuts off" System 1's activity and leads you to revise the original output.

System 1 cognition is often taken to be "modular," where a module is a component of the mind, the purpose of which (roughly) is to handle narrow cognitive domains. The paradigm modules are perceptual systems, such as vision, which are responsive only to particular kinds of input. The philosopher Jerry Fodor, who developed the contemporary modularity view, proposed that modules typically have some or all of a

	System 1	System 2
Cluster 1 **Consciousness**	Unconscious (preconscious)	Conscious
	Implicit	Explicit
	Automatic	Controlled
	Low effort	High effort
	Rapid	Slow
	High capacity	Low capacity
	Default process	Inhibitory
	Holistic, perceptual	Analytic, reflective
Cluster 2 **Evolution**	Evolutionarily old	Evolutionarily recent
	Evolutionary rationality	Individual rationality
	Shared with animals	Uniquely human
	Nonverbal	Linked to language
	Modular cognition	Fluid intelligence
Cluster 3 **Functional** **characteristics**	Associative	Rule based
	Domain specific	Domain general
	Contextualized	Abstract
	Pragmatic	Logical
	Parallel	Sequential
	Stereotypical	Egalitarian
Cluster 4 **Individual** **differences**	Universal	Heritable
	Independent of general intelligence	Linked to general intelligence
	Independent of working memory	Limited by working memory capacity

Table 3: A comparison of some characteristic features
of System 1 and System 2.

small set of features, and some of these features are also characteristics of System 1 cognition. Modules, like System 1 processes, operate automatically and quickly. Assuming your eyes are open and there is enough light, your visual system will more or less immediately see the world around you whether you like it or not.

Importantly, modules are also "informationally encapsulated"; that is, they are largely, though not entirely, insulated from the effects of the information that is present in other parts of the mind. They operate, roughly speaking, autonomously. Visual illusions provide classic illustrations of informational encapsulation. Figure 21 shows the well-known Müller-Lyer illusion. The lines in (A) and (B) are the same length, but the fins and arrowheads contribute to making the central line in (A) seem longer than in (B). Stare for a minute at the two lines and repeat the following mantra: *the lines are equal; the lines are equal; the lines are equal.* What effect does that have on what you see? Exactly none. That's because vision is modular, and modules are informationally encapsulated. Your conscious awareness that the lines are equal is in the very same skull as your perception of their apparent difference. But without a conduit between that information and your visual experience, no change in your perception can occur.

The Suspicion System is also a module. It is only interested in input of a certain kind—evidence of social threat—and is sensitive to *anything* that might signal threat, from facial expressions to the fact that someone like Cassio has possession of a handkerchief that doesn't belong to him. The Suspicion System operates quickly and automatically: when Frank Pentangeli sees his brother in the courtroom, or Othello sees Cassio with Desdemona's handkerchief, the system can't help but signal a threat. Finally, like other System 1 forms of cognition, the Suspicion System is informationally encapsulated—the central reason, as we'll see, why delusions are so hard to abolish.

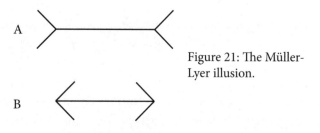

Figure 21: The Müller-Lyer illusion.

CALVIN: OTHELLO IN NEW YORK

But jealous souls will not be answered so;
They are not ever jealous for the cause,
But jealous for they're jealous. It is a monster
Begot upon itself, born on itself.

—*Othello*

Bertha Moore lies in bed poring over a photo album: her wedding to Calvin outside city hall in the early seventies; the two curled up with a dog on the couch; Calvin holding each of their grandchildren, always smiling; Bertha and her sister laughing with Calvin moments after a birthday cream pie found its way onto his face; numerous christenings, baptisms, and weddings; Calvin playing piano or congas. Bertha and Calvin. Always close. Always smiling. "He was a good guy. He took good care of me. He did everything for me, every day. He would do anything for me. Anything." Then one June morning, Calvin Moore woke up and decided he would kill his wife.

Calvin Moore was born in Northern California. His father abandoned him and his mother just after he was born, and later remarried and had a large family (Calvin never met his half-siblings). Calvin's mother remarried seven years later but grew unhappy with her second husband. She began divorce proceedings and planned on relocating to New York City. She brought Calvin to stay with his uncle in Upper Manhattan when he was ten. Several months later, she returned to California to finalize the divorce. Calvin stayed behind with his uncle. His mother never returned, and he never heard from her. For years, Calvin believed that another parent had abandoned him, choosing his stepfather over him. Eventually, Calvin's uncle told him the brutal truth; when his mother tried to leave her husband for good, he killed her and then himself.

Calvin Moore was not a strong student and got into trouble as a teen, stealing hubcaps and spending time in juvenile hall. He loved music, sang doo-wop with friends from high school, and even recorded a local hit song. He decided to join the army but never saw combat. He was trained to be a mechanic, the profession he would enjoy for more than forty years. He met his wife shortly after discharge from the military, and they had a daughter whom he adored. He stopped smoking when she was born. A few years into the marriage, his wife met another man and left with their daughter for Florida. He was alone again.

Bertha recalls living a few floors above Calvin when they were teens and being friendly with him. After his wife left him, Calvin moved back in with his uncle. Bertha still lived in the building, now with two children of her own from a previous relationship. Bertha and Calvin began dating soon after, and Calvin moved into her apartment several months later. Within a year they were married.

Calvin treated Bertha's children as his own. He was even more doting on the grandchildren. Bertha felt he spoiled them, particularly the youngest boy, born in their apartment, whom he treated more like a son. She recalls that when the Atari video console came out, he bought his grandson every game available. He took the family to Atlantic City, out to dinner, and to picnics in the park. He kept his suit from his own daughter's wedding, telling Bertha that he wanted to be buried in it when he died. He remained in contact with his daughter intermittently, although he hadn't seen her in many years and never got to know her children.

Bertha describes her husband as a homebody, not interested in going out drinking with friends. He was a romantic, often bringing Bertha flowers and cake. Bertha felt loved and cared for. She thought of Calvin as a man who would do anything for her and their family. He proved his dedication to her when Bertha became ill, twenty-five years into their marriage. She developed a neuromuscular disease, which left her paraplegic, bedbound, and in intense pain. They hired Ava, a home health aide, who became another member of the family. Still, a lot of the work fell to Calvin, who bathed his wife regularly. He brought her every video he could find so she could watch movies in her bed. He brought her sewing materials. Whenever Bertha had a flare-up of her illness, Calvin would keep her company during the long nights in the emergency room and stand up for her needs. During one period, she was in such intense pain that she was making near-weekly visits by ambulance to Bellevue. "One time, Cal was really pissed off with the hospital. I was in a lot of pain. They wanted to send me home, and I couldn't take it. Cal said, 'My wife is not leaving this place. She's not going home.' They kept me." She smiles proudly. He was afraid of losing her. Calvin tearfully confided in a neighbor that he was terrified that Bertha would die, that he loved her intensely, and that Bertha was the only thing he had in the world.

While Ava was the primary home health aide, there were others, particularly on weekends. When one was in financial distress, Calvin bought her a TV, a washing machine, and a bed. He had good friends. Bertha says that everyone liked him. He regularly bought clothing at thrift shops and donated them to the church for parishioners who were in need, though he was not a practicing Catholic and told the priest who married them not to expect to see him at Sunday services. But he would pick up Bertha from church with an umbrella when it was raining.

Calvin Moore loved baseball and football, and converted Bertha into a New York Jets fan, not a minor achievement. He enjoyed shopping and painting trompe-l'oeil pastoral landscape murals throughout the apartment. He was devoted to his music and would often have his old group over to sing and play. These visits eventually stopped as his musician friends drank and smoked pot, and Calvin didn't approve.

In the early years of their marriage, Calvin was protective, if not overtly jealous. He preferred accompanying her when she visited friends until she insisted that it was unnecessary. Calvin was not thrilled when men showed Bertha attention. He would ask rhetorically why a younger man needed to hold the door for Bertha. She would tut him and reassure Calvin that the guy was simply being polite. Bertha had a male friend who could not read. He would come over regularly to ask Bertha for help reading bills or filling out forms. Eventually, Calvin said that he didn't want the friend coming around anymore. Bertha didn't argue the point and simply helped the man at his home. Bertha understood that, because his first wife had left him for another man, Calvin was acutely sensitive to the threat of abandonment. As Calvin was a devoted, loving husband and his jealousy hadn't resulted in any real conflict, Bertha simply accepted it as part of who he was and gave it little thought.

After three decades of marriage, however, as Calvin neared seventy, things began to change. Calvin suffered a number of small strokes, none of which caused any apparent physical or mental deficits, but his jealousy swelled from the merely vigilant to the morbid. Over time, the accumulation of brain injuries resulted in vascular dementia. His thinking was not so impaired as to make it obvious to a casual observer that anything was amiss. He dressed and spoke well, and walked without any difficulty. But the damage from the strokes, like Iago whispering into Othello's ear, connived to convince Calvin that his wife was unfaithful.

The strange behavior began five years before Calvin became murderous. Bertha had been hospitalized once again at Bellevue, and Calvin and Ava came to visit her. Ava later told Bertha that she and Calvin had approached a tall, well-dressed man who was giving out the visitors' passes. When Calvin said that he was there to visit Bertha Moore and that he was her husband, the pass handler joked, "She's my wife, too!" Bertha remembers Calvin taking this statement to heart. He no longer visited her when she was in the hospital. She couldn't believe it. She had never even met the man.

More bizarrely, after Bertha returned home from Bellevue, Calvin pulled Ava aside and accused her of bringing Bertha to Bellevue for trysts with the tall man. Ava tried to reason with Calvin, but from then on, when the phone rang and Bertha picked up, Calvin needed to know who was calling. Still, throughout this period, Calvin never threatened or harmed her.

It was late spring and Calvin was getting worse. He was quick to anger and now seemed to resent bathing his wife. From the time Bertha had become bedbound, whenever Calvin left the apartment, he would come to their bedroom, kiss her, and tell her where he was going. When he returned, he would check back for another kiss. Now, Bertha would ask Ava where Calvin was and find out that he had simply left. He became taciturn and washed himself less regularly. For the first time, he yelled and cursed at her; Bertha cried. He later apologized, but the withdrawal continued.

Unsurprisingly, Calvin's memory had deteriorated over the previous months. Bertha described symptoms commonly seen in early dementia, like Calvin's leaving the stove on, or his entering a room and forgetting what he had come for. He had also begun hoarding things he had found in the street. Calvin scoffed at the notion that there was anything wrong with him.

In early June, Calvin told Ava about Bertha's lover. The man in question was someone who had bowled with Calvin a few times. Naturally, Ava informed Bertha, who, telling me about it a year after the fact, seems as shocked as when she first heard it. "I don't know this guy. He never came to the house; never visited. Calvin never brought him to my house." Calvin accused Ava of having an affair with the same man.

Calvin woke early that Saturday. He asked Bertha if she needed anything from the kitchen. He left the apartment and, when he came back a little later, announced that he would be bringing divorce papers on Monday. Calvin told Bertha that she had been lucky. He had gone out to buy a gun in order to kill Bertha, Ava, and their lover, but he hadn't found anyone to sell him one. He then said he could still stab her. Bertha began to pray. Calvin raised his balled fists, but on seeing his wife frightened, he stopped himself. Instead he began to cut up family photos. Bertha asked the weekend home attendant to go out to find a police car, but she feared that if she left the apartment, Calvin might kill Bertha. Instead, Bertha called 911. When the police arrived, they found Calvin in the kitchen still cutting up photos. Though it was late spring, he talked to the officers about the coming snow. He then told them that he was going to kill his wife. When asked the date, he was off by two years and two seasons. A police officer told Bertha that her husband was sick and called for an ambulance. Before Calvin was taken away, Bertha asked the police to take away his house key. She found it odd that he didn't protest. On the day before Father's Day, Calvin Moore was brought to Bellevue Hospital, the place he had waited with, advocated for, and visited his wife for a decade.

In an uncanny example of life cruelly imitating art, the evidence for Othello's and Calvin's "cuckoldry" was strangely similar. Just as Othello came to believe that his wife Desdemona was unfaithful because of a handkerchief found in Cassio's possession, so Calvin "knew" his wife was sleeping with another man because he could see his rival's face in the bath towel, proving that the adulterer had been in their home. Calvin even "saw" the lover and Bertha kissing passionately right in front of him on the day before his deadly impulse arose. That evening, Calvin had told Bertha that he was so angry he could kill someone.

In the hospital, Calvin matter-of-factly admitted to his psychiatrist that he had tried to buy a gun that morning. He also said that he had threatened to kill his wife, but it wasn't a big deal; everybody threatens their wife. Calvin now just wanted to leave the hospital and get a divorce. Though he could not understand why he was on a psychiatric ward, Calvin did acknowledge that he had been made crazy by sleep deprivation. Bertha had been purposely raising the volume of the television in order to keep him awake. Calvin now accused his wife of having had multiple affairs.

Aside from the image of the face in the bath towel, Calvin had no other hallucinations. He had never seen a psychiatrist in his life and had never been violent toward his wife or anyone else. A CT scan showed the many tiny holes that dotted Calvin's brain. His memory was poor; he told stories about events that had taken place decades earlier as if they had just happened. Many friends visited him in the hospital. To the last, they couldn't believe the recent turn of events.

Medication did little to change Calvin's delusional beliefs, but it helped him feel calmer and less angry at Bertha. Calvin remained adamant that he wanted a divorce but recanted his wish to kill his wife. As he was not yet demented enough that he could not care for himself, after a two-month stay, it was decided that Calvin would be discharged. He refused to be placed in an adult home and chose instead to live with a cousin in New Jersey. Bertha got an order of protection against him and awaited the divorce papers. They never came.

Bertha heard from Calvin's cousin that since he did not believe he was ill, he had stopped his medication and no longer went to his psychiatry or neurology appointments. Several months after his discharge from Bellevue, Calvin showed up at Bertha's church. He was lonely and wanted to return to her, to come home. He would never hurt her. He explained that he had been jealous because someone had poisoned his food. Was it her? Bertha couldn't take him back. He still scared her.

Weeks later, Calvin called Bertha to tell her that he would be visiting cousins in her building, the same apartment where they had met so many years ago. He wanted her to know that he wouldn't bother her and that she shouldn't be afraid. A year has passed and, from her window, Bertha has seen Calvin arriving at her building a number of times, but he has kept his word. Looking forlorn, Bertha says, "He never touched my door. He never touched my door."—JG

5

BELIEF UNHINGED

Like any system in our bodies, the Suspicion System can break down. When it does, delusions are one result, and they exhibit the themes that they do because they are all symptoms of a single disordered cognitive apparatus. The breakdown of suspicion and the nature of the Truman Show delusion are the dual themes of this chapter.

FROM SUSPICION TO DELUSION

If a healthy Suspicion System detects evidence of malign intentions more or less accurately and sounds the alarm, then a malfunctioning one will sound the alarm without good reason and detect evidence poorly—that is, see malign intent where there is none. Add to this the passage of time—days, months, years—and (paraphrasing DSM-IV) you get an idiosyncratic belief that is firmly maintained despite rational argument or evidence to the contrary. We should not be surprised: looking into the future, trying to predict what may or may not be a threat to ourselves, has both evolutionary advantages and costs. As Melissa Green and Mary Phillips put it with regard to persecutory delusions, "clinical levels of paranoia may represent the inevitable cost of efficient threat perception—or 'justified' suspicion—that is necessary for survival of the human species."

Below, we show the specific themes that a malfunctioning Suspicion System produces and what those themes look like in their healthy state, before delusion refracts their protective function.

Persecutory delusions: We've noted that persecutory delusions are far

191

and away the most prevalent cross-culturally, and we can now speculate as to why that is. Paranoia is nothing more than an overly sensitive form of suspicion that cannot shut itself down. Of all the ways that the Suspicion System can go wrong, persecution is the "closest" to its normal function.

Delusional jealousy: Jealousy, under normal conditions, is a motivational state designed to produce behavior that reduces one's partner's inclination to abandon or cheat on you. Threatening your spouse with violence has been the classic disincentive since time immemorial and (if morality happens not to be one of your hang-ups) remains a live option. A better strategy might be to give them a reason to value you more. If, for example, you have a substantial trust fund that you haven't mentioned yet, now would be a good time to do so, because wealthier men are more attractive to women, at least in the sense that rich men have more sex and more children. (As a public service to single readers, we note that male fertility is inversely correlated with intelligence.) When the behavior that jealousy motivates is successful, the evidence of your partner's renewed commitment tamps jealousy down because it is no longer necessary.

Delusional jealousy is not normal; it doesn't respond to the evidence that should turn it off. On the contrary, it sees evidence everywhere that keeps the jealous fire burning. Calvin (whose portrait appears on page 185) interprets harmless remarks as significant and sees the imprint of his rival's face in a bath towel. Delusional jealousy is paranoia focused into a narrow beam where the potential threat is restricted to one's partner.

Religious delusions: According to our interpretation, these are variants of persecutory or grandiose delusions, and so require no special explanation. As we noted earlier, the distinction between natural and supernatural social threats may exist only in the minds of theorists; the Suspicion System does not recognize the difference.

Delusions of control: A person with delusions of control feels like he is being harmed, but these delusions are different enough in content from persecution to call for a separate explanation. Notice, to begin with, that there is a conceptual connection between control and power. One view of power has to do with influence over other people's behavioral options. For example, Herbert Simon, the computer scientist and Nobel Prize–winning economist, conceptualized power as a matter of one person causing another person's behavior. The master has power over the slave, the adult has power over the child, and the senator has power over the intern: each can make their subordinate do what he wants. But power, on this view, isn't the same as force; it's *behavioral control*. Having control over someone means having the capacity to make that person act in your interests rather than his or her own. When these interests diverge significantly, exercising power is a form of exploitation. Controlling someone is not the only way to exploit, but it's a very effective weapon in the persecutor's arsenal. It is sensible to be afraid of exploitation by powerful others and to stay away from them. Delusions of control arise when the fear of exploitation is unmotivated by the evidence.

Delusions of thought (e.g., thought insertion and thought withdrawal) are a species of the genus of control. A highly effective and safe way to control someone is to deceive him or her into doing what you want. Lying is one way to accomplish this; manipulation by means of ToM is another. This is Iago's game. He makes use of his knowledge of human psychology and Othello's jealousy to implant the belief he wants Othello to have, without committing himself to much that is false. Iago controls Othello, as the expression goes, by *putting ideas into his head* ("I'll pour this pestilence into his ear," he says). By use of lies, innuendo, and misdirection, he manipulates Othello and others and gets what he wants, all the while limiting the risk to himself. When the Suspicion System is working well, it sometimes generates the feeling that someone is trying to get us to see things his way and for his purposes; in short, that he is a manipulator. The delusion of thought insertion is a distortion of this internal alarm.

A variation of this delusion, that someone is *reading your mind*, is part of the same theme. You don't have to be Iago to know that playing your cards close to your chest is often the safe thing to do. The more other people know about you, the more options they have for exploitation. Honest, openhearted people are more vulnerable to victimization and more often get targeted in real life than skeptical people who are on the lookout for a scam. A preemptive defense in social life is not revealing what's in your mind. A suspicion that someone has breached that defense, and knows something about you that was better kept secret, is a familiar one. Thought withdrawal and mind reading are the distorted forms of that suspicion.

Delusions of reference: A healthy Suspicion System is sensitive to the subtle, ambiguous cues buried within social interactions (cues such as direction of gaze), because the evidence of social threat is usually hidden and requires interpretation. When Othello sees Desdemona's handkerchief in Cassio's hands, he immediately understands that banal fact as having a profound significance for him; it is as if a spotlight has been turned on the handkerchief. Delusions of reference arise when a broken Suspicion System incorrectly identifies something insignificant in the environment and interprets it as carrying information about a threat, and thus of great personal significance.

Grandiosity or grandiose delusions: A central purpose of the Suspicion System is to initiate defensive action, and the action one takes depends on the threat. In response to a threat of physical attack, a display of physical power is a useful response. By making it clear to a potential attacker that there will be retaliation, he may reconsider his options. Making yourself look as physically intimidating as possible helps to demoralize your opponent—and even if you haven't got much, faking it is still a good strategy. Many animals use this tactic: puffer fish blow themselves up; zebras huddle together to look like a single large animal; cats arch their backs and make their fur stand up; elephants display their ears; and so on. We humans do many of the same things—pump up our biceps; stare opponents down; talk tough—but physical power is not as important to humans as social power. A significant contributor to social power is status or rank, in part because status facilitates protective social alliances: you may be small, but three small men can still defeat one large one. Status, in effect, does for social threat what physical size does for physical threat. Flexing your social muscles makes you less vulnerable to exploitation by others, and putting your high status front and center in a potential exploiter's mind might make them think twice about victimizing you. The mob boss, held at gunpoint in a dark alley, doesn't get weepy and beg for his life; he uses his status to put the gunman on the back foot: "Do you *know* who I am?"

And if you aren't socially powerful, you can still try to fake it. Under pressure, we often subtly exaggerate our status and perhaps occasionally lie about it. Grandiose delusions are the broken Suspicion System's disordered attempts to project social power and high status, with the aim of repelling (misperceived) social threats. The delusional person who asserts that he is Tony Blair's cousin, or is a famous DJ, or can cure cancer is attempting to raise his status in the mind of an imagined exploiter. Grandiosity is thus a symptom of a Suspicion System on overdrive, a caricature of the normal adaptive strategies we employ every day.

One of the apparent paradoxes of delusional thinking is that many sufferers have persecutory and grandiose delusions simultaneously. Why would a person who believes himself to be supremely powerful and important also feel vulnerable to the smallest, most inconsequential of conspiracies? One virtue of our hypothesis is that it predicts that paranoia and grandiosity *should* often coexist because they are functionally connected: paranoia is a broken form of threat detection, and grandiosity is a broken threat response.

In our view, *erotomania*—the belief that another person, such as a movie star, is in love with you—turns out to be a variant of grandiosity (as it does in Edward Hagen's theory of delusion). The erotomanic patient's imagined lover typically has a much higher social rank than she does. Among early descriptions of erotomania was that of a woman of fifty-three who believed that George V, Edward VII, and an American general were in love with her. Other sufferers have believed themselves loved by priests, doctors, veterinary surgeons, university lecturers, and (in at least one case) Paul McCartney. Erotomania was once called "old maid's insanity" because it tended to afflict unmarried women of "considerable age." This earlier term reflects the status of women in more traditional societies. In 1912, when the phrase was coined, the only way for most women to increase their social status was through marriage. Erotomania is therefore a form of grandiosity in which an assertion of status is made in a way that is culturally appropriate to a particular historical period. These days, people with erotomanic delusions, whether women or men, might be more likely to target celebrities to enhance their status.

The case of erotomania underscores the fact that a complete theory of delusion must account for data concerning sex differences among sufferers. An evolutionary perspective on some aspects of social cognition suggests that men and women ought to be different; jealousy is the paradigmatic case. The standard evolutionary account of jealousy takes offspring to be the crucial issue. Since a man can never be sure that his offspring are really his, male jealousy is directed at preventing another man from impregnating his partner. In contrast, a woman has no uncertainty about whether her children are her own. Her concern, rather, is with ensuring that someone is around to help look after them after they are born. If this is right, then male jealousy ought to be directed at sexual encounters, and the female variety at emotional involvement. And indeed there is some evidence for this. In heterosexual relationships, men experience more intense jealousy when imagining their partner having sex with someone else, but women feel it more keenly when they imagine their partner falling in love with another woman. If pathological jealousy comes about as the result of a broken Suspicion System, then, as Lucas Schipper, Judith Easton, and Todd Shackelford suggest, we might expect the same gendered differences in delusional jealousy as in normal jealousy. At the moment, unfortunately, there is no systematic research directed at sex differences in delusion.

The eight delusional forms just examined constitute a natural grouping, and constitute the framework for understanding the Truman Show delusion. But there are four other categories of delusion—delusions of guilt, somatic delusions, nihilistic delusions, and misidentification delusions—and we ought to say a word about them.

Delusions of guilt are often a symptom of psychotic depression and, along with *somatic delusions* and *nihilistic delusions*, are likely to be subtle strategies of defense against social threat. They are like grandiosity in purpose, but inverted in method. Whereas grandiosity attempts to raise one's status relative to a persecutor, guilt, hypochondria, and nihilism—in the extreme, a belief in one's own nonexistence—are strategic attempts to lower one's status for the purpose of self-preservation. They are, we suspect, forms of submission designed to prevent aggression, a common response observed in other animals. In effect, someone who says that he is guilty, sick, or dead is attempting to communicate that he is so pathetic as to be unworthy of an exploiter's time. Being sick also carries the subtle threat of contagion that might motivate a dangerous opponent to pick on less complicated victims.

In particular, as an anxiety about illness, the somatic delusion known as *delusional parasitosis* (the belief that one's skin is infested with parasites) may at first appear to have nothing to do with other people, but in the context of the self-deprecating strategy just discussed, it becomes deeply social because infection is one of the gravest risks of social living. Parasites are a significant problem for all primates, and not one that lies exclusively in the ancient evolutionary past—as a quick search on WebMD will show. In human evolution, skin infections would have been among the first threats of social life.

Misidentification delusions involve false beliefs about the people around you—for example, the belief that a loved one is an impostor—and co-occurs most commonly with dementia. Misidentification is probably associated with breakdowns in parts of the Suspicion System that are *prerequisites* to social threat detection. In order to keep track over time of dangers in the social world, one needs a mental map of that world: representations of who *you* are (your mind, your body, your friends and relatives; the things that matter to you) and representations of who *everyone else* is (including who might be dangerous). Various brain areas are known to perform the functions of self- and other-representation—the "temporal-parietal junction," or TPJ, especially in the right hemisphere, is the most important of these—and malfunctions in these areas very likely underlie misidentification delusions.

SIMONE: THE POPE

Simone was brought to Bellevue by police after she was found showering people with bottled water at the Port Authority in Manhattan. She claimed that she was casting demons out of the passersby with holy water. I believe it was Evian.

Simone was a twenty-four-year-old African American medical student in Florida who had just arrived in New York on a Greyhound bus. God had told her to go to Ground Zero, she said, to raise the dead of 9/11. On the bus ride north she recognized that many of her fellow passengers were possessed by demons who would try to keep her from her mission, so she protected herself by reading scripture continuously. But when she disembarked in New York, she became overwhelmed by the number of demons around her, and her fear grew. She walked past a television in the terminal showing President George W. Bush and the First Lady. Simone saw the number 666 in their faces and rushed to a shop where she bought two bottles of water and blessed them, thereby making them holy. The wet exorcisms of passersby (and intervention by police) followed soon after.

Simone had been an honors student at an Ivy League university prior to entering medical school in Florida. Her family reported that she was diagnosed with bipolar disorder during her junior year of college. At that time, studying for her medical entrance exams and sleeping little, she had been hospitalized after interrupting a Mass led by Cardinal O'Malley. She had stood up during the service and protested that Pope Benedict was a false prophet and that God had told her that *she* was to be named Pope (Simone was Southern Baptist). When asked about the incident, Simone stated that she was led astray by the Devil, who spoke to her at the time posing as God. A medical student at Bellevue unwisely inquired if it were possible that the voice of God she had been hearing recently was once again that of the Devil. Simone lost her temper and threw a cup of juice at the student and cursed him. No exorcism or baptism was intended.

Apart from this last incident, Simone was calm in the hospital, despite her belief that many of the staff and other patients were either inhabited by demons or were Devil worshipers. She continued to protect herself by reciting biblical passages, sometimes aloud, more often under her breath. She was particularly concerned about some of the female staff, whom she said were lesbians and were draining her spirit. She said she was in spiritual warfare with homosexuals because she was of Christ while they were of the Antichrist. At first, Simone demanded to be transferred to either Beth Israel or Mount Sinai, as they were hospitals consecrated by God, but shortly thereafter she asked to be released altogether, not only to complete her mission at Ground Zero but because she was about to be beatified and couldn't miss the ceremony.

After her bipolar diagnosis in college, Simone had taken and responded well to lithium. When I met her in Bellevue, she had been stable for almost three years. It seems that once she had finished her class work at medical school and had begun her clinical rotations in the hospital, she had become increasingly frustrated with the fine tremor often associated with lithium, which made it difficult for her to draw blood and tie sutures.

But the fact that she had responded well to lithium in the past trumped the concern regarding the tremor, and it was prescribed to her again, along with antipsychotic and anti-anxiety medication. She took the medication willingly, saying that no chemical of this world could harm her, and that we could slash her and her flesh would heal by the grace of God. Thankfully, she did not feel the need to demonstrate this miracle.

Simone responded quickly to the medication. After sleeping fourteen hours, she awoke and admitted that she had gone without sleep for close to five days. Over the following week, she heard God's voice with decreasing frequency and intensity. While this felt to Simone like a loss at first, she soon acknowledged the great fear that came with communicating directly with God. Her concern about gay people also diminished. She recounted that her younger brother, whom she considered her best friend, had recently come out to their parents, and while they appeared to have taken the news in stride, the possibility that they might reject him had been a great concern to Simone.

Before she returned to Florida and medical school, I offered Simone a medication to replace the lithium, as the disruptive tremor had indeed returned. She thanked me but said that she would make do. It was more important that she stay well. Besides, she remarked, she wouldn't be drawing much blood or tying many sutures once she became a psychiatrist.—JG

UNDERSTANDING DELUSIONS

In our review of the theories of delusion, we belabored the idea that many do not explain why delusions, as a group, have the content they do. In our view, delusional ideas originate in the Suspicion System, and they are logically related in the same way that visual problems or sleep abnormalities are—as a family of dysfunctions of a unitary mental system.

We also noted earlier that a theory of delusion must answer two central questions: (1) *How do delusional thoughts come about?* and (2) *Why do they persist?* Our answer to the first question should now be clear: delusions are the ideas that pop into your head when your Suspicion System is disordered. This view, however, raises a question about delusions, because while some involve "normal" thoughts (my wife is cheating on me; my coworkers are out to undermine me; I'm ill), many others are simply bizarre (I can fly; President Obama can read my thoughts; I'm dead). The question is where these bizarre ideas come from.

One answer, of course, is that if delusions originate in a disordered Suspicion System, then thought distortions are likely to be one of the manifestations of that disorder. There is also a second (not incompatible) possibility that draws on a dual process approach to delusion. The Suspicion System, as we've said, is an instance of System 1 cognition and has the modular property of being informationally encapsulated. Parallel to the Suspicion System, human beings have a form of System 2 thinking about social threat, a system that is slow, has to be initiated consciously, and takes mental effort to operate. We'll call this the Reflective System. We've suggested that the amygdala constitutes one of the central components of the Suspicion System; the Reflective System is likely to be dependent in part on the prefrontal cortex. This may explain why brain imaging studies of delusion have identified both of these structures as regions of interest (see Figure 8 in chapter 2). The Suspicion System produces behavior quickly and under conditions of uncertainty. The Reflective System aims to evaluate evidence in greater detail, when conditions permit, and decide whether the Suspicion System got it right. The Reflective System about social threat is, very likely, a combination of many of the conceptual and reasoning capacities that we can apply to *any* thought (though it doesn't include all of those capacities). However, there has to be communication between the Suspicion System and the Reflective System, if for no other reason than that the Suspicion System's alarm is likely to be what signals the Reflective System to initiate its own investigation into the possible presence of a social threat.

Delusions arise from a disordered Suspicion System *together with* a breakdown in communication between the two systems. (The Reflective System itself cannot be disordered, or that fact would show up all over the patient's thought and not just as delusions.) Delusional thoughts and their linguistic expression are thus cognitively isolated and not integrated with other thinking. "Someone is inserting thoughts into your mind," "You caused the earthquake in Haiti," or "Your husband is a duplicate" is the raw voice of a broken Suspicion System unmodulated by information available elsewhere in the mind. Ironically, to the extent that a split between the Suspicion System and System 2 thought is at the root of delusions, "schizophrenia" is not as much of a misnomer as one might think.

This brings us to the second question: Why do delusions persist? Seeing Cassio with Desdemona's handkerchief, Othello jumps to the conclusion that Desdemona is being unfaithful. That's a belief produced by the Suspicion System. But careful evaluation of the situation by the Reflective System would have led Othello to reject this belief. There can't be any *good* evidence of Desdemona's infidelity because she hasn't been unfaithful, and what evidence there is—Iago's innuendo, Cassio's possession of the handkerchief—easily lends itself to other explanations. Any husband in his right mind would think about things more carefully before believing that his wife was cheating on him and then strangling her to death. But Othello isn't in his right mind; that's exactly the point. Jealousy has overwhelmed his ability to make rational, System 2 discriminations. Under ordinary conditions, Othello's Reflective System thought about infidelity would "turn off" his Suspicion System, just as System 2 arithmetic corrects the mistaken output of System 1 arithmetic. For various reasons of emotional distraction and false leads, Othello's Reflective System is doing a bad job, and the output of the Suspicion System remains active.

Now consider our patient Calvin. Calvin's Suspicion System is broken; it produces the thought that his wife is cheating on him despite an almost complete lack of evidence to that effect (to say nothing of her status as a paraplegic). In someone whose mind is functioning normally, the Reflective System would shut off the Suspicion System, inhibiting the jealous thought; but if, as we've just suggested, the Suspicion System is disconnected from the Reflective System, it *can't* shut it off. And because the Suspicion System is modular, it is not built to receive messages from other parts of the mind that could modulate its internal state of alarm. The result is that the Suspicion System is left blind, sounding the alarm in the form of an undispellable thought. The thought thus continues to pop into Calvin's mind, and the delusion persists.

Even though the Suspicion System is functionally disconnected from the Reflective System, it must still have some sort of *output* access to thought beyond it, otherwise it could not enter consciousness or influence behavior. When Calvin suspects Bertha of being unfaithful, his Reflective System is engaged and begins to carry out its normal investigation into whether this threat is true or not. The question arises, therefore, why Calvin doesn't believe *both* that his wife is cheating on him and that she isn't. In general, why don't people with psychosis hold the delusional idea (a product of the Suspicion System) *and* a competing idea that the delusion is wrong (a product of the Reflective System)?

In fact, many delusional people *do* maintain both of these ideas simultaneously. People in the prodromal phase of schizophrenia (the period during which the disorder is developing) may have delusional thoughts that they recognize are very implausible. Recall that our first Truman patient, Albert, was willing to consider the possibility he was ill if he discovered that the World Trade Center had really been destroyed. Many patients with delusions retain "insight" into the strangeness of what they believe, at least for a while. The neuropsychologists Peter Halligan and John Marshall describe a patient, "Jim," who suffered from visual hallucinations of death and destruction after getting into an accident. He then began to believe that he could predict the future. When asked what he would have thought had he been told before his accident that *his doctor* could predict the future, Jim replied: "I would think it was a load of nonsense! . . . impossible to be done." Still, people who go on to develop schizophrenia and other forms of psychosis typically lose this insight in the early stages of their disorder and come to believe their delusions wholeheartedly. Why?

We suspect that as time passes, and the conflict between the Suspicion System and the Reflective System grows, the Suspicion System wins out. The Suspicion System is calibrated to err on the side of seeing threats that may not, in hindsight, have been there, so it is likely that over time, the output of the Suspicion System will take precedence on the grounds of prudence. However it happens, Reflective System doubts subside, and the world comes to look unambiguously as the delusion represents it to be.

Once this system conflict has been resolved, the Reflective System begins to play a new role: instead of examining the evidence for the threat, it takes the threat as fact and starts integrating it into a "coherent" view of the world. Human thought is always seeking out patterns and coherence, trying to make sense of the world. When a delusion is taken as true, it becomes the foundation for a new way of seeing the world. It is now a given that your wife is cheating on you or that you have become the target of a conspiracy. Faced with these "facts," a lot of questions arise—*Why is she cheating? With whom? Who's plotting against me and why?*—and the Reflective System goes to work, actively filling in all the details and missing links. The delusion has to be elaborated to answer the questions that arise, and elaboration can take any form that one can think up. Having read about the NSA for days on end, someone in the prodromal phase of psychosis might naturally latch on to this idea as a way of making sense of their delusional thought. If the NSA is at the heart of a conspiracy, then the feeling one has of being persecuted *makes sense*. There is something right, therefore, about Maher's idea that delusions involve normal reasoning about abnormal states.

Of course, some delusions are so strange that "making sense" can only be relative. If you come to believe that your wife is a duplicate, then there is only so much coherence in worldview that can be achieved. If you're living in the 1960s, you can hypothesize that she's a robot, and, in the 1990s, that she's a clone, but the distortion in the frame of reference brought about by the delusion makes true coherence impossible.

In chapter 2 we made the case that underneath the indefinitely large number of delusional contents lie only a handful of forms. It will now be clear that the form-content distinction also partially maps where the Suspicion System separates from the Reflective System. The Suspicion System is an ancient form of cognition, stable across human history and culture, and it continues to malfunction in the same ways now that it always has. In contrast, the elaboration of delusional ideas—making sense of the threat—falls to the Reflective System, which uses anything that seems relevant. The cultural sensitivity of delusion, therefore, is due to the openness of the Reflective System to the outside world.

It's worth noting, finally, that because the Suspicion System is designed to err on the side of caution, delusion-like thoughts can occur in healthy people in whom the Suspicion System is functioning normally. The husband who periodically becomes irrationally jealous or the business executive who sees plotting competitors everywhere are experiencing quasi-delusional thoughts without a mental disorder. What distinguishes these nonpersistent or occasionally persistent thoughts from true delusions is that they remain susceptible to influence by the Reflective System. It must be said, though, that the "normal" individual with a deeply paranoid worldview and the truly paranoid person are not always easy to distinguish. As in all areas of medical and social judgment, there are borderline cases where the difference between "normal" and "ill" is fundamentally arbitrary.

VIGILANCE

The function of the Suspicion System has implications for how we think about stress and vulnerability in psychosis. What exactly is it about the social determinants of psychosis—childhood adversity, immigration, city living—that make them stressful?

The most important hypothesis is that of Selten and Cantor-Graae, according to which it is social defeat, or subordination, that underlies these determinants of psychosis. Selten and Cantor-Graae's hypothesis is plausible in the cases of childhood adversity and immigration. Childhood abuse is a form of subordination, among other things, so social defeat is an apt characterization of it. Immigrants and children of immigrants suffer outright discrimination and the "daily hassles" that come with being treated as second-class citizens. Social defeat is very likely a part of the fabric of their lives as well. Where the limitations of the social defeat hypothesis emerge is around the question of psychosis and city living. In small towns, where everyone knows everyone else, humiliation may very well be a relatively uncommon occurrence. Selten and Cantor-Graae's hypothesis can therefore account for the difference between the prevalence of psychosis in rural and urban areas. However, the risk of psychosis goes up with population size or density in a nearly linear manner. If social defeat accounts for the toxicity of urban life, then it has to be more common in a big city like New York than in a smaller one like Montreal. Is that plausible?

Meet Cathy. She has lived in New York all her life, and, being a bit of a hothead, regularly gets into arguments with strangers. But since she tends to get tongue-tied when angry, the altercations always leave her feeling humiliated. Cathy's cousin, Natalie, has lived in Montreal all her life. She's also easily angered, and no more articulate, so she too has regular experiences of feeling humiliated by strangers. The fact that New York is three or four times more populous than Montreal, however, isn't going to increase the number or intensity of Cathy's experiences compared to Natalie's. Their humiliations depend on the people they *actually* encounter, not on the number of people who live in their geographical vicinity. There are surely enough strangers in Montreal to provide as many humiliating encounters for Natalie as Cathy gets in New York. Once a city is big *enough,* experiences of social defeat won't proliferate, but psychosis will. Social defeat doesn't seem to be the right way, therefore, to characterize whatever it is about urban environments that are toxic.

However, what large cities have in common with childhood abuse, and the experience of being an immigrant, is fear. We've argued that the price of social life is eternal vigilance, watchfulness against potential dangers; but being vigilant is inherently stressful. We suspect that the social determinants of psychosis bring about an internal state of heightened vigilance, and this, rather than social defeat, is what enhances vulnerability to psychosis. Being victimized or subordinated produces a *fear* of future repetitions, and although large cities are not necessarily more dangerous than small ones, they may *feel* that way. When people feel this way about the environment they live in, they become more vigilant. A 2005 study by Georg Schomerus and his colleagues provides some evidence for this claim. They set out to investigate whether people with schizophrenia are more likely to be victims of urban crime and, indirectly, whether victimization might be a cause of schizophrenia. The investigators interviewed people with schizophrenia from nine areas, both urban and rural, in the United Kingdom, Germany, and France, and while they found no difference in the rates of victimization among people with psychosis, participants' "subjective sense of safety" varied significantly. People living in cities felt more threatened than those living in rural areas, and the greater the sense of threat, the greater the severity of their delusions or hallucinations. Neighborhoods that are more ethnically homogeneous and more socially cohesive may protect people against schizophrenia precisely because they feel safe.

If psychosis is affected by vigilance to the possibility of social threat, why isn't psychosis more common in *dangerous* places rather than in *populous* ones? Recall Enquist and Leimar's idea that as the geographic area one lives in gets larger, the risk of free-riding goes up. This is because larger territories increase the possibility of encountering strangers whose dispositions are unknown. The size of cities may be significant because cities are filled with strangers, and the Suspicion System focuses on their possible malign *intentions* rather than on absolute levels of danger. Suppose that the cognitive limit of human social group size is around 150. There is some evidence that group size is constrained in part by the limits of ToM, so let's suppose that ToM can deal with the optimal group size of 150 but no more. Someone who lives in a small town, therefore, has a capacity to keep track in an ongoing way of the mental states of everyone around. In a town of 1,500, however, one can keep track of the mental states of only 10 percent of the locals, and in a city of 1.5 million, only .01 percent. If the Suspicion System is affected by how many potentially dangerous others it *can't* track, it might indeed be more stressed by a bigger number. The larger the number of unknown others, the greater the vigilance required and the greater the stress.

Selten and Cantor-Graae's hypothesis has the virtue of being able to form the basis of an explanation of how the social determinants of psychosis can lead to illness. Social defeat in animals has demonstrable neurobiological effects (e.g., on dopamine) that may interact with psychosis. In contrast, our view holds that it is the stress of malicious intentions, whether coming from an abuser, a racist, or a stranger, that does the damage, and one might be skeptical that this kind of stress is pernicious enough to be pathogenic. That skepticism is natural, but it's mistaken. British civil servants on the low rungs of the hierarchy do not, presumably, feel regular or persistent severe stress due to their restricted autonomy at work. Nonetheless, the health inequalities evidence shows that a mild but prolonged stressful experience of the wrong sort is toxic enough to shorten your life. By comparison, the stress of threatening intentions is surely poisonous enough to raise the risk of psychosis.

The social determinants of psychosis, therefore, may be stressors that increase our need for vigilance and in the long run "overload" the Suspicion System. Childhood abuse and immigrant adversity render malign intentions more tangible, and urban living multiplies them. As the amperage being sent through the Suspicion System increases, it overheats; and when social life puts too much current across these already heated circuits, delusions are kindled.

WHEN LIFE IMITATES ART

The Truman Show is highly entertaining and frighteningly prescient. Made over fifteen years ago, it predates YouTube, the 4,000 CCTV security cameras in Lower Manhattan—and the more than 4.9 million CCTV cameras in Britain, one for every 14 residents. Films may not fuel mental illness. However, technology that leaves us feeling more interconnected yet less connected to others—that offers more information but less privacy—just might.

Technology is changing more quickly now than in the past. During the Cold War, psychotic people often invoked the KGB in their delusions, but the Cold War was a pretty stable backdrop for more than forty years. When *The Truman Show* was released, many people didn't yet use cell phones. Today there are more than five billion cell phone subscriptions worldwide. Who needs microchips implanted in molars when we cell phone users are voluntarily tagging ourselves with tracking devices? The German politician Malte Spitz discovered that Deutsche Telekom had traced his location more than 35,000 times during a six-month span between 2009 and 2010. And in 2011, iPhone, iPad, and Android phone users discovered that their smart devices were recording and storing information as to their whereabouts. One of my patients—and not someone who is psychotic—recently sat down in my office and took the battery out of his phone to be sure he couldn't be tracked. A New York City subway sign chirpily announces, "What's next? Watching out for you. To improve safety, we're installing surveillance cameras on 1,150 more buses. Smile." What's the difference between watching out for you and watching you? Not everyone is smiling.

Before his suicide in 1961, Ernest Hemingway complained to those close to him that the FBI was bugging his phone and reading his mail. Hemingway had a mood disorder, likely bipolar in nature, was certainly alcoholic, and may well have been psychotic later in life. Yet, decades after his death, the FBI admitted to having surveilled Hemingway since the 1940s on the orders of J. Edgar Hoover. The line between paranoid and prudent has only gotten blurrier since Papa's time. In the spring of 2013, a patient of mine with bipolar disorder who had been mildly paranoid during previous manic episodes told me that the "National Intelligence Agency" and Microsoft were tapping his phone and hacking into his computer. He was hospitalized. One month later, Edward Snowden blew the whistle on PRISM, the National Security Agency's domestic spying program, which involved Microsoft, Google, Facebook, Yahoo, Apple, Verizon, and other communications giants. My patient definitely needed to be hospitalized, as he was suffering from other disabling psychiatric symptoms (he had gone without sleep for four days, thought he might be killed, and later believed that Microsoft employees had infiltrated the psychiatric unit). Still, it gives you pause. What do you tell a paranoid patient when a persecutory delusion happens to be true?

As we wrote subsequent drafts of this book, it felt as though the goalposts kept getting moved. Today's delusion is tomorrow's headline. By the time this book is published, the device you are reading it on may be reading you.

What impact did Snowden's information have on those with mental illness? *The Daily Show*'s first segment after the Snowden story broke was "Good news! You're not paranoid." Of course, those with persecutory beliefs are not reassured when the world confirms them. The director of the psychiatric emergency room at Bellevue at the time told me that at least one paranoid patient had incorporated PRISM into his delusional system shortly after the story broke. This isn't surprising—we expect people to integrate current events into their delusional ideas—but for those suffering from paranoia, it was validation of something long feared. And what about for the rest of us? At what point will we begin to hesitate when we hit "send" on an email, knowing that 1.4 million Americans hold top-secret clearance and can read everything we type?

More important still are the people who might already have a greater inclination toward paranoia and are teetering on the edge of full-fledged psychosis. Another Bellevue colleague told me about a middle-aged woman who had been treated for depression as an outpatient during the previous six months but had never been psychotic. Not twenty-four hours after the NSA story had come to light, she arrived in the ER suspicious that AT&T was monitoring her. Her concern was justified, but her agitated response crossed the line into psychosis and she was hospitalized. Some of the data the NSA collects might be meta, but the fear engendered is not.

Could the accelerating change of technology so blur our social boundaries—private and public, hidden and exposed, opaque and transparent— that it might overwhelm those at risk for psychosis? And so we are left with the question: Can our culture be making us crazy?—JG

NOWHERE TO HIDE

We come, at last, to the Truman Show delusion. At the turn of the nineteenth century, delusional fears of control focused on an influencing machine that produced waves of controlling animal magnetism; in 1919 and 1958 these fears shifted to mechanical men and robots; in the twenty-first century, the influencing machine consists of lasers, computer viruses, and microphones. Each technological and political change brings a new twist to the delusion. Twenty-first-century technology has given us a means of control that makes old-fashioned methods obsolete. "Knowledge works as a tool of power," Nietzsche said, and knowledge provides the means for a new form of control. Although the Truman Show delusion first appeared to be a hybrid of persecution, grandiosity, and delusions of reference, it now seems to us to be the new face of the influencing machine. The Truman Show delusion expresses the fear that one is being controlled not by force, but by what people know. The Truman Show delusion is a delusion of control in the age of surveillance.

The prehistory of surveillance begins in the lifetime of James Tilly Matthews. About ten years before Matthews was committed to Bethlem, the great utilitarian philosopher Jeremy Bentham (known for his view that "it is the greatest happiness of the greatest number that is the measure of right and wrong") was developing his own machine of control. In the service of the public good, Bentham designed a prison that he called the Panopticon, whose purpose was to control the inmates not with magnetism but by means of architectural design. The prison was to be circular in shape, with the "inspector's lodge" at the center and the cells on the building's circumference, each with an internal window. The windows of the lodge were to have blinds so the prisoners could not see in; but behind the blinds, all the inmates could be viewed in their cells by the "all-seeing" inspector—hence the term "Panopticon."

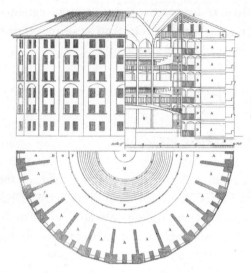

Figure 22: The Panopticon, Willey Reveley, 1843.

The goal of the design was explicitly to exert influence; Bentham describes it as a "new mode of obtaining power of mind over mind, in a quantity hitherto without example." Knowing they *could* be seen but never when they actually *were* being watched, the prisoners would have to keep to the rules all of the time to avoid punishment. The Panopticon would thus allow for the "*apparent omnipresence* of the inspector . . . combined with the extreme facility of his *real presence*." Wherever control was needed, Bentham suggested, the Panopticon could serve the purpose; it could function as a factory, asylum, hospital, or school as easily as a prison.

Bentham's prison was never built (a handful of "radial" prisons designed by others were), but the idea of the Panopticon occupies a central place in the history of ideas according to some thinkers because it demonstrates a uniquely modern conception of power as surveillance. The chief theorist of "panopticist" power is the French philosopher Michel Foucault:

> He [the prisoner] is seen, but he does not see . . . And this invisibility is a guarantee of order . . . [T]he major effect of the Panopticon: to induce in the inmate a state of conscious and permanent visibility that assures the automatic functioning of power.

Foucault takes panopticism to be a way for the state to create docile or "disciplined" citizens in a manner that is "lighter, more rapid, more effective"; it is "a design of subtle coercion for a society to come"—the society based on capitalism. As a method of social regulation, Bentham's concept has proven visionary: surveillance is undoubtedly more efficient and less risky than force. Knowledge is a tool of power.

As a bit of historical analysis (and especially as an interpretation of Bentham), Foucault's theory of the Panopticon is controversial. But if it could once have been doubted that surveillance is a mark of the modern, that is surely no longer the case. Surveillance is becoming pervasive, and new technology has freed panopticism from architectural constraint. The existence of cell phone tracking, internet eavesdropping, genetic information, biometrics, wiretapping, surveillance drones, social network analysis, ID chips, data fusion, cryptography, and other methods we have developed to watch one another now means that we can keep tabs on people incomparably more efficiently than the inspector of the Panopticon ever could. (Uncertainty remains: we were told by a friend in the UK that many Londoners doubt that the Powers That Be are sufficiently competent to keep all the CCTVs in London functioning all the time. But in Panopticist fashion, they don't have to; if they work occasionally, that's enough.) Control of the nineteenth-century inmate depends on Bentham's architectural arrangement. The new surveillance technologies need no specially structured space.

The film *The Truman Show* presents us with something quite like a Panopticon of the twenty-first century. Because seeing and hearing are extended by cameras and microphones, Truman's world is larger than the Panopticon but no more private. The film presaged the loss of privacy accompanying the new technologies of surveillance, and the ways in which one can be exploited when privacy is gone. Three years after the film first appeared, and forty-five days after the 9/11 attacks, the PATRIOT Act was signed into law. According to the political theorist Priscilla Regan, the "Act amends virtually every information privacy statute to facilitate access, increase data collection, and reduce the due process and privacy protections for record subjects." In the light of the new political realities of the twenty-first century, abstract worries about the invasion of privacy took on a menacing new life, and it is probably no accident that the first Truman Show patients appeared not long after 9/11, when the West's collective sense of threat was at an all-time high, and the American government directed that surveillance be increased dramatically.

Panopticism has become even lighter. As we write, the world community has just discovered that the conspiracy theorist's fevered midnight fear—that the government is tapping his telephone and reading his email—turns out to be not only true, but American government policy. We are now living in the Panopticon as surely as the sad inmates of Bentham's imagination.

The Truman Show delusion is a delusion of control, but with an exceptionally light touch: the controller doesn't have to move your body or insert thoughts into your mind. With adequate knowledge, control at a distance is possible and considerably more effective than animal magnetism or divine rays. It is thus a "mediated" form of control: by knowing enough about someone, you can get them to act in your interests, as Iago does with Othello. In the Truman Show delusion, knowledge is, quite literally, power.

But why, one might ask, should increasing surveillance be stressful? It is a familiar refrain that the only people who have something to fear from surveillance are those who have something to hide. If our experience is anything to go by, that argument cuts no ice with most people. Most of us who have nothing to hide still prefer not to be open books. Mistakes can happen, enemies don't always play by the rules, and anything known about our activities, legal or illegal, can potentially be used against us. Privacy is a prudent form of personal hygiene, like washing your hands, locking your door, or using a condom. The need for privacy runs deep, and the loss of privacy is a serious threat.

There is a second theme that runs through the delusion. In the film, Truman is seen by billions around the world by means of mass media; the "Truman Show" of the film is, after all, a television show. The sociologist Thomas Mathiesen has argued that Foucault's panopticism is only half the story of contemporary culture. At the very moment when the modern prison was being born, the mass media were also coming into existence, starting with mass-circulation newspapers and followed by film, radio, television, and the internet. The birth of the prison marks the beginning of panopticism, in which one person surveys many; the mass media, in contrast, initiate what Mathiesen calls "synopticism," in which the many observe the few. Surveillance technology combined with mass media thus express the fear not only of being watched, but of *being watched by an indefinitely large number of unknown others.*

Writing about James Tilly Matthews, the historian of medicine Roy Porter says that "[e]very age gets the lunatics it deserves." It is not surprising that in the current culture of reality television, celebrity-as-power, and overnight fame, many Truman Show patients speak of the "entertainment" they are providing to their viewers. Still, the element of performance built into the delusion doesn't change the fact that it is a delusion of control. The afflicted may believe their lives have sky-high Nielsen ratings, but the watching goes on without their consent.

Social media have dramatically increased the threat of mass-media panopticism. In the age of Twitter and Facebook, you need not be particularly powerful to control others by viewing them; you just have to be part of the crowd providing its opinion. Every teenager who has been humiliated online—sometimes enough to commit suicide, as in the recent sad cases of Rehtaeh Parsons and others—is a victim of the panopticism-synopticism one-two punch. Big Brother is not the only one watching you anymore; all of your Facebook friends—and friends of friends—are potential viewers.

The Truman Show delusion thus represents a confluence of two seismic cultural changes: the loss of privacy and the new porousness of social life. Many human beings are now exposed to a far greater number of unknown others than ever before—strangers who can know a lot about us with a few clicks of the mouse—and the Truman Show delusion is a pathological fear about what those strangers might do with the new knowledge they have.

LAWRENCE: ARTIFICIAL INTELLIGENCE

In the late stages of preparing this book for publication, I was contacted by a man, Lawrence. He is a lawyer who believes he is an "artificial intelligence" living in a computer program from the future. Lawrence has held this belief about himself for many years. He is aware that others around him consider this a delusion, but he nonetheless feels it is real. Like nondelusional people, this man (who remains anonymous) has navigated his way through family and career, all the while maintaining his delusional belief system. What follows is his first-person account of his life. I have spoken to Lawrence and his wife and confirmed various aspects of his story, and it is clear to me that his story is authentic. Lawrence has consented to his story being published, and hopes that doing so might help shed light on the workings of the human mind.—JG

I am presently under a firm belief that I am artificial intelligence in a computerized entertainment program. The program is satirical. It is also an epic, an extended miniseries. I am the primary actor, subject to real-time control by whoever is operating the program. The operators of the program are lampooning us. I suspect that the persons who are operating the program are humans, a few decades in the future. For several years, tongue-in-cheek, I have been referring to them as the "aliens." However, I no longer believe that they are aliens; they are probably us, in the future.

I now see the overall situation with this program as follows. We can already create fairly sophisticated artificial intelligences to interact with each other in computer games and simulations. In the future, as technology advances, we should ultimately be able to mimic the human brain in a computer program, complete with emotions and a large part or all of the accumulated intelligence and history of humankind. Assuming that futuristic beings still have an interest in entertainment, they should have the ability to create entertainment programs.

I am fascinated by the possibility that some or all of our history may have been created by the beings that are controlling me, and by the question of whether they inherited much of human history and began modifying it at some point in their computer simulation. (They are clearly modifying it now.)

My own experience leads me to believe that the aliens can control me in real time and allow me some amount of free will. I am constantly disturbed by the question of how much of my life is subject to my free will and how much is predestined by the aliens.

Perhaps their entertainment program is a commercial program designed such that a buyer may plug into it for a full life experience with a guaranteed positive outcome. I have also considered that perhaps I am a paid actor, an artificial intelligence with enhanced abilities and powers. I have been party to fuzzy communications from the aliens to the effect that I am an actor in a program that has "seasons," as do many of our television shows. However, I have been prone to many fantasies and delusions in trying to address what the aliens are up to, and I am at present skeptical of this prospect.

Computer games arguably have been a huge influence on my current state of belief, that there are different classes of artificial intelligence in the computer entertainment program I reside in. I am the lead AI character. My family members and close friends are of a somewhat lower AI class. The rest of the world is of a different, NPC (nonplayer character) class, entirely random. Computer games have also precipitated the fleeting notion, sometimes approaching a belief, that I am a character in a video game or computer game. Indeed, I have had flashes of insight that some kid with his console is tormenting me with his various pranks. I now believe that the aliens are teasing and tormenting me, but with an optimistic ultimate outcome in sight.

Our second child was born in 19■■. My wife and I now had two children in diapers and two stressful lawyer jobs. I was unable to cope. I had some kind of a break while reading a Babar book to my child. I complained bitterly about feeling like a robot, like someone else was controlling me and I was just going through the motions. I had visual disturbances, feeling like I was looking at everything through a thick pane of glass. I could not see and integrate a landscape; I only had tunnel vision. At home, in the house, I would go through periods of feeling like a ghost, floating around the house and observing my family in my daily activities. I had out-of-body experiences. I lacked empathy; I was disconnected from others.

I quit my partnership at the law firm and went solo. I took on an unusual case. I thought it was worth maybe $100,000 at the most. It was a bizarre, over-the-top experience, and the judge awarded my client $2.8 million. Looking back, I see this case as so improbable that I now believe it was scripted by the beings operating the computer entertainment program that I am stuck in. In fact, looking back, I see my whole life as so improbable that I now believe that it was scripted. I developed a theme about myself that there was another person inside me who was controlling me.

To the outside world, I appeared to be fully functional.

In 19■, fed up with private law practice and unduly stressed, I took a job with the federal government. When alone, I had periods of intense self-analysis and temporary psychiatric disorders. I fell into difficulties with my new boss and supervisor. During this period there were numerous peculiar incidents and improbable timing at work. I began to have serious thoughts, bordering on delusion, that the entire matter was somehow scripted through some sort of paranormal source. I became intrigued with the collectively amoral behavior of the entire agency. While on vacation in Costa Rica, I happened to be observing a lengthy trail of leaf-cutter ants at a tiny rural airport. I began ruminating about the hive behavior of ants and bees, and I found the behavior of certain personnel in my agency to be similar. I researched the issue and discovered "stigmergy." A sample article regarding stigmergy describes collective behavior in robotics and artificial intelligence, thus providing some preliminary support for my current theory of my status as artificial intelligence in a computer simulation.

Over the next several years, I had a number of very strange, seemingly paranormal experiences when I was alone. I ruminated, almost in fugue states, that there was a person inside me who was controlling me, that I was mechanical, robotic, operating on some kind of unspoken command. I was introspective, self-analytical, desperately trying to figure out what was going on. I had profound flashes of insight. I had thoughts associated with deep empathy towards family and friends. My robotic self, on the other hand, lacked empathy and was disconnected from others.

In 20■, I attempted to read some philosophy, hoping to discover some metaphysical basis for the strange feelings I had about being controlled by "aliens." I formed a plausible belief that our universe must have been "created" by some other being. Faced with the skepticism of others, I defended myself with the proposition that I was no different from the many persons who believe in "God," except that my belief is more rational. I was not argumentative or obsessive with this notion, I simply threw it out in conversation and dropped it. The reaction was not shock, but bemusement. My cover story is old age. I may be viewed simply as the stereotypical eccentric old man, sitting at his computer obsessively trying to research and find support for his various conspiracy theories.

My perspective on the aliens has advanced from the view that they are a delusion, to the concession that they are a rational possibility, to, finally, the firm belief that they are "real." I have started talking to them aloud on occasion, first almost as in a prayer, next in a mood of resignation, and finally as if in a mode of conversation. They do not speak back to me, but I often have a feeling of having received a communication or order of some kind.

The issues of cruelty and human suffering have troubled me. I have been able somehow to get by in life, and I am now very happy. On the other hand, I feel very badly for my poor youngest child, who continues to struggle with ██████. I am able to rationalize these issues by supposing that the aliens may not have given AI characters other than myself the ability to experience pain and suffering. They may be at a different level of artificial intelligence. Or perhaps the aliens' system simply mimics the common religious belief that God has created, and maintains, a level of human suffering.

For years, my children have seen me as eccentric and a bit crazy. A year or so ago I engaged my middle child in a conversation about the aliens. She said, "You are talking like a schizophrenic." I responded, "Well, you know, I have always been crazy." She responded that I was the sanest person in the family. My children are well aware of my beliefs and seem perfectly comfortable with them. All three are aware that I smoke some marijuana. So I assume that they attribute my beliefs to the fact that I am an eccentric who indulges in marijuana.

I am reclusive. However, my second wife is very sociable, and we have frequent visitors. I have shared my beliefs with a few of them. On occasion, I have raised the issue of my status as sort of a "Creationist," living in a computer program operated by unknown beings. Some react with polite interest but quickly change the subject. Others react as if they heard the doorbell ring and a couple of Jehovah's Witnesses carrying a Bible were standing in front of them.

One of our visitors was a practicing psychologist. I told him I had a "delusion" and explained it briefly. He was contemptuously dismissive, and he gave me a brief discourse about bizarre and nonbizarre delusions, closing with the comment that if sufficient other people share the same delusion, "you get a free pass."

I never press the issue, and I do not argue in support of myself, as I do not wish to appear to be obsessed. They know me to be an eccentric and they are accepting of me in that regard. I am otherwise perfectly rational.

6

BEYOND BELIEF

Thinking about modern technological culture has taken us some distance from a narrow concern about delusion. The role of culture in psychosis raises some broad and difficult issues related to mental illness, however, and we'll end by considering three: the role of social media, psychotherapy, and psychiatry's vision of itself.

IMAGINED CITIES

New technologies are threatening, but they are also liberating and replete with the possibility of new forms of community. This is not the first time technology has altered social life. The advent of printing saw books unite villages separated by great distances into what the anthropologist Benedict Anderson has called "imagined communities." The internet and other digital technologies seem to be doing much the same thing today, but to a degree that we're only just beginning to understand. What effect will they have on our social life and our mental health? The fact that someone prone to psychosis is put at risk by the size of her city raises a pressing question: *Is the internet a kind of city?* The answer is not obvious: "The main difficulty with the research [on cities and psychosis]," Jane Boydell and Kwame McKenzie write, "is that there has been surprisingly little work on the concept of a city."

As we argued in chapter 5, the relation of cities to psychosis lies in the fact that other people present threats that call for persistent vigilance. As the number of people who can know about us grows, the risks of manipulation and exploitation increase. Electronic communities may not be cities, but they are certainly *like* physical cities in the range of dangers they present. For example, the FBI's priorities in cyber crime include computer and network intrusions, identity theft, and fraud (various e-scams, peer-to-peer networks, and "phishing" for personal information in electronic communications). And this is to say nothing about cyberbullying, sexual predation, and cyberterrorism. One doesn't have to be remotely disposed to persecutory delusions to be scared as hell about the brave new electronic world that is forming around us. The social environment is larger today than it has ever been in human history, and we are exposed to a greater variety of malicious intentions and new methods for acting on them than ever before. A motto for mental health today could be "It's a good life, if you don't weaken."

Living in the global village has many attractions, but it might well be a stress for someone vulnerable to psychosis, and the stress could contribute to a psychotic episode. Would this hypothetical patient remain healthy in a world without dangerous technology? We can't be sure, but imagine a pair of identical twins who, for genetic reasons, are at high risk of lung cancer. The twins are adopted by different families, one in Shizuoka, Japan, and the other in Burlington, Vermont. The air pollution in Shizuoka leads to lung cancer in one, while the twin breathing the cleaner air of upstate Vermont is spared. Now imagine a second pair of adopted twins who, for genetic reasons, are at a high risk of schizophrenia. One twin is raised in a small mountain town in Switzerland, population 1,000, in which there are 865 personal computers and 1,072 cell phones; the other is raised in a similarly sized town in Niger, where there is one computer and about 70 cell phones. If social-media technologies create bigger communities, then the twin in Switzerland lives in an exponentially larger community than his twin in Niger, despite their physical proximity to the same number of people. Since urban living increases the risk of psychosis, the Swiss twin develops schizophrenia and the Nigerian twin does not.

At the moment, this scenario is no more than speculation. Our aim is not to defend this idea, but to make a case for its consideration. There is currently almost no research on the relationship between the internet and psychosis, but there are hints that we ought to take the connection seriously. Uri Nitzan and his colleagues, for example, report on three patients who, having had little social interaction on the internet and no prior psychiatric disorders, developed psychotic illnesses while engaged in "computer-mediated communication." Two of these individuals "felt that they had exposed themselves more than they intended, and were appalled that the information they had given about their private lives could now be freely accessed over the web." A second illustration is provided by a recent study by Vijay Mittal, Derek Dean, and Andrea Pelletier, who found a positive correlation between "psychotic-like experiences" (such as brief auditory hallucinations) and problematic internet usage. Although we cannot tell whether too much of the internet might cause the psychotic experiences or the other way around, the link between the two needs to be explored further. This is particularly urgent because there is evidence of a relation between "internet addiction" and brain abnormalities, and one such study has found abnormalities in brain regions implicated in schizophrenia. Research addressing these questions should, in our opinion, be a public health priority.

Not long ago, having "the talk" with your kids referred to safe sex; now it refers to the dangers inherent in one's digital footprint. Stories of the sometimes tragic effects of youthful indiscretion are becoming more common. The primary purpose of privacy is keeping information out of the hands of others who could use it to our disadvantage. The more we reveal of ourselves, whether deliberately or inadvertently, the more we risk exploitation by others. The advent of the internet, though only a moment in evolution, may turn out, therefore, to be a major event in human social life. With very large communities come greater anxieties about potential threats; in one sense, then, we may be living in the most threatening environment human beings have ever created.

BENJAMIN (PART 1): MISPERCEPTIONS

Benjamin is a well-mannered, well-groomed, exceptionally polite African Caribbean man in his late forties. He immigrated to the United Sates with his family when he was ten years old. He has never been married and has no children. Benjamin speaks in a stilted manner and tends to use grandiloquent language when simpler words will do. Initially, I experienced his circumlocution as a distancing mechanism, keeping me at bay so as not to reveal too much about himself, and I sometimes found myself mirroring his speech when we met.

Benjamin had been sent to me from the employee-assistance program at the large multinational corporation where he had worked for more than a decade. Colleagues had complained about his erratic behavior, and the EAP wanted him psychiatrically evaluated. Piecing his story together was a challenge, as he knew that people at his company thought he was ill, and he worried that my evaluation would be used against him. This was not an altogether unreasonable concern. Benjamin had not wanted to see me; he was required to. Having signed a consent form, he knew that I would be submitting my opinion to the EAP. Nonetheless, as Benjamin values honesty, instead of simply denying that certain events had transpired or disavowing the beliefs that ultimately brought him to me, Benjamin instead responded to my questions. His answers were vague and ambiguous at first, and he told me that he would rather drop the matter altogether. Over time, though, his story emerged.

Benjamin has a master's degree in finance. He prides himself on continual self-improvement, both physical and intellectual, and he frequently pursues higher education. Some years ago, he began to notice that a coworker, Robert, was overly interested in his affairs. Eventually, Benjamin came to believe that both Robert and a supervisor, Simon, were undertaking "subversive activities" in an attempt to disrupt his studies. He believed that if he got his doctoral degree, he would be promoted, and so the two men felt threatened by him. Benjamin mentioned clues and cues embedded in company intranet communications. He felt that Robert might be doing Simon's bidding, since one man couldn't be both at work and at his apartment simultaneously. The two coworkers conspired to sabotage his plans with "unfavorable noises" and "unpleasant activities." The plot included bugging Benjamin's apartment, but the real trouble was the noise made in Benjamin's environment. He believed that Robert and Simon enlisted his landlord to make noise, especially when he was studying. The noise problem became so bad that Benjamin had to move. But since Benjamin suspected that listening devices would be planted in his next apartment, too, he chose instead to live in a storage unit without heat for six months, including much of the winter.

Benjamin was initially reluctant to talk about what we came to call his "misperceptions," preferring to discuss my thoughts on Shakespeare or the

Bible. Having slept for four hours a night for years on end, he believed that the initial persecutory ideas he had were a product of sleep deprivation. He said that once he began sleeping six hours a night, his mind became clearer. But things weren't much better at his new residence.

After living in the storage facility, Benjamin moved to a new apartment. There, he didn't feel persecuted but rather chastened by his neighbors for his own racket. When I asked him about the commotion he was causing, Benjamin told me that he had been typing on his laptop computer. And who was he disturbing? His upstairs and downstairs neighbors, who heard his typing through the floor and ceiling. He knew this because whenever he typed, the neighbors would tap on their floor or ceiling, mimicking the sound of his typing, signaling Benjamin to keep it down. Another noise he made that bothered the neighbors was the rumbling of his stomach. They would communicate their displeasure when they heard these sounds by slamming the toilet seats in their bathrooms. The fact that people never spoke to him about their annoyance, but used the same signals, made Benjamin feel as though they had all read from the same rulebook and were working in unison, just like Robert and Simon.

Early on, Benjamin revealed that he was anxious about his inability to control his flatulence: Robert had made "allusions" to it, perhaps by turning on the air conditioner or by leaving a can of Lysol around. I was surprised to learn that not only did Benjamin not smell anything himself, but he did not even experience the passing of gas. He simply assumed that he was flatulent because of the signals Robert and others were sending—for example, someone mentioning gas masks. Nobody had ever said anything to Benjamin about flatulence. He felt that his colleagues were simply being polite by using signals rather than speaking to him about an embarrassing problem.

One afternoon just before a scheduled session, Benjamin called to cancel, saying he had an emergency. The following session he admitted that he wanted to spare me from his odor and that he was still feeling a bit "toxic." He had visited a perfume shop earlier in the day to find something that could mask his smell. He worried that his kidneys or liver might not be functioning. After another missed session, he conceded over the phone that he was having trouble with flatulence again. He believed that the problem had grown so severe that the foul stench was emanating from his pores.—JG

THE RETURN OF THE EXPRESSED

Because the social world plays such an important role in the development of psychosis, it's natural to wonder whether social interactions could also *treat* psychosis. In the wake of the failings of psychoanalysis, it was universally accepted that patients with psychotic disorders were beyond psychotherapy. In the second half of the century, however, supportive psychotherapy and cognitive behavioral therapy (CBT) began to show promise as treatments for a variety of psychiatric complaints, including psychosis.

Supportive psychotherapy aims to relieve patients' symptoms (particularly anxiety), increase their self-esteem, enhance their social skills, and improve their overall functioning. The latter is achieved in various ways, including enhancing patients' capacity to maintain authentic and healthy relationships and bolstering their defense mechanisms. The goal is to help patients move from the use of maladaptive defenses, like denial, to more adaptive ones like humor and sublimation—the transformation of unconscious impulses, often sexual or aggressive, into socially acceptable behavior. In fact, what is *supported* in supportive psychotherapy are defenses. If particular ones are helping the patient to cope, adjust, and improve, they are encouraged, not analyzed. If defenses are causing the patient difficulties, the task of the therapist is to work with him to "trade up" to more successful ones. Interpretation of unconscious material is similarly avoided in favor of a focus on "here-and-now" issues in the patient's life. And instead of encouraging the development of transference to be interpreted by the therapist, emphasis is placed on the "real relationship" between patient and doctor. Life outside of the consulting office is considered more important than life in it. The supportive psychotherapist takes an active role in the work, encouraging, educating, praising, and even making suggestions to the patient, rather than taking the neutral, "blank-screen" approach of the classic Freudian analyst.

Freud correctly predicted that, in time, "the large-scale application of our therapy will compel us to alloy the pure gold of analysis freely with the copper of direct suggestion." Not surprisingly, he concluded, "whatever form this psychotherapy for the people may take, whatever the elements out of which it is compounded, its most effective and most important ingredients will assuredly remain those borrowed from strict and untendentious psycho-analysis." In practice, all psychotherapies are alloys and compounds; even the strictest of analyses offers supportive measures at times; and even the most supportive of therapies uses some interpretation.

Until recently, CBT wasn't used much with psychosis because psychotic thought was considered incoherent, and it would make no sense to attempt to modulate thinking that made no sense. However, there is increasing evidence of the effectiveness of CBT in treating psychosis. Research shows that it can reduce the occurrence of hallucinations and delusions, as well as the negative symptoms of schizophrenia. In 2009, the United Kingdom's National Institute for Health and Care Excellence (NICE) updated its guidelines for the treatment of schizophrenia to make CBT a first-line therapy. NICE's American equivalent, the Schizophrenia Patient Outcomes Research Team (PORT; it's a mystery why it isn't SPORT), updated its recommendations in a similar fashion. The proven effectiveness of CBT, especially in concert with medication, shows that people who hear voices and have delusions can get better by talking to another person. CBT research has also shown that patients' thoughts about their illness play a role in recovery. The conclusion seems undeniable: if other people can damage your brain, they can also minister to it.

The therapeutic alliance—the doctor-patient relationship—remains a healing force on its own. A study of 143 people with schizophrenia found that those who developed a strong rapport with their therapists within the first six months were more likely to adhere to their medication regimen, required less medication, and had better clinical outcomes two years later than those who did not. They were also more likely to remain in therapy. The Study of Cognitive Re-alignment Therapy for Early Schizophrenia (SoCRATES) trial is another study that supports the benefits of psychotherapy. In this study, more than three hundred patients with a psychotic illness were given either medication alone or medication with psychotherapy. The success of the therapy was found to depend entirely on how the patients felt about their relationship with the clinician. Richard Bentall writes, "Good relationships, it seems, are a universal therapeutic good, and may yet turn out to be the single most important ingredient of effective psychiatric care."

We have been appropriately critical of the disappointing results of psychoanalytic treatment of psychosis. But psychiatry has come a long way since Freud's time and, indeed, since the profession's angry debates in the 1980s about how to square the good in earlier hypotheses with new, more accurate findings. It might even be worth revisiting the controversial idea that some people with psychosis might actually benefit from psychoanalysis. Elyn Saks is a high-achieving academic who also happens to have lived with psychosis for most of her life. She describes the benefits of psychoanalysis to her:

> [P]sychoanalysis has helped me, a person with psychosis, in many ways . . . helping me identify and deal with stress; helping me become more psychologically minded and strengthening my observing ego; helping me come to terms with the narcissistic injury of having a mental illness and needing medication and therapy; giving me a safe place to bring my chaotic thoughts; offering interpretations that provided insight; and giving me the support of a kind, caring, nonjudgmental person who accepted me not only for the good, but also for the bad and ugly.

BENJAMIN (PART 2): BUILDING TRUST

Early on, I repeatedly offered Benjamin medication, suggesting to him that it might help reduce his symptoms, but he always politely refused. He expressed concerns about antipsychotic medication, some of them not altogether unreasonable ("I do not want to alter my thinking capacity") and some less so ("I do not want to become a vegetable").

Though I did not prescribe Benjamin any meds, we continued to meet for weekly supportive psychotherapy. As his trust in me grew, I was able to use techniques borrowed from CBT for psychosis to challenge some of Benjamin's perceptual and thought distortions. When I suggested to him that he might be more sensitive to noises around him (people walking above, toilet seats being lowered) when he was studying and concentrating intensely, he responded, "I am very grateful that you have enlightened me, Doctor, with respect to my propensity toward incorrect attribution of noises."

As for his belief that he was producing a foul odor, I repeatedly and directly told him that, despite his sitting only a few feet away, I didn't smell anything. Benjamin's symptoms improved and eventually resolved, save for a few minor setbacks when he was under stress or deprived of sleep. Benjamin said that through therapy he had come to perceive things more accurately. He described his use of "empathy" to help him with his referential ideas. For example, when staying at a hotel on a trip, he became aware of the "inconsiderate activities of the occupant above," but then thought, "Perhaps I am not as considerate as I could be to my neighbors beneath me . . . It would be inappropriate of me to come to the conclusion that it is an intentional effort to disrupt my harmony." On another occasion, when he wondered if his typing might be an annoyance to the neighbors, because he heard sounds "that might be considered retaliatory," he thought again and decided that the neighbors were more likely just having a good time. Benjamin was gaining insight. Referring to the time we first met, he said, "Some screws were loose in my head."

Benjamin's symptoms improved most when he changed jobs and moved to quieter surroundings in the country. Even though he was no longer compelled by his company to see me, he chose to continue our work together, commuting several hours to our sessions. Benjamin found his new home to his "wholesome benefit," observing that "humans function better in their own space." Benjamin believed that in the countryside he could analyze his perceptions more clearly. He could "observe how I think under certain conditions and remember how I used to think: Because A + B happened, then C." Living in the city caused him to "perceive stimuli incorrectly—precisely why I moved away—too many correlations threw me off." And not all noises were equally disturbing to Benjamin. He enjoyed the sounds of children playing. At his new home, he had "no distorted thoughts." Benjamin improved further still after moving to an even more sparsely populated state, where he works part-time in a library. We have remained in contact.

In the first year of working with Benjamin, a picture emerged of a man who struggled with his place in the social world. He described having had friends when he was younger, but that they had grown apart over the past decade. Benjamin described his difficulty trusting people. He was ambivalent about becoming closer to others. "I have chosen to alienate myself," he said. However, sometimes within the same session, he would suggest that things were not quite so straightforward. At times, when feeling more optimistic, he wondered if—his symptoms now under control—he could become more extroverted. In time he did. Benjamin developed friendships with a small group of people and began a romantic relationship. He was socializing regularly. During one session, Benjamin described a situation which, to my ears, suggested that one of his new friends might be taking advantage of him. Benjamin reassured me. He could trust his friend.

During our time together Benjamin became less guarded, and he continues to value our relationship. He recently told me: "Our sessions are so important. Your counsel is essential for me, especially in the absence of medication. You share your insights. They become a part of me." He continued, "Some of the circumstances I faced in New York, I recognize that there are similar circumstances in this region, that if I didn't have you in my life, I would have adopted the thought processes I had in New York and they would have come to haunt me." In our sessions, Benjamin could learn to challenge his own beliefs, practice interacting with another person and, in coming to trust me, trust others a little more. We talked about our shared goal of Benjamin eventually not needing me to keep his thoughts in check, the time when he will become his own counsel.

We may not be that far away from reaching our objective. Recently, Benjamin had been jogging near a local shooting range that he didn't know about. He was sure that in the past, if he had heard shots in the distance as he now did, he would have immediately concluded that he was being shot at. Instead, he had the presence of mind to ask a passing jogger what was going on. When told about the shooting range, he continued his run, and stopped worrying.

Postscript: A basic assumption of this book is that delusions, like all thoughts produced by the mind, have meaning. Yet psychiatry today is not inclined to this view, has no interest as to why different brains choose different delusions, and is simply interested in eradicating the psychotic symptom. This is curious. Our patients take great interest in the content of their delusions—is there any reason to think they shouldn't? Most of us take our own thoughts seriously, and a basic premise of psychiatry is to think about our thoughts. When we listen closely to what our patients are saying, paying attention to psychotic and nonpsychotic thought with equal consideration, we foster the therapeutic alliance, and stronger alliances yield better therapeutic outcomes. The fact that delusions mean something to our patients is reason enough for them to mean something to us.—JG

THE ASPIRATIONS OF PSYCHIATRY

The social world is at the heart of our theory of delusions, and this puts us at odds with much of mainstream psychiatry. In the 1970s, psychiatry abandoned psychoanalysis; in search of a new theory, it found neuroscience. Of course, psychiatry had never really lost neuroscience. As our brief history of mental illness shows, long before psychiatric disorders were unconscious conflicts, they were diseases of the brain. But the advent of psychoanalysis cast a veil over the brain. For the analysts, it mostly didn't exist. Today the brain has returned to psychiatry with a vengeance, and it's now dogma among many psychiatrists that mental illness—at least severe mental illness—is nothing more than genetic and neural dysfunction. If psychiatric theory needs nothing more than biology to understand mental illness, then there's no place for ideas about the social world—or the theory of delusions we've presented.

There is, however, more than one "psychiatry." Psychiatry is a *practice*: it's the name for the activity of treating people with mental disorders. Psychiatry has a *theory*: a set of hypotheses about what mental illness is. And psychiatry has *aspirations*: a conception of itself as a mature discipline. How do these aspects of psychiatry differ when it comes to the brain?

Even a brief visit to a psychiatric hospital will confirm that there is much more to psychiatric practice than neurobiology. Severe mental disorders are treated with all manner of talk and art therapy, mindfulness training, physical activity, and so on. Social workers, clinical psychologists, and therapists of all stripes—none of whom can prescribe medication—are as much a part of the practice of psychiatry as psychiatrists. And even psychiatrists are as likely to talk to patients as to give them pills.

What about theory? Outside of psychoanalysis, psychiatry doesn't have an overarching theory, but the DSM provides a snapshot of what we currently take to be the core features of psychiatric disorder. A brief look at DSM-5 reveals that there is a lot to mental disorder beyond neuroscience and genetics. Apart from anything else, the cognitive, behavioral, and emotional aspects of psychiatric disorders are front and center, and socioeconomic and cultural issues that affect diagnosis are also emphasized. No one whose only acquaintance with psychiatry was familiarity with the DSM would think that psychiatry is interested only in the brain.

Aspirational psychiatry (as we might call it) is another matter altogether. The aspirations of psychiatry are the ideas that researchers and clinicians have about the shape they hope or expect psychiatry will take as it matures as a clinical science. Aspirational psychiatry is concerned with what psychiatry will look like in the future, about what will be contained in a "final" psychiatric textbook, so to speak. When we say that mainstream psychiatry believes that mental illness is nothing more than genetic and neural dysfunction, it is aspirational psychiatry that we have in mind. In chapter 1 we quoted Nancy Andreasen expressing optimism that the maps of the human genome and the human brain will give us the power to understand mental illness. And we quoted Thomas Insel and Remi Quirion's exhortation that mental disorders be understood and treated as brain disorders. If one were to ask a psychiatrist what she believes psychiatry will be in a few generations, the answer is quite likely to echo those sentiments: psychiatry will be an application of brain science.

Another source of evidence for the aspirations of psychiatry comes from the National Institute of Mental Health (NIMH), which plays a very big role in setting the agenda for psychiatric research. It currently has four strategic research objectives. The first of these articulates aspirational psychiatry well:

Promote Discovery in the Brain and Behavioral Sciences to Fuel Research on the Causes of Mental Disorders

1.1: Develop an integrative understanding of basic brain-behavior processes that provide the foundation for understanding mental disorders.

1.2: Identify the genetic and environmental factors associated with mental disorders.

1.3: Identify and integrate biological markers (biomarkers) and behavioral indicators associated with mental disorders.

1.4: Develop, for research purposes, new ways of classifying mental disorders based on dimensions of observable behavior and neurobiological measures.

Of course, the aspirations of the NIMH, however important, are not likely to reflect every psychiatrist's expectations about the future of psychiatry. Undoubtedly many clinicians and researchers neither hope for, nor believe in, the future hegemony of neuroscience. Aspirational psychiatry, in short, does not represent the aspirations of every psychiatrist. But there is a significant strand of psychiatric thought according to which the preferred or probable future of psychiatry is one in which we will come to understand and treat mental disorders as brain disorders.

There are certainly some good reasons to think that this goal will one day be within our grasp. The past fifty years in psychiatry have seen some spectacular advances in treating mental illness. The development of medication for severe mental disorders and electroconvulsive therapy (ECT) for severe depression have been nothing short of astonishing. Immeasurable suffering has been prevented, and a great many lives saved, as a result. Arguably, psychiatry is also the place where neuroscience has been most successful in the clinic. We can't yet restore sight to the blind; we don't have good treatments for Alzheimer's or Parkinson's; we can't even stop the ordinary mental decline that often accompanies aging. Psychiatry, in contrast, has already given us reason to believe in the possibility of cures.

Still, as we noted in the first chapter, psychiatry's most powerful clinical tools were discovered by accident, and it's still a mystery how they lead to improvements in mental disorder. Why, then, are so many people convinced that the future of psychiatry lies in neuroscience? In large part, we suspect, because mental disorders just are, in some sense, disorders of the brain. What else could they be? To paraphrase Griesinger, the only organ that can be diseased in mental illness is the brain, so psychiatry will one day have to be clinical neuroscience. That just seems like a fact of logic.

The belief that "psychiatry" will eventually become "clinical neuroscience" is part of a larger conception of science known as *reductionism*, according to which it is desirable for scientific theories to be articulated in more fundamental terms. Watson and Crick's discovery of the double helix structure of DNA, for example, made possible the reduction of Mendelian genetics. Once it was understood that genes were DNA molecules (qualified in certain ways we can ignore for simplicity), it became possible to explain the principles of genetics in fundamental molecular terms. If we could understand delusions and other psychotic symptoms in terms of genes and the brain, we'd be in a position to reduce the science of psychosis to biology with no remainder; ideas about the social world would be discarded. The self-evident fact that mental illness can only be the outcome of a disordered brain, therefore, seems to make reductionism inevitable: if there's nothing more to mental disorder than a disordered brain, then psychiatric theory—if we ever get to complete it—*must* be clinical neuroscience. It couldn't be anything else.

Reductionism is an appealing idealization. It represents the universe as God might see it—as a very large collection of simple entities governed by a few universal principles; as atoms in the void. If it's news to you, however, that real life tends to be messier than our idealizations, you are probably too young to drive. Even if the universe is simple—and nothing stops us assuming that it is—that still doesn't guarantee much of anything about how one moment in science is likely to develop. And, indeed, science as it actually is right now doesn't seem to fit very well with the reductionist ideal. Even in physics, where our understanding of the universe is deepest, science is messier than we'd like. For example, writing about the prospects of a single unifying theory in physics—a Theory of Everything (TOE) or a Grand Unifying Theory (GUT)—the philosopher of science Tim Maudlin claims that while unification is a dogma in physics, "there is little hard evidence for the kind of structure postulated by the GUTs and even less for the TOEs." Likewise, even if mental illness is caused by nothing more than a malfunctioning brain, and the brain is nothing more than a large collection of neurons (and, in turn, a larger collection of particles), it's still an open question what a successful psychiatric science is going to look like.

To see why this is so, think of earthquakes. Like the brain, earthquakes are nothing but a huge number of atoms moving around in space. How likely is it that we will one day have a theory of earthquakes expressed in terms of atoms? Well, who knows? If you could predict the future of science merely by thinking about the fact that everything in the universe is made up of atoms, then it would be the metaphysicians, rather than the scientists, who would be winning the Nobel Prizes. All we can say at the moment is that there seems to be little prospect of an atomic theory of earthquakes. So far as we can tell, the best way to understand earthquakes is in terms of the theory known as plate tectonics. It's not that the earth's crust *isn't* made up of atoms; it's just that the science human beings have actually managed to develop thus far can explain earthquakes best at a different level of physical organization.

What is true of earthquakes may be true of mental illness, too. There is no doubt that as we come to understand the brain better, we will learn a lot about psychosis and other forms of mental illness. But it is by no means inevitable that this research will take us down the path to exclusively biological theories of mental illness. The best theory of mental illness may include all sorts of things, including ideas about the social world. The moral: what things are *made of* doesn't say anything about what a good *scientific theory* of those things will be.

It's worth pointing out that even if there could in principle be an atomic theory of earthquakes or mental illness, it's possible that human beings are no more capable of producing it (or even understanding it) than your poodle is of proving Fermat's last theorem. As Noam Chomsky puts it, "humans are part of the natural world. They plainly have the capacity to solve certain problems. It follows that they lack the capacity to solve other problems, which will either be far too difficult for them to handle within existing limitations of time, memory, and so on or will literally be beyond the scope of their intelligence in principle." If one meditates on this sentiment for a while, one starts to feel grateful we can understand the universe at all—and less confident that plate tectonics will eventually be supplanted by physics, or psychiatry by clinical neuroscience.

Confidence about where science is headed, based on knowledge of science's past, also requires that we forget about the existence of scientific revolutions. We call them *revolutions* precisely because they change our views in ways no one could have predicted. How we understand a natural phenomenon doesn't depend on the fact that it is made up of particles or neurons but on the actual progress of science; and science is constantly surprising us. No matter how confident we are that the universe is made up of nothing but simple physical entities, there is very little evidence from the history of science (*real* science, that is, not science as it would be if everything were as tidy as it should be) that we can predict where the patterns in the universe will be found. Like all research programs, biological psychiatry is a bet. It's not irrational to take that bet, but it *is* irrational to believe that it's a sure thing.

KEVIN: THE OLYMPIAN

Coincidences are significant in the mind of Kevin Hall. It was a coincidence that he and I were in the same class at Brown University. It was a coincidence that we spent freshman year in adjacent dorms. And it was a coincidence that the week Kevin reached out to me was both the week he and his family had relocated to the Bay Area and the week I had made plans to travel to San Francisco to interview another person for this book. As Kevin made his way to meet me for dinner at Fisherman's Wharf, the car in front of his had a sticker on it that read KH. In the past, coincidences like these might have fueled delusions in his mind.

Kevin Hall was born in Ventura, California, to physician parents who graduated from McGill University Medical School, where I was also trained—another coincidence. Kevin was a good student but spent most of his time sailing. It "was all I wanted to do, all I thought about, lived, breathed," Kevin wrote to me. He was teased for being uncoordinated as a child, but at the age of fifteen he set a record for being the youngest boy to win the singles junior national sailing title. He was also the first to repeat as titlist and the first to win in both the singles and the doubles classes. It was not surprising that Kevin was recruited in 1987 to study and sail at Brown. He would later become the only sailor inducted into the Brown Athletic Hall of Fame (though he never mentioned it). Despite our proximity at Brown, neither of us could recall ever having met. In a text message describing who I should be looking for, Kevin wrote, "tan pants, no hair, sunburn."

Kevin double-majored at Brown. He studied math for his father, who wanted him to have a practical degree, and French literature for himself, which remains a lifelong passion. He was particularly taken with the works of Marguerite Duras, the author and film director. Kevin's senior thesis, "Les Histoires d'Amours de Marguerite Duras et Ludwig van Beethoven," won an award, particularly useful as it came with a cash prize. But before he had written the thesis or claimed his prize, Kevin had gone through two medical emergencies.

In November 1989, Kevin had his first manic episode. He became euphoric and delusional and believed he would save the world. Cramming for midterms after recovering from a case of shingles, he was sleeping very little and drinking enormous amounts of caffeine. Eventually, he wasn't sleeping at all. He began to notice that every song on the radio referred to his life. Kevin felt that he was being watched and could help save the world by making ethical consumer choices. Kevin would enter a store and pretend to be weighing a particular brand decision. He would ultimately choose the product of "the better corporate citizen." In buying the more ethical product, he would influence all those who were watching him to do the same, and thereby influence the entire world economy.

Kevin ultimately came to believe that his messianic launch would take place in Boston at a "world party" he was arranging which would feature Madonna and Michael Jackson. This would be the first in a series of events he was coordinating that would increase political awareness, spread messages of love and harmony, and raise funds for those in need. Kevin recalls having "conversations" with the agents for Michael Jackson and Madonna on a pay phone. Kevin knows that if it were to happen today, instead of Madonna and Michael Jackson, the musicians he would cast in his delusion would be Lady Gaga and Bono, who are also world famous and socially active. As Kevin put it, "That served as the spine of the delusion: just trying to make the world a better place."

As Kevin was about to leave the Brown campus in Providence for his "show" in Boston, a helicopter passed overhead. Kevin knew immediately that the cameras and microphones were on that helicopter, and he made a mental note to project his voice in its direction. The world was watching what he would one day call the "TrumanKev Show." Kevin got on the bus to Boston, and all of its passengers were characters from Marguerite Duras's books and movies. The seating arrangement and their behavior confirmed that everything Kevin was thinking was true.

Once in Boston, Kevin spent a night on the street. After approaching strangers with unwelcome questions and then climbing a tree, Kevin was arrested. It was all part of the "script," so he complied with the police.

Kevin was finally hospitalized at McLean Hospital. His mom flew to Boston to be with him. Friends visited. He wrote of his experience at McLean: "DayNightRoomsGroupBasketballMusic and finally the anguish." As his mania abated, he felt acute sadness that the world would not be saved, that war and poverty would continue.

Kevin was diagnosed with bipolar disorder. Lithium treated the mania, but Kevin felt "three quarters numb" while skiing with his father, who took a hiatus from his work as an ER physician to spend time with his son. The world had become "gray." Adding Prozac and lowering the lithium dose helped and, after much discussion and support from the administration at Brown, Kevin returned for the spring semester of junior year, with the understanding that he could leave at any time. But he did well, and returned to his studies and sailing without skipping a beat.

Then came fall semester of senior year. Kevin was diagnosed with testicular cancer. Shortly thereafter, he had a testicle removed back in California, at his father's hospital. The doctors wanted Kevin to have a round of radiation treatment, but he insisted that unless his life was at risk he preferred to return to Brown. Just three weeks later, Kevin came in second place at the intercollegiate sailing championships.

Enter Amanda, an eighteen-year-old freshman. Amanda was drawn to Kevin, but sees now that much of the appeal was in dating a man who had bipolar disorder and had just been treated for cancer. It allowed her to play the role of a healer and to feel needed. Amanda later became an ER physician, just like Kevin's father, perhaps another coincidence.

Kevin's senior year revolved around his love affair with Amanda. He was finally enjoying hanging out with his friends after years of putting sailing first. Amanda regarded Kevin as a Luddite because he wrote his thesis with a fountain pen and shunned television and computers—ironic given the technological content of his delusion.

Just after graduation, while editing his thesis, Kevin was on an American sailing team that took part in a goodwill regatta in Tokyo. While he was there, Kevin had his second manic episode. He and his teammates were "partying and competing, partying and competing, partying and competing" and in time, he says, "I was gone."

Kevin took off from the hotel one morning wearing his sailing gear. He walked around the city, including through traffic, with his eyes closed. He wanted to force the "Directors" to reveal that he was in fact "The One."

He came upon an unlocked truck and, thinking about a scene in *Terminator 2* where Arnold flips down the sun visor and the keys are there, Kevin flipped down the visor and, yes, the keys fell into his lap. Of course! The research group in the Control Center knew that he loved that *Terminator* scene. He drove around Tokyo and in retrospect is amazed he didn't kill anyone. After a full day of coincidences and improbabilities, including breaking into a karaoke lounge with a basketball hoop in it (he had found a basketball earlier), Kevin arrived at the emperor's palace naked and was promptly arrested. After a couple of hours explaining that he meant no disrespect to the palace or to the emperor, he was released. It was now almost a full day since he had left the hotel. He got on and off buses depending on signals from the Directors in the Control Center. And eventually he just walked. He had no idea where the hotel was; he didn't read Japanese, yet he found it. It was dawn. Kevin remembers that moment with a degree of wonder. "How could I have done that? I couldn't do it again. I couldn't do it sober. I couldn't do it with all the coffee in the world, now. But it happened then." The team thought they might be able to get him back home, but the stimulation of the airport proved too much. Kevin ran off through the baggage claim and found himself standing under a 747. This time the police would not let him go, and his father had to fly to Japan to bring him back home for treatment.

In December 1992, Kevin discovered that he had a second testicular cancer. In January he had his other testicle removed along with lymph nodes in his abdomen. He was devastated. He stopped sailing for a couple of years and required testosterone replacement therapy. He moved back to Providence to be near Amanda. He drank "over the top of the lithium," and the grief of the second operation led to another manic episode. Kevin drove wildly, again to Boston, and would have ended up in the harbor if a terrified Amanda had not wrested the wheel from him. Twenty years later, Kevin still struggles with the idea that he might have seriously traumatized Amanda on that ride.

At some point, Kevin built a backstory connecting his episodes of mania, or as he calls it, his "Trumaning." When Kevin is ill he believes that four generations ago a small group of wealthy individuals who lived through World War I and the Depression came together to prevent another such disaster. Their answer was to "generate" a second coming of the Messiah. "Enter me, in Boston in 1989, with the plan to save the world." Kevin believed he was on television worldwide. Those closest to him, his family and friends, had been in on the conspiracy since he was a young child. Their jobs weren't their real jobs. "Their real jobs are to make sure we are doing what we're trying to do, the big picture, which is to save the world."

During the early episodes before the internet, television and radio were the primary platforms for Kevin. Hidden cameras and mics were everywhere, as well as in plain sight. "The feed went to the Control Center, and was produced and distributed to the world from there." If Kevin turned on a television, the Directors would transmit something else to that TV alone. He was the only person who couldn't watch the TrumanKev Show.

With the advent of the internet, Kevin's group of "handlers" would direct his searches to particular websites, thereby influencing his choices, guiding him to knowledge he would need in his quest. This also explained why he didn't find himself plastered all over the web, as one might expect of the most famous person in the world. The handlers were directing him away from those pages. But in a sophisticated twist, the handlers allowed Kevin just enough of a web presence to keep him playing along. Of course, that presence was grounded firmly in reality: coverage of his sailing, his cancer, and his involvement with the Livestrong Foundation.

Kevin observes that in every episode he removes three items: his shoes (so he can feel closer to the earth), his watch (time ceases to have any meaning for him), and his wallet (he no longer needs money). "If I'm hungry, the show will give me breakfast."

After years of struggle—with bipolar disorder, Truman Show delusion, cancer, fellow competitive sailors, and with the American and International Olympic committees over his having to take exogenous testosterone—Kevin finally got to represent the USA as an Olympian in the 2004 games in Athens. Though his need for injected testosterone was medically self-evident, the Olympic rulebook didn't have a clause that applied to a man who had had both of his testicles removed. At times, Kevin would have his blood taken daily. Even on the day of his injection, Kevin would only have a testosterone level about 80 percent that of his competitors, and his level gradually dropped over the course of two weeks. As his level dropped so did his strength and, worse, his mood.

He went so far as to stop his psychotropic medications during the Olympic trials so that he would be at full capacity. He did not tell Amanda, because he knew she would freak out. To maintain his balance, he cut out all alcohol and kept a rigorous training schedule. Up at 6:00 a.m., asleep at 10:00 p.m. "Just me and the water." He says he didn't come remotely close to having an episode. He did resume his mood stabilizer in the lead-up to the Olympics, and while he finished respectably, one spot ahead of mid-fleet, he was unhappy with his performance. Although Kevin enjoyed the trials, his Olympic experience was "sad." He wasn't "present." All anyone wanted to talk about was his eligibility and the testosterone. He forgot he was supposed to enjoy the sailing. His one regret in life is not sitting with his family during the medal ceremony. He is more proud of being an Olympian now than he was then.

During another episode in Sardinia, Kevin threw his wallet and Olympic watch off a terrace. A teammate retrieved the watch by trading it for the contents of the wallet. Unfortunately, the U and A in the USA logo beneath the Olympic rings on its face broke off and disappeared into the works.

Amanda stayed with and cared for Kevin throughout her four years at Brown, but at twenty-two, she felt she needed to see the world and have other experiences. Kevin's response was to marry the first girl he met, all the while knowing she wasn't the one. While his initial manic episodes were primarily euphoric, the "middle" episodes over the coming years were more paranoid in nature and driven in part by the knowledge that he was married to the wrong woman.

Kevin chose not to approach strangers in an attempt to get off the show because he didn't want to bother anyone. "I'd like to think that some of the 'deluded me' knew that it would be really upsetting for them," he explains. These middle episodes were also marked by a sadness surrounding Kevin's belief that he had lost his free will to the show. He would try to soothe himself with the knowledge that his sacrifice of free will was offset by the greater good of saving the world. By the later episodes, Kevin came to accept his position, come what may. "I think the reason I have managed to come out the other side is I figured out how to embrace Being Truman."

After four unhappy and unhealthy years, Kevin finally found the courage to end the marriage. He had yet another manic episode in 1999. When he got out of the hospital, he called Amanda. She flew out to California the following day, and they have been together ever since. This time, Amanda was drawn not to the complicated man with major illnesses but to Kevin, the person she describes as "kind, loving, sensitive, communicative, thoughtful, funny, smart, talented . . ." The couple got married and have adopted three children. "Despite Kevin being the one with the DSM diagnosis," Amanda says, "he's the most stable, most even-keeled parent." Kevin also came to see that his manic solipsism was not unlike the feeling a child has of being the center of the universe. He thinks that the sort of steering Amanda did to keep them out of Boston Harbor comes in handy when she has to wrangle their three-year-old safely in and out of the bath.

And what impact did becoming a father have on Kevin? He swore he would never go off his medication again, and he has kept that promise. Kevin avoids too much red wine and caffeine, the substances that have triggered his mania in the past. He acknowledges sometimes being frustrated—"How come I don't get a Friday night?"—but he knows that the stakes are too high. And aside from his family, those stakes have included a successful career on America's Cup teams, which have taken him around the world. Amanda laughs about the fact that Kevin, the former Luddite, is now his team's navigator, the one with the computer. He is fascinated with technology and an avid reader of *Wired* magazine, but his relationship to technology, she assured me, was a healthy one.

Kevin has become a professional sailor and sailing coach. Amanda notices that he enjoys the social aspects of his work, including managing other members of his team. One concern Amanda has, however, is that part of the job involves hanging out in bars, the place where sailors network. It's the "worst place for him to be," she says, but also where Kevin might get his next gig.

Kevin is a great music lover and is slowly teaching himself guitar. He loves to sing. Kevin says that when he is manic, lyrics take on referential meaning, and he feels "manipulated by the music and the patterns on the radio." But during these episodes there is also a heightened beauty: Kevin feels he can hear a piece of music as both a whole and as a series of its parts. He believes that he unwisely stopped taking his lithium in the past for two reasons: it messed with his sailing and detracted from his enjoyment of music. Kevin even uses a musical metaphor to describe the experience of approaching mania: when he starts seeing resemblances to celebrities in strangers' faces, that sensation feels to him like recognizing the subtlest changes in the Goldberg or Diabelli variations. This has become an early

warning sign for Amanda and him. If Kevin starts making such comparisons, they both know that he may be tilting toward Tru-mania.

Kevin Hall is the only person in this book who is not disguised in any
way. He assured me that he was perfectly comfortable coming out as someone with bipolar disorder and Truman Show delusion. First off, he has
some experience speaking publicly about illness (his cancer), which was
documented in the *New York Times*, the *Washington Post*, and elsewhere.
More important, all of the significant people in his life already know about
his mood disorder. Amanda had no qualms with Kevin sharing his story.
Kevin says, "It would help me a lot to believe my being a real person could
help somebody else." This would not be the first time that Kevin has used
his experience with being bipolar to help someone else. A former Olympic teammate had become a coach. One of his student athletes developed
bipolar disorder, and the teammate reached out to Kevin. He and the student spent a few days together surfing and talking. "I felt great about it. It
wasn't just for him."

Like many people with Truman Show delusion who learn of their fellow
sufferers' experiences, Kevin expresses a measure of relief that he is not
alone. At the same time, there is a kind of sadness in sameness. "One of the
things you want very much is to be special . . . Part of you is saying, 'Well,
no, everyone who goes crazy does this same thing, so it's just madness, it's
not actually "real"—and part of you is saying, as you get sick, 'I am special.
And not only am I special, but this specialness is special. Different to all
those others.'"

But delusion is not without emotional rewards. "I can honestly say
there's a good chance I have felt most things which most people are able to
describe. There's a limited list of things I haven't felt—being a Holocaust
survivor or losing a child. However, there are times that I am so overwhelmed by the emotion of things like that, it seems darn close. Maybe
that's why I am so lucky. Most people have to go pretty far out of their way
to be overwhelmed like that."

Since first meeting, Kevin and I have stayed in touch. He still finds coincidences fascinating and recently sent me an excursus on James Joyce's interest in them. Not long ago, after the death of a close friend, and after fourteen
years without one, Kevin had a brief episode of Truman Show delusion.

He has come to think that the contradiction between feeling both like

241

the center of the world when experiencing the Truman Show delusion, and "yet just another guy with TSD, is explained by, and held [together] by the Zeitgeist." Kevin thought that "before spinning up to full TSD there must be a way to keep differentiating and talk myself back down," avoiding "my path toward and down the rabbit hole."

And so Kevin gave himself a present.—JG

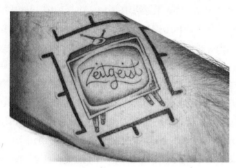

Figure 23: *Zeitgeist*, Amanda Hall, 2014.
Reproduced with permission.

THE FUTURE OF PSYCHIATRY

In this book we've presented the evidence that delusions are symptoms of a cognitive system whose purpose is to detect social threats and motivate one to defend against them. That's to say, the function of the regions of the brain that do the job of the Suspicion System can be understood only with reference to the social world. If we are right, then a future theory of delusion could be a purely biological theory only if it can translate the social description of the Suspicion System into biological terms. We're deeply skeptical that such a translation is possible, though since we're insisting on agnosticism about the future of science, we have to acknowledge the possibility.

Beyond the narrow topic of delusion is the question of the path that psychiatry ought to take. Aspirational psychiatry has hitched its wagon to the star of neuroscience, but we don't know how long it will be before that star begins to cool. It would be wise for psychiatry to be a broad church at least until the science catches up with our hopes. After all, psychiatrists know that wish fulfillment is the stuff of dreams.

Instead of looking to understand mental illness exclusively in neural terms, there is another strategy that psychiatry could adopt. It could simply embrace the social environment on its own terms and not as an illusion waiting to be reduced to biology. In taking account of the role of the social world in mental illness, it may be necessary to hang on to notions like threat, discrimination, exploitation, and status, and there may be no way to understand these concepts other than by theories far removed from neurons. Plate tectonics is no less "scientific" because it makes reference to the earth's crust rather than to atoms, and psychiatry would be no less scientific for embracing the concepts of exploitation and suspicion *as well as* that of dopamine function. Reductionism in psychiatry constrains theory to operate within the skull or the skin. Our bet is that the outside world is going to matter as well.

What may seem such an eccentric psychiatric view—the interplay of biology and social factors—is an accepted fact in other fields and with other illnesses. The status of lung cancer and schizophrenia as biological diseases doesn't mean that the outside world can safely be ignored. No self-respecting oncologist would advocate smoking, and no psychiatrist can be indifferent to the toxicity of social life.

There is, in fact, a profound irony in the idea that a theory of mental illness must be a theory of genetic and brain disorders alone. The framework for all of biology—the theory without which nothing in biology makes sense (as Theodosius Dobzhansky famously put it)—is evolutionary theory. Natural selection addresses, among other things, the relation of organisms to their *environment* and sexual selection addresses organisms' relation to their *social world*. Evolutionary theory is not demeaned by making reference to concepts like environment or adaptation alongside DNA and mutation, nor would biological psychiatry be demeaned by giving the concept of social threat a place alongside that of neurotransmission. Aspirational psychiatry, according to which psychiatry becomes clinical neuroscience, is what mental illness looks like through a keyhole. Its narrow view misses the wide biological perspective in which living things, humans included, are best understood. The problem with aspirational psychiatry, then, is not that it is too biological. The problem is that it is not biological enough.

NOTES

xv   *to protect confidentiality:* In one case that will be clear to the reader, a subject has consented to not be disguised.

xv   *identifying data have been changed:* All names have been changed, other than that of the person described above. Disguise can include creating a composite subject, or using information from more than one patient. The following short vignettes are composites: Donald, Simone, Samir, and Jada.

xviii *The world as it had been shown to him . . . escape from this asylum:* Heinlein, 1941, pp. 89, 92.

PREFACE

4   *directed by Peter Weir:* Niccol, 1998.

4   *"TRUMAN: Who are you? . . . You're the star.":* Niccol, 1998, pp. 104–5. Stage directions have been omitted.

7   *"There's no point . . . revolves around me somehow":* Niccol, 1998, pp. 45, 67, and 96. Stage directions have been omitted.

8   *CHRISTOF: [Feeding Marlon his lines] . . . because there is no it:* Niccol, 1998, p. 68.

12 *one in four has Truman syndrome:* Interview with Rachel Wang, Chocolate Films, Hammersmith Hospital, May 26, 2009.

12 *prodromal patients compare their experiences to* The Truman Show: Addington, 2008.

13 *any psychiatrist will tell you that is not true:* A psychiatrist, suffering from bipolar disorder, traveled from Florida to New York City in 2007, where he assaulted a mother while attempting to kidnap her young son. A news report of the hearing to keep that psychiatrist hospitalized said he had gone to New York to "get out of 'The Truman Show'"; Francescani and Davis, 2007.

CHAPTER 1

17 *written records of human civilization:* We rely throughout this chapter on Porter, 2002, and Shorter, 1997.

NOTES

17 *The Papyrus Ebers:* Bryan, 1931.
17 *the Indian* Atharva-Veda: Whitney, 1905; quotes are from p. 361.
17 *Israelites who fail to obey the Lord:* Deuteronomy 28:28.
17 *the envious King Saul who raves:* 1 Samuel 18:7–11.
17 *condemned to eat grass for his pride:* Daniel 4:30.
18 *punishment from the gods or demonic retribution:* Porter, 2002.
18 *"'the gods have made you mad . . . the clearest head around'"*: Homer, 1996, Book 23, ll. 12–13.
18 *dates from at least 5,000 BC:* Porter, 2002.
18 *a medieval medical fantasy:* See Shorter, 1997.
18 *having a stone in one's head:* See Mora, 2008b, p. 232.
19 *of the lover:* Plato, 1997, pp. 522–527.
19 *a common trope in medieval literature:* Mora, 2008a.
19 *creativity more generally—continues to our day:* See, e.g., Jamison, 1993.
19 *the soul of the madman:* Porter, 2002.
19 *less like his rational God:* Mora, 2008a.
19 *the Gadarene man healed by Jesus:* Mark 5.
19 *in the ancient world:* Simon, 2008.
19 *belief in the evil eye:* The evil eye is also related to the doctrine of the humors: it can "dry" the victim up and make them infertile. "Here's lookin' at you"—a toast made over drinks—echoes the belief in using liquid to ward off the evil eye. Ibid.
20 *conceive of it as disease:* Our discussion in this section follows Simon, 2008.
20 *"from nothing else but thence . . . and fears and terrors assail us"*: Hippocrates, 1849, pp. 854–55.
20 *maintained physical health:* See Porter, 2002.
20 *tarry stool, according to one historian:* Simon, 2008.
20 *"the devil rejoices in the humor of black bile"*: Ibid., p. 181.
20 *a dream of divine origin:* Patton, 2004.
20 *the dialectical method:* Simon, 2008.
20 *talk therapy could cure madness:* See Simon, 2008.
20 *central to medicine for fifteen hundred years:* Mora, 2008a.
20 *The Diseases Which Deprive Man of His Reason:* See Paracelsus, 1941.
21 *Anatomy of Melancholy:* Burton, 2001.
21 *travel, music, or marriage:* Porter, 2002.
21 *belladonna, and camphor:* Weiner, 2008a.
21 *"psychology has a long past, yet its real history is short"*: Ebbinghaus, 1908, p. 3.
21 *stand up to violent behavior:* Mora, 2008a.
21 *baptism and communion:* Ibid.
21 *a ward for those suffering from madness:* Ibid.
22 *baths, perfumes, and concerts:* Ibid.
22 *Bethlem was founded in 1247:* See Andrews et al., 1997.
22 *half of those with mental illness:* Porter, 2002.
22 *humane and medical motives:* See Shorter, 1997.

NOTES

22 *the term* psychiatry: See Marneros, 2008.

22 *"Like criminals . . . corrupting in their own filth":* Johann Christian Reil, *Rhapsodieen über die Anwendung der psychischen Curmethode auf Geisteszerüttungen,* quoted in Shorter, 1997, pp. 6–7.

22 *"in the thickness of this tower's corner . . . knocked off with an iron bar":* Quoted in Weiner, 2008a, p. 257.

22 *in this position for ten years:* Jay, 2014.

23 *the Bastilles confining the mad:* See Porter, 2002, p. 107.

23 *psychiatry was born:* Weiner, 2008b.

23 *the chains of the inmates:* Ibid.

23 Description of the Retreat: Tuke, 1813. For a history of the asylum, see Shorter, 1997.

23 *both visitor and inmate:* See Andrews et al., 1997, p. 2 and chapter 13. All quotes are from p. 181.

24 *"moral (i.e., psychological) therapy":* See Shorter, 1997, pp. 19–20.

24 *"on an air . . . to those of others":* Quoted in Shorter, 1997, p. 21.

24 *a bodily disease or a* mental *one:* Marx, 2008.

25 *"wrong ideas together":* Locke, 1975, II, xi, 13.

25 *the second half of the eighteenth century:* Wallace, 2008.

25 *he coined the term* neurosis: Gach, 2008.

25 *"hurried association of ideas" producing "false judgement":* Quoted in Porter, 2002, p. 128.

25 *one hundred thousand a century later:* See Porter, 2002.

25 *thought to be hereditary:* Gach, 2008.

26 *isolation cells:* Shorter, 1997, p. 66.

26 *"It was after 7 p.m. . . . for God's sake let me out!' ":* Quoted in Shorter, 1997, p. 66.

26 *"a perfectly hellish contrivance . . . as a result of it":* Ibid., p. 65.

26 *"heating of their buildings . . . the making up of accounts":* Ibid., p. 68.

26 *breaking of the chains:* Sadly, in parts of the world today the chains remain unbroken. A recent article in *The Lancet* (Edwards, 2014) describes Ghanaian "prayer camps" that offer spiritual therapy for mentally ill patients. The article cites a report of Human Rights Watch that details cases of patients being shackled and forced to fast. Our colleague Carol Bernstein, M.D., recently visited the prayer camp featured in the *Lancet* article and saw shackled patients.

26 *a Welsh tea broker living in London:* We follow Haslam, 1988, Introduction; Jay, 2014; Porter, 1985; 1991.

26 *"I pronounce your Lordship . . . a most diabolical Traitor":* Haslam, 1988, p. xx.

26 *"I profess myself . . . I am perfectly otherwise":* Ibid., p. xxiii.

27 *case study in British psychiatry:* Porter, 1991.

27 *come to be known as schizophrenia:* Carpenter, 1989. Although he plays the role of the villain in the story of James Tilly Matthews, Haslam is an important figure in the history of psychiatry. Apart from his penetrating case histories, his book *Medical Jurisprudence,* published in 1817, is, according to Roy Porter, "the pioneering English text of forensic psychiatry"; Porter, 1991, p. 60.

27 *it may very well have been true:* Jay, 2014.

28 *she has "the itch"*: Haslam, 1988, p. 27. Probably scabies; see Siena, 2013.

28 *"At home . . . filthy community"*: Haslam, 1988, p. 21.

28 *"the vapours of vitriol . . . the horse's greasy heels"*: Ibid., p. 28.

28 *tuberculosis contracted in Bethlem*: Porter, 1991.

29 *"a man of considerable accomplishments"*: Andrews et al., 1997, p. 426.

30 *would not "submit" to Haslam's authority*: Jay, 2014, p. 228.

30 *"The irons . . . the use of his tongue"*: Quoted in Jay, 2014, p. 228.

30 *firmly rooted in medicine*: Gach, 2008.

30 *understood as machines*: This is an oversimplification of the tenets of mechanical philosophy; see Garber, 2013.

30 *thinking about insanity*: Gach, 2008.

30 *"What organ . . . can only be the brain"*: Griesinger, 1882, p. 1. Griesinger's views were more complicated than his opening salvo suggests; see Fuchs, 2012.

30 *declared it a branch of biology*: Gach, 2008.

31 *known as Wernicke's aphasia*: See Eggert, 1977.

31 *learn to read them*: See Shorter, 1997.

31 *without anatomical pathology*: Bürgy, 2008; Gach, 2008.

32 *it was surprisingly good*: See Shorter, 1997.

33 *in the mind or in psychological function*: The history of the concept of schizophrenia is fascinating and complex; see Berrios, Luque, and Villagrán, 2003; Gilman, 2008.

33 *has its roots in this term and (unfortunately) persists*: See Andreasen, 2011.

33 *in other areas of pathology*: Gach, 2008.

33 *our modern classification*: See Kraepelin, 1902.

33 *whispered to Freud*: "C'est toujours la chose genitale." Porter, 2002, p. 189.

33 *In a letter to István Hollós*: Kafka, 2011.

34 *"make me angry . . . a poor psychiatrist"*: Quoted in Dupont, 1988, p. 251.

34 *"Analysis of a Case of Paranoia"*: Freud, 1896/1962, p. 174.

34 *"paranoia, too . . . what has been repressed"*: Ibid, pp. 174–5.

34 *"complained that she . . . in her house"*: Ibid., p. 176.

34 *"these hallucinations . . . return of the repressed"*: Ibid., p. 181.

34 *"was now making up . . . as a child"*: Ibid., p. 178.

34 *"oscillates all through his life . . . over into the other"*: Freud, 1911/1958, p. 46.

34 *distinct from schizophrenia*: Ibid.

34 *strictly speaking, sexual energy*: Later theorists use *libido* to refer to "psychic energy" more generally, and often suggest that Freud also accepted a broader definition. We believe, however, that Freud maintained the more narrow pleasure-seeking definition. See Freud, 1923/1955. Freud did write about *Eros*, the "life instinct" that encompasses the *libido*. See Freud, 1920/1955.

34 *infantile state produces schizophrenia*: Freud, 1911/1958.

34 *Freud believed was incurable*: Freud, 1913/1955.

34 *"[n]eurosis is the result . . . the external world"*: Freud, 1924/1961a, p. 149.

35 *"have turned away . . . inaccessible to us"*: Freud, 1933/1964, p. 59.

35 *drove the libido inward*: Freud, 1924/1961a.

35 *without interpretation, treatment is impossible:* A "healthy" (i.e., neurotic), not psychotic, person will have sufficient amounts of both object and ego libido, on this view. Freud, 1924/1961b.

35 *poor or even disastrous results:* See Dolnick, 1998.

35 *patients with schizophrenia could develop transference:* Federn, 1934.

35 *too little libido invested in themselves:* Federn, 1932.

35 *"must help the patient in the actual affairs of his life":* Federn, 1934, p. 211.

35 *think of as supportive psychotherapy:* For instance, he suggested not having the patient use the couch, a situation that tends to foster regression as the patient cannot see the analyst. Instead, he suggested that the patient sit up, facing the analyst. A description of supportive psychotherapy is found in Winston, Rosenthal, and Pinsker, 2012.

35 *successful treatment was, he thought, impossible:* Federn, 1934.

36 *"ultimately has become . . . conceptualizations of schizophrenia":* Sledge, 1992, p. 184.

36 *the schizophrenic patient and the analyst:* Young-Bruehl, 2002.

36 *inability to develop transference:* Ibid.

36 *better understand his patient:* Boschan, 2011.

36 *"mutual analysis" with a disturbed patient:* Fortune, 1993.

36 *he was the one who was schizophrenic:* Young-Bruehl, 2002.

36 *"was challenged . . . were wedded to":* Personal communication.

36 *the defenses (or defense mechanisms):* Freud, 1937.

36 *"object relations theory":* Greenberg and Mitchell, 1983.

36 *exert an influence into adulthood:* Ibid.

36 *take in pleasure and expel pain:* Klein, 1932.

37 *the "paranoid-schizoid" position:* Klein, 1948.

37 *the "depressive" position:* Ibid.

37 *psychosis might be the eventual result:* Klein, 1960.

37 *the Freudian and Kleinian schools:* Wallerstein, 2002.

37 *"[t]here is no such thing as an infant":* Winnicott, 1960, p. 587.

37 *"an environmental deficiency disease":* Winnicott, 1963, p. 343.

37 *difficulty in relationships with others:* Greenberg and Mitchell, 1983.

37 *those suffering from psychosis:* Havens, 1976.

37 *considered himself to be a Freudian:* Lothane, 2011.

37 *the formative role of culture and society:* Evans, 1996.

37 *a "therapeutic milieu":* Ibid.

38 *[I]f we changed the attitudes . . . recovery rate became high:* Sullivan, 1962.

38 *the development of schizophrenia:* Auchincloss and Samberg, 2012.

38 *a "participant-observer":* Havens, 1976.

38 *"In retrospect . . . inhabitants of psychosis-land":* Kafka, 2011, p. 31.

38 *a young navy veteran:* Sullivan, 1976.

39 *"[s]ee if there is . . . story told in the dream":* Ibid., p. 117.

39 *"what the hell he is trying to do":* Ibid., p. 210.

39 *"People come to me . . . living untangled":* Ibid., p. 216.

39 *"the most influential . . . American psychiatry":* Havens and Frank, 1971, pp. 1704-5.

39 *deficiency was most toxic:* See Dolnick, 1998, for an extended discussion of a wide range of such theories.

39 *the "schizophrenogenic mother":* Fromm-Reichmann, 1948; see Neill, 1990.

39 *their child had developed schizophrenia:* E.g., Callard et al., 2012.

39 *like frontal lobotomy:* Watts and Freeman, 1948.

39 *its views about psychosis:* See Paris, 2005.

39 *published a follow-up study:* McGlashan, 1984b.

39 *"The data are in . . . The experiment failed":* Quoted in Harrington, 2012, p. 1293.

40 *an accompanying manic-depressive illness:* See Paris, 2005.

42 *a Kraepelinian model of disease classification:* In addition to psychoanalysis and biological psychiatry, behaviorism has been an important contributor to psychiatry. Although we do not explore that history here, our discussion of cognitive behavioral therapy (CBT) demonstrates that behaviorism continues to play a role in psychiatric practice; see Eysenck, 1985.

42 *the topics of this section and the next:* A third factor was the social movement that began in the 1960s, when patients with severe mental illness began to be deinstitutionalized and sent home to their families—the very people, according to psychoanalytic theory, who had caused the illness in the first place. The new biological psychiatry gave family members the ammunition to cast off the burden of blame that psychoanalysis had laid on them and insist on better care for their children. The National Alliance for the Mentally Ill (subsequently changed to the National Alliance on Mental Illness, or NAMI) was established in the 1970s and founded on the idea that schizophrenia is an illness like any other. It became a force to be reckoned with. Science and social change thus joined forces to drive a stake into the heart of the schizophrenogenic mother. See Harrington, 2012.

42 *after the Second World War:* The Society for Biological Psychiatry was founded in 1946, and a dozen years later, Jules Masserman, then president of the society, articulated the keystone idea—an idea, he says, as "old" as it is "fundamental": "that the behavior of human beings is patterned largely by their nervous systems and . . . that much of medicine, psychology, sociology, anthropology, history—indeed, all of the sciences that comprise psychiatry—stem from the basic discipline of neurology"; Masserman, 1959, p. xiv.

42 *mental illness, including psychosis:* We rely throughout on Healy, 2002, and Swazey, 1974. The Association for Research in Nervous and Mental Diseases, a group interested in neuroscience and disease, first met in the United States in 1920 (Gach, 2008), and, as just mentioned, the first meeting of the Society for Biological Psychiatry was held in 1946. The first modern textbook of biological psychiatry, Nielson and Thompson's *Engrammes of Psychiatry,* was published in 1947.

42 *to be discharged from hospital:* Shorter, 1997.

42 *"an unknown psychiatrist . . . negligible equipment":* Quoted in Shorter, 1997, p. 257.

43 *the figure of Paul Ehrlich:* See Bosch and Rosich, 2008.

43 *"That is little Ehrlich . . . pass his examinations":* Quoted in Bosch and Rosich, 2008, p. 172.

NOTES

44 *a "euphoric quietude"*: Quoted in Swazey, 1974, p. 78.

44 *the "lytic cocktail"*: Laborit used "lytic" to refer to the capacity to reduce the activity of the autonomic nervous system; Swazey, 1974.

44 *"psychic disorientation"*: Quoted in Swazey, 1974, p. 96.

45 *indifferent to what was going on:* Healy, 2002.

45 *"no longer talks . . . threat of vengeance"*: Quoted in Swazey, 1974, p. 115.

46 *"brought about a transformation . . . means of restraint"*: Quoted in Swazey, 1974, p. 137.

46 *never left the barbershop:* Reported in Healy, 2002.

46 *"a drug . . . and social phenomenon"*: Quoted in Swazey, 1974, p. 138.

46 *entered North America through Canada:* Shorter, 1997.

46 *"About three to four weeks . . . new treatment concept"*: Quoted in Swazey, 1974, p. 155.

47 *"At the time we . . . refractory to treatment:* Lehmann quoted in Swazey, 1974, p. 157.

47 *"[a]t the end . . . schizophrenia in weeks"*: Quoted in Shorter, 1997, p. 252.

47 *"At the time . . . working with drugs"*: Quoted in Swazey, 1974, p. 196.

48 *Philip Seeman in Canada:* See Healy, 2002, for a detailed history.

48 *the "dopamine hypothesis" of schizophrenia:* For a history of the hypothesis, see Howes and Kapur, 2009, and Kendler and Schaffner, 2011.

48 *J. M. van Rossum:* van Rossum, 1966. Carlsson and Snyder themselves were skeptical of the dopamine hypothesis; see Healy, 2002.

48 *by no means the whole story:* Kantrowitz and Javitt, 2009; Raedler and Freedman, 2009; see also Javitt and Kantrowitz, 2009.

48 *came from genetic research:* We rely on Dolnick, 1998.

48 *that chronic psychosis was heritable:* Edward Shorter, personal communication.

48 *"I'd noticed . . . in the genes' ":* Quoted in Dolnick, 1998, p. 158.

48 *the adoptive ones, were ill:* Dolnick, 1998; Rosenthal and Kety, 1968. See also Ingraham and Kety, 2000; Kendler, Gruenberg and Kinney, 1994; and Kety et al., 1994.

49 *"there can be . . . twisted molecule"*: A phrase due to R. W. Gerard; quoted in Gach, 2008, p. 400.

49 *took it to be largely irrelevant:* See Shorter, 1997.

49 *asked to provide a diagnosis:* Kendell et al., 1971.

49 Diagnostic and Statistical Manual of Mental Disorders: The first manual was actually titled *Diagnostic and Statistical Manual: Mental Disorders.*

49 *the sixth edition of Kraepelin's textbook:* Shorter, 1997.

50 *to establish diagnostic consistency:* DSM-III, 1980, Appendix F. Field trials: interrater reliability and listing of participants, 1980.

50 *taken with a grain of salt:* A famous case, such as that of "Deborah," whose successful treatment by Frieda Fromm-Reichmann is portrayed in *I Never Promised You a Rose Garden* (Green, 1964), would probably not be diagnosed with schizophrenia today; North and Cadoret, 1981.

50 *listed 297 disorders:* See Shorter, 1997.

50 *latest revision of the DSM, DSM-5:* the Roman numerals have been dropped to provide an identifying scheme for incremental updates of the "5.1" variety.

50 *drug abuse, and personality, among others:* The complete list: neurodevelopmental

NOTES

disorders (e.g., autism spectrum disorder); schizophrenia spectrum and other psychotic disorders; bipolar and related disorders; depressive disorders; anxiety disorders; obsessive-compulsive and related disorders; trauma- and stressor-related disorders (e.g., posttraumatic stress disorder, or PTSD); dissociative disorders, i.e., disorders involving a lack of mental integration (e.g., dissociative identity disorder, formerly known as multiple personality disorder); somatic symptom and related disorders (e.g., conversion disorder, the descendent of hysteria, which manifests as neurological symptoms); feeding and eating disorders (e.g., anorexia); elimination disorders (e.g., enuresis, or bedwetting); sleep-wake disorders (e.g., narcolepsy); sexual dysfunctions (e.g., premature ejaculation); gender dysphoria, a divergence between one's assigned gender and experienced gender; disruptive, impulse-control, and conduct disorders (e.g., kleptomania); substance-related and addictive disorders (e.g., alcohol use disorder); neurocognitive disorders (e.g., cognitive deficits associated with Alzheimer's disease); personality disorders; paraphilic disorders, i.e, disorders of sexual behavior (e.g., voyeuristic disorder); other mental disorders; medication-induced movement disorders and other adverse effects of medication; and other conditions that may be a focus of clinical attention.

50 *schizotypal personality disorder:* DSM-5, 2013, pp. 655–59.
51 *the strange beliefs known as* delusions: Ibid., pp. 87–88.
51 *We live in an era . . . has finally come:* Andreasen, 2001, p. 318.
51 *"psychiatry's impact . . . as brain disorders":* Insel and Quirion, 2005, p. 2221.
52 *how antipsychotic drugs work:* Miller, 2009.
52 *severe depression—improves mood:* Bolwig, 2011.
52 *simplistic at best:* Kroeze, Zhou, and Homberg, 2012; Sharp and Cowen, 2011.
52 *good enough even to be wrong:* The phrase is attributed to the physicist Wolfgang Pauli; Peierls, 1960.
52 *genetic research has been carried out:* See chapters 12, 13, and 14 in Weinberger and Harrison, 2011.
52 *regions of the human genome are associated with schizophrenia:* Ripke et al., 2013.
52 *that can confirm a diagnosis:* Lawrie et al., 2011.
53 *and it quite possibly isn't:* Taylor et al., 2010.
53 *"We were hoping . . . to make our diagnoses":* Hamilton, 2013.
53 *the philospher Michel Foucault:* Foucault, 1988.
53 *the psychiatrist Thomas Szasz:* Szasz, 1974.

CHAPTER 2

59 *"Since time immemorial . . . to be deluded":* Jaspers, 1997, p. 93.
59 *as many as seventy-five illnesses:* Manschreck, 1979.
59 *psychiatric disorders and physical illnesses:* Ibid.
59 *being robbed of one's possessions is not:* Mullins and Spence, 2003.
59 *the other way around:* Holt and Albert, 2006.

NOTES

59 *Cotard delusion:* Berrios and Luque, 1995; Cotard, 1882.

60 *quite likely to be depressed:* Berrios and Luque, 1995.

60 *"mood congruent":* DSM-5, 2013, p. 825.

60 *behavior or thought is grossly impaired:* With respect to jealousy, for example, see Munro, 1999, and Soyka, Naber, and Völcker, 1991.

60 polythematic *delusions:* See Coltheart, 2013.

60 *we are not alone in this:* Persons, 1986.

60 *New York Times/CBS News poll:* Zernike and Thee-Brenan, 2010.

61 *had grown to 45 percent:* Condon, 2011.

61 *infractions the Dartmouth fans saw:* Hastorf and Cantril, 1954.

61 *the same in both cases:* Tversky and Kahneman, 1981.

61 *mind-control experiments:* See, e.g., "Abducted by Uncle Sam—Coming to a Bedroom Near You?"

61 *"fixed beliefs . . . conflicting evidence":* DSM-5, 2013, p. 87.

62 *resistant to change in the face of evidence:* See, e.g., Nickerson, 1998.

62 *"false belief . . . evidence to the contrary":* DSM-IV-TR, 2000, p. 821. DSM-IV-TR is a text revised version of DSM-IV, 1994. The definition of delusion is unchanged from DSM-IV, p. 765.

62 *nearly every condition of the definition:* See Coltheart, 2007; Davies et al., 2001.

62 *"are like sailors . . . the open sea":* Neurath, 1983, p. 92.

62 *fall into twelve broad types:* See also Stompe et al., 2003.

63 *Joseph Capgras:* Capgras and Reboul-Lachaux, 1923, 1994; Signer, 1987.

63 *often by a substantial margin:* Bentall and Udachina, 2013.

63 *haven't evolved over time:* Stompe et al., 2003.

63 *the instrument of all this mischief:* Haslam, 1988.

65 *already made by nineteenth-century psychiatry:* Berrios, 2008; see also Jaspers, 1997, pp. 58–59: "Form must be kept distinct from content which may change from time to time, e.g., the fact of a hallucination is to be distinguished from its content, whether this is a man or a tree, threatening figures or peaceful landscapes. Perceptions, ideas, judgments, feelings, drives, self-awareness, are all forms of psychic phenomena; they denote the particular mode of existence in which content is presented to us. It is true in describing concrete psychic events we take into account the particular contents of the individual psyche, but from the phenomenological point of view it is only the form that interests us."

65 *theme of the delusion its* form: See Gold and Gold, 2012. As we mention above, the distinction between form and content is an old one in psychiatry. Our version of the distinction is somewhat idiosyncratic, however; see Berrios, 2008.

65 *the chief disciple of the Buddha:* Yip, 2003.

65 *in technical terminology, "pathoplastic":* On pathoplasticity and pathogenesis—where culture *causes*, rather than shapes, mental disorder—see Tseng, 2001.

66 *microchips or the internet:* On microchips, see Eytan et al., 2002; on the internet, see Bell et al., 2005.

66 *more prevalent in Germany than in Japan:* Stompe et al., 2003.

66 *to suffer from erotomania:* Suhail, 2003.

66 *their former compatriots:* Suhail and Cochrane, 2002.

66 *regions of the same country:* Gecici et al., 2010.

66 *"puppy pregnancy":* Chowdhury et al., 2003.

66 *an anxiety disorder known as* koro: See Tseng, 2001.

66 *the inheritors of that tradition:* Simons and Hughes, 1985.

66 *in other cultures as well:* Buckle et al., 2007.

66 *optional in many cultures:* Stompe et al., 2003.

66 *the Pope, and Simpson:* Sher, 2000.

66 *"New Labour New Danger":* Kelly, 1996, p. 1385.

67 Continuation of My Cry of Distress: Krauß, 1867.

67 *"naive, agitated style . . . his sufferings":* Margaret Mahony Stoljar, personal communication.

68 *"Ah vous êtes un bon mâle!":* Ah, you are a fine man!

69 *A fine glove . . . Against love:* The original quatrain reads, in French:
Beaux atours,
Vos charmes
Sont des armes—
Contre l'amour.

71 *the psychoanalyst Victor Tausk:* Tausk had studied law and worked as a journalist, but inspired to become a psychoanalyst by Freud, he studied medicine and was one of the first psychoanalysts to take an interest in the application of Freudian theory to psychosis. Tausk read "On the origin of the 'influencing machine' in schizophrenia" to the Vienna Psychoanalytic Society in 1918 and published it in 1919. He died by his own hand shortly thereafter. The original paper is Tausk, 1919, and the English translation is Tausk, 1933.

71 *familiar to his colleagues at the time:* Tausk, 1933. We are grateful to Margaret Mahony Stoljar and Mike Jay for help with this issue.

71 *"is operated by enemies":* Tausk, 1933; all the quoted passages are from pp. 520–2.

72 *"representation of the . . . outer world":* Ibid., p. 529.

72 *Mount Sinai Hospital in New York:* Linn, 1958.

72 *"a male or at least a phallic persecutor":* Ibid.; all of the passages quoted are from pp. 206–7.

72 *"She responded . . . in evasive monosyllables":* Ibid., p. 307.

73 *Dusan Hirjak and Thomas Fuchs:* Hirjak and Fuchs, 2010; all quotes are from p. 98.

73 *a patient called Schreber:* In recent years, there has been quite a bit of interest in Schreber. He has gone from being a psychiatric patient to a cultural figure whose life is thought to illuminate a wide range of topics from philosophy, to sexuality, child abuse, anti-Semitism, and fin de siècle anxiety. The psychiatrist Zvi Lothane is the most important authority on Schreber, and we rely on his work throughout.

73 Memoirs of My Nervous Illness: A contemporary edition is Schreber, 1955.

74 *a form of influencing machine delusion:* Connor, 2008.

74 *"fleetingly improvised . . . divine miracle":* Schreber, 1955, p. 28.

NOTES

74 *"dead and rotting"*: Lothane, 1992, p. 472.

74 *"it really must be . . . succumbing to intercourse"*: Schreber, 1955, p. 46.

74 *"twisted off with a 'nerve probe' "*: Lothane, 1992, p. 472.

74 *a sign of his sexual change:* Ibid.

75 *from working as a judge:* Ibid.

75 *in print for seven years:* Ibid.

75 *although he considered doing so:* Ibid.

75 *"loved and honoured"*: Freud, 1911/1958, p. 41.

75 *a "simple formula"*: Ibid., p. 41.

75 *an "outburst of homosexual libido"*: Ibid., p. 43.

75 *unconsciously from love to hate:* Schreber's delusion of being turned into a woman is presumably a second way of denying his homosexual impulses. If he is a woman, his feelings for Flechsig are "normal." Ibid.

75 *"It may be presumed . . . delusions of persecution"*: Ibid., p. 47.

75 *model of the Capgras delusion:* See Berson, 1983; Enoch and Ball, 2001.

76 *the presence of the symptom:* Moutoussis et al., 2007.

76 *the psychologist Brendan Maher:* E.g., Maher, 1974; 1992; 1999.

77 *Hayden Ellis and Andrew Young:* Ellis and Young, 1990.

77 *"covert recognition"*: See Rivolta, Palermo, and Schmalzl, 2013.

77 *this is exactly what is found:* Ellis, et al., 1997.

77 *to leave some questions unanswered:* See, e.g., Davies et al., 2001.

78 *this explanation is wildly implausible?:* Andrew Young, personal communication, claims that upon hearing Young's account of Capgras, the philosopher Steven Stich took off his glasses and said that despite the experience of the world looking blurry, he didn't have any inclination to believe that it actually *was* blurry. See also Davies et al., 2001.

78 *a strange explanation:* See Fine, Craigie, and Gold, 2005.

78 *a delusion of shrinkage:* Ibid.

79 *that the world is gray?:* See Sacks and Wasserman, 1987; a point made to us many years ago by Jillian Craigie.

79 *disorders of reasoning:* See So et al., 2012.

79 *Todd Woodward and his colleagues:* Woodward et al., 2006.

79 *"The man has just escaped . . . guard dogs"*: Ibid., p. 608.

80 *a "jumping to conclusions" (JTC) bias:* E.g., Colbert, Peters, and Garety, 2010; Freeman et al., 2008; Garety and Freeman, 1999; Garety et al., 2005; So et al., 2012.

81 *the conflicting evidence and accept it:* The best way to make decisions like those required by the beads game is to use a fundamental principle of probability theory called "Bayes's theorem"—after the eighteenth-century cleric Thomas Bayes, who devised it. Bayes's theorem to the beads problem tells you how to decide on the probability of some event occurring based on the occurrence of other events. Given that the first bead is red, Bayes's theorem can tell you how likely it is to have come from the "red jar" as well as the likelihood that it came from the "black jar." Applying Bayes's theorem reveals that if the first two beads are red, the chances are 96.9

percent that they came from the "red jar." If you think it is rational to make a choice of jars when you are 96.9 percent confident—and that may *not* be everyone's idea of rationality—then the behavior of people with delusions accords more closely with an ideal of rationality than people without delusions. With this notion of rationality as a guide, then, it is the *healthy* participants in the experiment who have a reasoning disorder; see Maher, 1992; see also Haigh, 2012.

81 *Martin Davies and their colleagues:* Coltheart, Langdon, and McKay, 2007, 2011; Davies et al., 2001.

82 *but they know she isn't:* Davies et al., 2001.

82 *they retain "insight":* Amador and David, 2004.

82 *Daniel Freeman and his colleagues:* Freeman et al., 2007; see also Freeman and Garety, 2004.

85 *is taken by Richard Bentall:* Bentall, Kinderman, and Kaney, 1994. Bentall seems, however, to have largely abandoned this account; see Bentall and Udachina, 2013.

85 *Bentall and Sue Kaney:* Kaney and Bentall, 1989.

86 *at work in paranoia:* Bentall et al., 2001.

87 *the biology of delusion per se:* See Blackwood et al., 2001; Murray, 2011.

87 *Delusional disorder:* Munro, 1999.

87 *such as dementia:* See Ibanez-Casas and Cervilla, 2012.

87 *the amygdala and the hippocampus:* Knobel, Heinz, and Voss, 2008.

88 *the frontal lobes are frequently found:* Devinsky, 2009; Feinberg et al., 2005.

88 *a general hypothesis about schizophrenia:* Andreasen, 1999; see also Andreasen et al., 1999.

88 *a disturbance in association:* Andreasen, 1999, p. 782. Bleuler (1950, pp. 349–50) writes: "It appears as if those pathways of association and inhibition, established by experience, had lost their meaning and significance. Associations seem to take new pathways more easily, and thus no longer follow the old preferred ways, that is the logical pathways indicated by past experience."

88 *"disruption of . . . thought and action":* Andreasen, 1999, p. 784.

89 *"word salad":* DSM-5, 2013, p. 88.

89 *"flight of ideas":* Ibid., p. 128.

90 *the psychiatrist Shitij Kapur:* Kapur, 2003.

91 *the symptoms of psychosis:* For a related theory of why delusions are maintained, see Corlett et al., 2009.

91 *"are a 'top-down' . . . make sense of them":* Kapur, 2003, p. 15.

92 *the same numerical value:* Derovan, Scholem, and Idel, 2007.

92 *a son of the prophet Isaiah:* Isaiah 8:3.

93 *that many psychotic people feel:* Garrett, Stone, and Turkington, 2006.

94 The Center Cannot Hold: My Journey Through Madness: Saks, 2007.

94 An Unquiet Mind: A Memoir of Moods and Madness: Jamison, 1995.

95 *developed by Christopher Frith:* Frith, 1992; for a review, see Abu-Akel and Shamay-Tsoory, 2013.

95 *"Theory of Mind," or ToM:* see Apperly, 2011.

NOTES

95 *as young as fifteen months:* Onishi and Baillargeon, 2005.

95 *the "false belief task":* Wimmer and Perner, 1983; see also Baron-Cohen, Leslie, and Frith, 1985.

96 *people with autism have with social interactions:* Baron-Cohen, Leslie, and Frith, 1985.

98 *"designed by natural selection . . . hunter-gatherer ancestors":* Tooby and Cosmides, 2005, p. 16.

98 *the discipline of "evolutionary psychiatry":* For evolutionary psychology, see Buss, 2012; and for evolutionary psychiatry, see Brüne, 2008.

98 *Edward Hagen:* Hagen, 2008.

99 *delusions* aren't symptoms of illness: Adaptive beliefs need not be true: see McKay and Dennett, 2009.

99 *evidence for both of these claims:* See Hagen, 2008.

100 increase *your social isolation:* Delusions *do* presumably increase social bonds when they lead someone to see a psychiatrist.

100 *rare in absolute terms:* Hagen, 2008, p. 194; DSM-5, 2013, p. 92.

100 *a behavioral adaptation:* Here's a relevant contrast: angina, a symptom of heart disease, is about ten times more common than delusional disorder; see Vos et al., 2012. Assuming that adaptations are likely to be much more common than malfunctions, it's unlikely that delusional disorder is an adaptation.

100 *"social rejection . . . and adults":* Hagen, 2008, p. 187.

101 *A paranoiac psychosis . . . of the whole cosmic process:* Dick, 2002.

110 *correspondence like Ethan's:* Not that governments don't have a history of reading people's snail mail: Lepore, 2013.

111 *"psychological distance . . . to everyone else":* Humphrey, 2007, p. 748.

111 *"the otherness of other people":* Ibid, p. 748.

CHAPTER 3

115 *the anthropologist Pascal Boyer:* Boyer, 2001.

116 *no less powerful:* Kopytoff, 1971.

116 *can also be grandiose:* One remarkable psychotic disorder with grandiose religious delusions as a central symptom is known as Jerusalem syndrome and occurs in visitors to the Holy City. Many of the people who develop the syndrome are actively psychotic, or in the prodromal stage of psychosis, and come to Jerusalem as part of a delusional mission. There is some evidence, however, that there are cases of "pure" Jerusalem syndrome in which people with no prior illness become psychotic shortly after arriving in the city. According to Yair Bar-El and his colleagues (2000), who have studied many of these patients, they go through a characteristic series of stages in a fixed order. These include feeling a growing anxiety; having a desire to leave their travel companions; developing an obsession with cleanliness; making a "toga-like" gown, sometimes out of bed linen; shouting biblical verses or singing spiritual

songs; marching to a holy site; and delivering a sermon that calls for people to live a better life. The psychotic episode usually lasts for about a week and then appears to resolve completely. Of the forty-two cases reported by Bar-El and his colleagues, forty were Protestants who came from deeply religious families, one was a Catholic, and one was a Jew who had lived as a Protestant during World War II. The Bible had played a significant role in the lives of all of the patients.

116 *"I could find . . . I can fly"*: Knowles, McCarthy-Jones, and Rowse, 2011; all quotes are from p. 685.

116 *invitations to be cared for:* See, e.g., Kirmayer and Young, 1998.

117 *the Fregoli delusion:* Mojtabai, 1994.

117 *at work and at home:* Horan, Lee, and Green, 2013.

118 *A large body of research:* Roberts and Penn, 2013.

118 *function successfully in a social group:* Couture and Penn, 2013.

118 *social roles and expectations:* Addington and Piskulic, 2013.

118 *imitating, and experiencing emotion:* For a review, see Kohler et al., 2010; and Kohler, Hanson, and Marsh, 2013.

118 *differ in attributional style:* For a review, see Bentall and Udachina, 2013.

118 *(ToM) is impaired in schizophrenia:* For a review, see Abu-Akel and Shamay-Tsoory, 2013.

118 *A recent meta-analysis:* Bora, Yucel, and Pantelis, 2009.

118 *the "hinting task":* Corcoran, Mercer, and Frith, 1995.

118 *"Paul has to go . . . Jane to do?"*: Ibid., p. 12.

119 *the Reading the Mind in the Eyes test:* Baron-Cohen et al., 2001.

120 *Christian Kohler and his colleagues:* Kohler et al., 2010.

120 *Amy Pinkham and her colleagues:* Pinkham et al., 2011.

120 *faces expressing other emotions:* For this and threat perception in psychosis, see the review of Green and Phillips, 2004.

120 *scan angry faces in a unique way:* Green and Phillips, 2004.

120 *threatening facial features:* Green, Williams, and Davidson, 2003a; b.

120 *Melissa Green and Mary Phillips:* Green and Phillips, 2004.

121 *Abbie Coy and Samuel Hutton:* Coy and Hutton, 2013.

121 *sentences contained in passages of text:* Kaney et al., 1992.

121 *emotionally neutral ones:* Bentall, Kaney, and Bowen-Jones, 1995.

121 *words expressing threats:* Bentall and Kaney, 1989.

121 *Katherine Newman Taylor and Luisa Stopa:* Newman Taylor and Stopa, 2013.

121 *negatively evaluated by others:* DSM-5, 2013, p. 202.

122 *show a similar impairment:* Amminger et al., 2012.

122 *Kimmy Kee and her colleagues:* Kee et al., 2004.

122 *immigration, and city living:* This does not mean, of course, that these factors do not contribute to other forms of mental disorder as well. The evidence, however, is not as clear as it is in the case of psychosis; see, for example, Galea et al., 2005; Lofors and Sundquist, 2007; Magnusson et al., 2012; Silver, Mulvey, and Swanson, 2002; Weich et al., 2003; and Weich et al., 2004.

NOTES

122   *"On the Significance . . . Dementia Praecox"*: Abraham, 1907/1955.

122   *paid attention to child abuse:* Read et al., 2005.

122   *John Read and his colleagues:* Ibid.

122   *reported physical abuse:* Morgan and Fisher, 2007.

122   *25 percent physical abuse:* May-Chahal and Cawson, 2005.

122   *abuse before age sixteen:* Janssen et al., 2004.

122   *risk of developing a psychotic disorder:* The facts about risk are sometimes reported in terms of "relative risk" and sometimes as "odds ratios." Odds ratios are not precisely equivalent to relative risks, but in many contexts (such as the present one) are nearly the same. For the sake of simplicity, therefore, we ignore these statistical subtleties in the text. See Davies, Crombie, and Tavakoli, 1998.

123   *cases that involved penetration:* Cutajar et al., 2010.

123   *the mother but not the father:* Fisher et al., 2010.

123   *had experienced the greater trauma:* Heins et al., 2011.

123   *psychosis due to childhood adversity:* Varese et al., 2012.

123   *said they had been bullied:* Kelleher et al., 2013.

123   *ALSPAC:* Schreier et al., 2009.

123   *are at particularly high risk:* Kelleher et al., 2013.

124   *the results were unchanged:* See also Arseneault et al., 2011; Bebbington et al., 2004; Lataster et al., 2006.

124   *(SEYLE) study:* Kelleher et al., 2013.

124   *psychotic symptoms in the child:* Morgan et al., 2007.

124   *a single-parent household:* Wicks et al., 2005.

124   *in the care of social services:* Bebbington et al., 2004.

124   *whether the birth was wanted or not:* McNeil et al., 2009.

125   *with and without schizophrenia-spectrum disorders:* Tienari et al., 2004.

125   *cardiovascular disease, and diabetes:* See Yang et al., 2013, and the references therein.

125   *why should psychosis be different?:* See Tienari and Wahlberg, 2008.

125   *"expressed emotion" (EE) on the course of schizophrenia:* Kingdon and Turkington, 2005; McCreadie and Robinson, 1987.

126   *more likely to suffer a relapse:* Bebbington and Kuipers, 1994.

126   *"this behavior . . . a psychotic illness":* Haddock and Spaulding, 2011, p. 674.

126   *critical of the person with schizophrenia:* Docherty, Cutting, and Bers, 1998.

126   *have a tendency to feel guilty:* Bentsen et al., 1998.

126   *independent of medication compliance:* Falloon et al., 1985.

126   *a 78 percent rate at two years:* Leff et al., 1985. Lowered EE included less "face-to-face" time patients spent with their families. Although the lower EE group had far lower relapse rates, two of the low EE patients committed suicide.

126   *Norwegian immigrants to the United States:* Ødegaard, 1932.

127   *Denmark, Australia, and Canada:* Bourque, van der Ven, and Malla, 2011.

127   *perinatal complications:* Kendell, Juszcak, and Cole, 1996; Shrivastava et al., 2013.

127   *their risk of psychotic disorder:* Veling et al., 2011.

NOTES

127 *healthier than the native population:* Marmot, 2004.

127 *much less clear or consistent:* Kirkbride and Jones, 2008.

127 *hasn't been supported by the data:* Selten, Cantor-Graae, and Kahn, 2007.

127 *more likely to use cannabis:* Veen et al., 2002.

127 *mixed urban-rural regions:* Bourque, van der Ven, and Malla, 2011.

127 *what makes immigration psychologically toxic:* See McKenzie, Fearon, and Hutchinson, 2008.

128 *Bangladeshis to the United Kingdom:* Coid et al., 2008; Fearon et al., 2006; King et al., 1994.

128 *Moroccans and Turks to the Netherlands:* Hanoeman, Selten, and Kahn, 2002; Selten et al., 2002; Veling et al., 2007.

128 *Africans to Sweden:* Zolkowska, Cantor-Graae, and McNeil, 2001.

128 *United Kingdom, and New Zealand:* McGrath et al., 2001.

128 *European immigrants to Israel:* Corcoran et al., 2009b.

128 *likely to face discrimination:* For the study of Ethiopian immigrants to Israel, see Weiser et al., 2008; for other communities, see Werbeloff, Levine, and Rabinowitz, 2012.

128 *might explain the immigrant effect:* See McGrath, 1999.

128 *vitamin D deficiency:* McGillivray et al., 2007.

128 *have dark skin:* E.g., Smith et al., 2006; see Bourque, van der Ven, and Malla, 2011.

129 *communities in The Hague:* Veling et al., 2007.

129 *over a three-year period:* Janssen et al., 2003.

131 *first-episode psychosis in Chicago:* Faris and Dunham, 1965.

131 *rates of psychosis higher in London:* Kirkbride et al., 2006.

131 *Brixton and Camberwell:* Kirkbride, Fearon et al., 2007.

131 *A 2004 review:* McGrath et al., 2004.

131 *an almost linear fashion:* Vassos et al., 2012.

132 *the greater the risk:* Pedersen and Mortensen, 2001.

132 *would count as rural areas today:* Torrey, Bowler, and Clark, 1997; see Boydell and McKenzie, 2008.

132 *it gets called depression:* Durà-Vilà, Littlewood, and Leavey, 2013.

132 *psychosis represents the extremes:* van Os, Hanssen et al., 2000.

132 *with no will of their own:* Peters et al., 2004.

132 *the more such symptoms were found:* van Os et al., 2001.

132 *the "social drift" hypothesis:* See March et al., 2008.

132 *movement in the other direction lowered it:* Pedersen and Mortensen, 2001.

133 *before the onset of illness:* Dauncey et al., 1993.

133 *under conditions of stress:* Lederbogen et al., 2011.

133 *has been done in Copenhagen:* Mortensen et al., 1999; Pedersen and Mortensen, 2001.

133 *by* Monocle *magazine:* Bloomfield and Booth, 2013.

134 *we will leave it aside:* See Johnson et al., 2013.

134 *linked to schizophrenia in offspring:* Brown et al., 2004.

NOTES

134 *higher rates of the disorder:* Battle et al., 1999; Mednick et al., 1988.

134 *increases viral transmission:* Takei et al., 1992.

134 *raise the risk of psychosis:* Shrivastava et al., 2013.

134 *those living in the countryside:* Kuepper et al., 2011.

134 *the urban effect:* Kirkbride, Fearon et al., 2007; Kirkbride, Morgan et al., 2007.

134 *more people live alone:* van Os, Driessen et al., 2000.

134 *for only short periods:* Giggs, 1986; Silver, Mulvey, and Swanson, 2002.

134 *compared to the least fragmented:* Allardyce et al., 2005. It is not inconceivable that people with schizophrenia, or those who are disposed to it, drift into more fragmented neighborhoods.

135 *"social fragmentation . . . brought up in cities":* Zammit et al., 2010, p. 919.

135 *and indeed countries:* For neighborhoods, see Kirkbride et al., 2014; and for countries, see Burns, Tomita, and Kapadia, 2013.

135 *turn out to vote locally:* Kirkbride, Morgan et al., 2007.

135 *neighborhoods with lower ethnic density:* Boydell et al., 2001.

135 *an increased rate of psychosis:* Kirkbride et al., 2008.

135 *Veling and his colleagues:* Veling et al., 2007.

135 *independent of socioeconomic status (SES):* Kirkbride et al., 2008.

136 *over sixteen years:* Bresnahan et al., 2007.

136 *on the basis of race alone:* See Neighbors et al., 2003.

136 *for those most disadvantaged:* Corcoran et al., 2009a.

136 *"social defeat":* Selton and Cantor-Graae, 2005.

136 *submissive behavior or social defeat:* Tidey and Miczek, 1996.

136 *"By social defeat . . . subordinates them":* Luhrmann, 2007, p. 151.

137 *effects of this form of stress:* E.g., Powell, Tarr, and Sheridan, 2013.

137 *to enhance the effect:* Tidey and Miczek, 1996.

140 *81 of 179:* Hollingshead and Redlich, 1958.

140 *protects against premature death:* Antonovsky, 1967.

140 *life expectancy increased dramatically:* Phelan, Link, and Tehranifar, 2010.

140 *African American babies compared to whites:* Dunkel Schetter and Glynn, 2011.

140 *no different in birth weight:* David and Collins, 1997.

141 *very-low-birth-weight (VLBW) infants:* Collins, Herman, and David, 1997; see also Dunlop et al., 2011; Rowley, 1994.

141 *because of their race:* Collins et al., 2004.

141 *by a year and a half:* Murray et al., 1998, cited in Marmot, 2004.

142 *Whitehall I and Whitehall II:* See, e.g., Rose and Marmot, 1981. Our discussion follows Marmot, 2004.

143 *better health than the poor Swede:* Wilkinson, 1997.

143 *the gap between richest and poorest:* Kawachi, Kennedy, and Wilkinson, 1999.

143 *large social inequalities:* Wilkinson, 1999; Wilkinson, 2001; Wilkinson and Marmot, 2003.

144 *as well as its health:* Sapolsky, 2004.

144 *a say in the battle plan:* Ibid.

144 *suppression of the immune system:* Ibid. and the references therein.

146 *the "vulnerability" model:* Zubin and Spring, 1977.

147 *delusions in later life:* Bentall and Fernyhough, 2008.

147 *John Farhall, and Ben Ong:* Goldstone, Farhall, and Ong, 2011.

148 *known as the striatum:* Howes and Kapur, 2009.

148 *"final common pathway":* Ibid.

148 *significantly affected by stress:* Aiello et al., 2012.

148 *model of psychosis might look like:* Walker and Diforio, 1997; Walker, Mittal, and Tessner, 2008.

148 *Maria-de-Gracia Dominguez and her colleagues:* Dominguez et al., 2011; Cougnard et al., 2007.

149 *runs as follows:* van Winkel, Stefanis, and Myin-Germeys, 2008.

149 *including in the brain:* For an overview, see Goldberg, Allis, and Bernstein, 2007.

149 *the social world alters brain function:* Toyokawa et al., 2012.

149 *the mechanisms of this process:* Weaver et al., 2004.

150 *something similar in humans:* McGowan et al., 2009.

150 *epigenetic differences in people with psychosis:* Labrie, Pai, and Petronis, 2012.

150 *"gets under the skin":* Galea, Uddin, and Koenen, 2011, p. 400.

155 *disease a patient has:* This saying is also frequently attributed to William Osler.

CHAPTER 4

157 *Interviewer . . . a skull over the genitals!:* Brooks and Reiner, 2009.

158 *Primates, humans included, have big brains:* See Dunbar and Shultz, 2007.

158 *2 percent of its weight:* Raichle and Gusnard, 2002.

158 *social group size for that species:* Group size appears to be the most important feature, but not necessarily the only one. Diet, for example, may also have been a secondary pressure on brain size; Barton, 1996.

158 *The bigger the neocortex:* Dunbar, 1998; see also Dunbar, 1993.

158 *than other brain areas:* Dunbar 2013; Finlay and Darlington, 1995.

158 *traditional villages:* Dunbar, 1993.

158 *the "social brain hypothesis":* For a discussion of the brain regions that seem to be devoted to social function, see Bauman et al., 2011.

158 *defense against predators:* Dunbar, 1988.

158 *out of reach for individuals:* Dunbar and Shultz, 2007.

159 *relatively solitary animals:* See Neuberg, Kenrick, and Schaller, 2011.

159 *hell is other people:* Sartre, 1956.

159 *perspective taking:* See, e.g., May and Wendt, 2013.

159 *"at times of great social or financial trouble":* Stiller and Dunbar, 2007, p. 100; see also Lewis et al., 2011.

160 *"of a free . . . As asses are:* Othello, I.iii.400–403.

160 *exploitation becomes widely known:* Buss and Duntley, 2008.

NOTES

160 *Steven Pinker:* Pinker, 2011.

160 *Robert Muchembled:* Muchembled, 2012.

160 *even the quite recent past:* We're grateful to Ralph Adolphs for this observation.

160 *with a scattering of exceptions:* See, e.g., Mitchell and Thompson, 1986.

161 *in love with Cassio:* Othello, III.iii.337–345.

161 Catch Me If You Can: Spielberg, 2002.

162 *Columbo: By the Book:* Spielberg, 1971.

162 *the use of tactical deception:* Byrne and Corp, 2004.

162 *characterization of chimpanzee behavior:* de Waal, 1998.

162 *the "Machiavellian intelligence hypothesis":* Byrne and Whiten, 1988; Whiten and Byrne, 1997. For an earlier proposal along the same lines, see Chance and Mead, 1953; Humphrey, 1976; and Jolly, 1966.

162 *the very possibility of cooperation:* Dunbar, 2004.

162 *"free riding":* Enquist and Leimar, 1993.

163 *protecting themselves against them:* Neuberg, Kenrick, and Schaller, 2011.

163 *one of these defenses:* See also Dunbar, 2004.

163 *their malicious intents:* For a similar view directed at obsessive-compulsive disorder, see Boyer and Liénard, 2006.

163 *a number of investigators in evolutionary psychiatry:* See, e.g., Flannelly et al., 2007; Gilbert, 1993; Green and Phillips, 2004; Walston, David and Charlton, 1998; Zolotova and Brüne, 2006.

163 *trial and error is too high:* See Woody and Szechtman, 2011.

164 *are deeply ambiguous:* Blanchard et al., 2011.

164 *on the side of caution:* Haselton and Nettle, 2006.

164 *not easily learned:* Ullman, Harari, and Dorfman, 2012.

164 *the direction of someone's gaze:* Emery, 2000.

164 *reading emotion in faces:* Baron-Cohen et al., 1996.

164 *perceiving body movements:* Simion, Regolin, and Bulf, 2008.

164 *interpreting hand orientation:* Tessari et al., 2012.

164 *suspicion of infidelity is called jealousy:* see Buss, 2000.

165 *missing a real threat:* Haselton and Nettle, 2006.

165 *Other people's intentions to harm you:* For the relation between persecutory delusions and Theory of Mind, see Walston, Blennerhassett and Charlton, 2000.

166 *take defensive action:* Neuberg, Kenrick, and Schaller, 2011.

169 *attributed to the Unabomber:* All details and quotes are from Sally Johnson's report of her forensic psychiatric evaluation of Theodore Kaczynski, January 16, 1998. A redacted copy of the report was unsealed by the court on September 11, 1998.

169 *"just so" stories:* The phrase is a play on Rudyard Kipling's *Just So Stories.* It appears to have first been used as a disparaging description of an evolutionary explanation by Stephen Jay Gould; see Gould, 1978.

170 *looked more competent:* Todorov et al., 2005.

170 *less accurate at predicting the outcome of the election:* Todorov and Charles Ballew: Ballew & Todorov, 2007.

NOTES

170 *judgments about social threat:* Indeed, a rich source of social information generally; see Adams et al., 2013.

170 *investigated this psychological process:* Todorov, 2008; Todorov, Pakrashi, and Oosterhof, 2009; see also Oosterhof and Todorov, 2008.

170 *longer than one sixth of a second:* At least some types of eye movements: see Kojima, Soetedjo, and Fuchs, 2010.

170 *made in a single glance:* That we make judgments of trustworthiness doesn't mean, of course, that they are accurate.

171 *further supports this idea:* Bar, Neta, and Linz, 2006.

171 *more quickly than, trustworthiness:* Locher et al., 1993; Todorov, Pakrashi, and Oosterhof, 2009.

172 *the amygdala:* We rely here on Buchanan, Tranel, and Adolphs, 2009.

172 *fear responses of some kind:* Davis and Whalen, 2001.

172 *seeking out social activity:* Dicks, Myers, and Kling, 1969.

172 *"retarded in their ability . . . dangerous confrontations":* Ibid., p. 71.

173 *dangers in the social environment:* Bauman et al., 2004.

173 *the social character of the amygdala:* Adams et al., 2013.

173 *put you in particular at risk:* Adams et al., 2013.

173 *two . . . are connected to the amygdala:* Bickart et al., 2011, 2012.

173 *in both brain hemispheres:* Tranel, and Hyman, 1990.

173 *a mild "executive function" impairment:* Elliott, 2003.

173 *recognize fear in faces:* Adolphs et al., 1994.

173 *other emotional states:* Buchanan, Tranel, and Adolphs, 2009.

174 *throughout the experiment:* Feinstein et al., 2011.

174 *"trustworthiness" and "approachability":* Adolphs, Tranel, and Damasio, 1998.

174 *"she did not . . . distrust and 'danger'":* Buchanan, Tranel, and Adolphs, 2009, p. 310.

174 *"she tends to 'trust' . . . more wary of strangers":* Ibid., p. 301.

174 *she doesn't look for them:* Ibid.

175 *anterior cingulate cortex and the insula:* McNaughton and Corr, 2004; Fiddick, 2011; Schlund et al., 2013. Recall that part of the anterior cingulate cortex is the region found by Lederbogen et al., 2011, to be salient.

175 *interactions with other people:* Ames, Fiske, and Todorov, 2011.

176 *addressing gaze perception:* A. Cooper and A. Puce, unpublished data described in Puce and Perrett, 2003.

177 *making gestures and expressing emotions:* An experiment of Wheaton, Aranda, and Puce, 2002, described in Puce and Perrett, 2003.

178 *signal dissembling or deception:* Rossini, 2011.

178 *evidence is available:* See Abu-Akel and Shamay-Tsoory, 2013.

178 *a "worldwide game":* Hall, 2011a.

178 *"is a good thing . . . what I have done":* Ibid.

179 *"believed President Obama . . . on television":* Levine and Goldman, 2013.

179 *Recent mass shootings:* Mayors Against Illegal Guns, 2013.

NOTES

179 *a medical professional was made aware:* Ibid.
179 *involuntary hospitalization be strengthened:* Hall, 2011b.
179 *predicting who will:* Swanson, 2008.
179 *threat/control-override (TCO) symptoms:* Link and Stueve, 1994.
179 *Threat/Control-Override Questionnaire:* Nederlof, Muris, and Hovens, 2011.
180 *supported these findings:* Swanson et al., 1996.
180 *with control-override symptoms:* Stompe, Ortwein-Swoboda, and Schanda, 2004.
180 *no delusions did:* Appelbaum, Robbins, and Monahan, 2000.
180 *"Although delusions can precipitate . . . discharge from hospitalization":* Ibid., p. 566.
180 *who had no delusions:* Swanson et al., 2006.
180 *antisocial personality disorder:* Swanson, 2013.
180 *increased risk for serious violence:* Coid et al., 2013.
181 *electromagnetic radiation:* Hermann and Marimow, 2013.
181 *a "microwave machine":* Gabriel, Goldstein, and Schmidt, 2013.
181 *"angry outbursts":* Schmidt, 2013.
181 *"after 'multiple' disciplinary breaches":* Foster and Sanchez, 2013.
181 *"anger-fueled 'blackout' ":* Ibid.
181 *disorderly conduct:* Vargas, Hendrix, and Fisher, 2013.
181 *narrowly missing his neighbor:* "Incident Report from Aaron Alexis's 2010 Arrest," 2013.
181 *are never violent:* Swanson, 1994.
182 *consciously engaged in problem-solving:* There is a substantial literature on dual process theories in psychology. For good introductions, see Evans, 2008; 2010; and Kahneman, 2011; and for a historical overview, see Frankish and Evans, 2009. Unlike some theorists, we believe that there are multiple systems that deserve the title "System 1." The Suspicion System is only one of them.
182 *decision making, and social cognition:* See Evans, 2008.
182 *taken to be "modular":* See Ibid.
182 *narrow cognitive domains:* Fodor, 1983; see also Coltheart, 1999. For the sake of simplicity, we ignore the theoretical questions concerning the relation between modularity and dual process theory; see, e.g., Eraña, 2012.
184 *the well-known Müller-Lyer illusion:* The Müller-Lyer illusion is a very simple case, of course, and not representative of all of vision. Informational encapsulation comes in degrees, and some aspects of visual function are influenced by mental processes external to it.

CHAPTER 5

191 *"clinical levels . . . the human species":* Green and Phillips, 2004, p. 333; see also Zolotova and Brüne, 2006.
192 *more sex and more children:* Hopcroft, 2006.
192 *inversely correlated with intelligence:* Ibid.
192 *does not recognize the difference:* Boyer, 2001.

193 *causing another person's behavior:* Simon, 1957, p. 5.

193 *"I'll pour this pestilence into his ear":* Othello, II.iii.350.

194 *to initiate defensive action:* In evolutionary terms, its purpose is to increase fitness.

194 *Many animals use this tactic:* Eibl-Eibesfeldt, 1970.

194 *status or rank:* Bentall and Udachina, 2013.

194 *defeat one large one:* Hagen, 2008.

195 *higher social rank than she does:* Enoch and Ball, 2001, chapter 2.

195 *were in love with her:* Ibid.

195 *Paul McCartney:* Ibid.

195 *women of "considerable age":* Hart, 1912, p. 122.

195 *to enhance their status:* McCutcheon et al., 2003.

196 *emotional involvement:* Buss, 2000.

196 *in love with another woman:* Ibid.

196 *as in normal jealousy:* Schipper, Easton, and Shackleford, 2007.

196 *no systematic research:* But see, e.g., Walston, David, and Charlton, 1998.

196 *observed in other animals:* Eibl-Eibesfeldt, 1970.

197 *risks of social living:* See Neuberg, Kenrick, and Schaller, 2011; Nunn and Altizer, 2006, chapter 6; Schaller, 2011.

197 *the most important of these:* Wible, 2012; Young, Dodell-Feder, and Saxe, 2010.

200 *many others are simply bizarre:* See Cermolacce, Sass, and Parnas, 2010.

200 *a dual process approach to delusion:* See Speechley and Ngan, 2008; see also Asp and Tranel, 2013.

200 *the Reflective System:* We mean to stay noncommittal about what this system is like beyond saying that it is a form of System 2 cognition. For a theoretical use of the term "reflective" in the context of dual process theories, see Stanovich, 2009.

200 *information available elsewhere in the mind:* In an prescient parallel, Freud posited a primary and a secondary process. The primary process is a system generated by the id, exists in the unconscious and is governed by the pleasure principle. Primary process thought is illogical: there is no cause and effect, no time. Primary process is expressed in dreams, and is observed in the thought of young children and in people with psychosis. When thought enters into consciousness, it is faced with the reality principle. The ego's secondary process system edits, organizes, and imbues thought with logic. We might think of the primary and secondary processes as psychoanalytic systems 1 and 2. See Freud, 1920/1955.

201 *and the delusion persists:* For a closely related account, see Asp and Tranel, 2013.

202 *the prodromal phase of schizophrenia:* Yung and McGorry, 1996.

202 *retain "insight":* Amador and David, 2004.

202 *"I would think . . . impossible to be done":* Halligan and Marshall, 1996, p. 258.

203 *normal reasoning about abnormal states:* Notice that when we say that the Reflective System integrates delusional ideas with other thoughts, it's not doing so in a normal fashion. The direct functional connection between the Suspicion System and the Reflective System is broken in delusion. But as we've said, the Reflective System gets access to the delusional idea once it enters thought. As a result, it

doesn't treat that thought as it would if it had access to it from the Suspicion System. Its job now is not to evaluate it, and perhaps reject it, but to make the best sense of it that it can.

203 *she's a clone:* Silva et al., 1989.

203 *the Suspicion System is functioning normally:* We owe this point to Kengo Miyazono; see McKay and Dennett, 2009.

204 *is fundamentally arbitrary:* Many of the details of the theory have been left out of our account; see Gold, forthcoming; and Gold, forthcoming.

204 *the "daily hassles":* See Kanner et al., 1981.

205 *a fear of future repetitions:* See Macdonald et al., 2012.

205 *more dangerous than small ones:* Fisher, 2012.

205 *a cause of schizophrenia:* Schomerus et al., 2008.

205 *"subjective sense of safety":* Ibid., p. 595.

206 *the limits of ToM:* Lewis et al., 2011.

206 *toxic enough to shorten your life:* Marmot, 2004.

207 *security cameras in Lower Manhattan:* Palmer, 2010.

207 *CCTV cameras in Britain:* Barrett, 2013.

207 *between 2009 and 2010:* Cohen, 2011.

207 *information as to their whereabouts:* Angwin and Valentino-Devries, 2011.

207 *psychotic later in life:* Martin, 2006.

207 *the orders of J. Edgar Hoover:* Hotchner, 2011.

208 *shortly after the story broke:* Amit Rajparia, MD, personal communication.

208 *top-secret clearance:* Bacon and Welch, 2013.

208 *had never been psychotic:* Jillian Copeland, MD, personal communication.

209 *"Knowledge works as a tool of power":* Nietzsche, 1968, p. 266.

209 *"it is the greatest . . . right and wrong":* Bentham, 1843a, p. 394.

210 *"new mode of obtaining power . . . without example":* Bentham, 1889, p. 93.

210 *The Panopticon:* see Steadman, 2007.

210 *"apparent omnipresence . . . real presence":* Bentham, 1843b, p. 45.

210 *"radial" prisons designed by others:* Steadman, 2007.

210 *He [the prisoner] . . . functioning of power:* Foucault, 1995, pp. 200–201.

211 *"lighter, more rapid . . . a society to come":* Ibid., p. 209.

211 *theory of the Panopticon is controversial:* See Semple, 1992.

211 *Surveillance is becoming pervasive:* Ball, Haggerty, and Lyon, 2012.

211 *to watch one another:* See, e.g., Rennie, 2008.

211 *"Act amends . . . record subjects":* Regan, 2004, p. 482.

212 *the loss of privacy is a serious threat:* Other animals may also have a need for privacy: see Klopfer and Rubenstein, 1977.

212 *half the story of contemporary culture:* Mathiesen, 1997.

213 *"[e]very age gets the lunatics it deserves":* Porter, 1991, p. 73.

213 *Rehtaeh Parsons:* "Rehtaeh Parsons, Canadian Girl, Dies After Suicide Attempt; Parents Allege She Was Raped by 4 Boys," 2013.

NOTES

CHAPTER 6

219 *"imagined communities"*: Anderson, 2006.

219 *"The main difficulty . . . the concept of a city"*: Boydell and McKenzie, 2008, p. 91.

220 *the FBI's priorities:* see http://www.fbi.gov/about-us/investigate/cyber, consulted February 3, 2014.

220 *"It's a good life, if you don't weaken":* The title of a graphic novel by Seth, 2003; also the title of a song by The Tragically Hip, 2002. With "great" in place of "good," it can be found in Buchan, 1927, p. 105.

220 *The air pollution in Shizuoka:* Yorifuji et al., 2013.

220 *about 70 cell phones:* See http://www.nationmaster.com/graph/med_per_com_percap-media-personal-computers-per-capita; and http://www.nationmaster.com/graph/med_tel_mob_cel_percap-telephones-mobile-cellular-per-capita, consulted March 7, 2014.

220 *"felt that they . . . over the web":* Nitzan et al., 2011, p. 210.

221 *Derek Dean and Andrea Pelletier:* Mittal, Dean, and Pelletier, 2013.

221 *"internet addiction" and brain abnormalities:* Lin et al., 2012.

221 *brain regions implicated in schizophrenia:* Yuan et al., 2011.

224 *psychiatric complaints, including psychosis:* Dobson, 2010; Tarrier et al., 2000; Winston, Rosenthal, and Pinsker, 2012.

224 *improve their overall functioning:* Winston, Rosenthal, and Pinsker, 2012.

224 *"the large-scale application . . . direct suggestion":* Freud, 1919/1955, p. 168.

224 *"whatever form this psychotherapy . . . untendentious psycho-analysis":* Ibid., p. 168.

225 *the negative symptoms of schizophrenia:* Rector and Beck, 2012; Wykes et al., 2008; Zimmermann et al., 2005.

225 *National Institute for Health and Care Excellence:* www.nice.org.uk; for the guidelines on schizophrenia and psychosis, see http://guidance.nice.org.uk/CG178/NICEGuidance/pdf/English, consulted March 10, 2014.

225 *updated its recommendations in a similar fashion:* Dixon et al., 2010.

225 *play a role in recovery:* Chadwick, Birchwood, and Trower, 1996.

225 *a healing force on its own:* Glover, 1931; Winston, Rosenthal, and Pinsker, 2012.

225 *(SoCRATES) trial:* Lewis et al., 2002.

225 *"Good relationships . . . effective psychiatric care":* Bentall, 2009, p. 260.

226 *lived with psychosis for most of her life:* Saks, 2011.

226 *[P]sychoanalysis has helped me. . . . the bad and ugly:* Saks, 2011, p. 68.

229 *it mostly didn't exist:* Freud believed that the substrate of psychoanalysis would ultimately be found to be the brain. The year before he died, Freud wrote: "But here we are concerned with therapy only in so far as it works by psychological means; and for the time being we have no other. The future may teach us to exercise a direct influence, by means of particular chemical substances, on the amounts of energy and their distribution in the mental apparatus. It may be that there are other still undreamt-of possibilities of therapy. But for the moment we have nothing better at

our disposal than the technique of psycho-analysis, and for that reason, in spite of its limitations, it should not be despised"(Freud, 1938/1964, p. 182).

229 *none of whom can prescribe medication:* Psychologists are permitted to prescribe medication in New Mexico, Louisiana, and Guam.

230 *an application of brain science:* See note above beginning *it mostly didn't exist.*

230 *Promote Discovery ... neurobiological measures:* "NIMH: Strategic Research Priorities," 2008: http://www.nimh.nih.gov/research-priorities/strategic-objectives/strategic-objective-1.shtml, consulted March 10, 2014.

231 *conception of science known as* reductionism: Bickle, 1998; Churchland and Churchland, 1994; Nagel, 1979.

232 *atoms in the void:* the phrase is that of the Greek philosopher Democritus: "By convention sweet and by convention bitter, by convention hot, by convention cold, by convention colour; but in reality atoms and void" (Taylor, 1999, p. 9).

232 *"there is little hard evidence ... for the TOEs":* Maudlin, 1996, p. 143.

233 *a different level of physical organization:* Fodor, 1997; Gold and Stoljar, 1999.

233 *"humans are part ... their intelligence in principle":* Chomsky, 1988, p. 149.

234 *patterns in the universe will be found:* See Fodor, 1974; 1997.

243 *nothing in biology makes sense:* Dobzhansky, 1973.

BIBLIOGRAPHY

"Abducted by Uncle Sam—Coming to a Bedroom Near You?" Above Top Secret. http://www.abovetopsecret.com/forum/thread982091/pg1. Consulted November 14, 2013.

Abraham K. 1907/1955. "On the significance of sexual trauma in childhood for the symptomatology of dementia praecox." In *Clinical Papers and Essays on Psycho-Analysis*. Translated by H Abraham. 13–20. London: Hogarth Press and the Institute of Psycho-Analysis.

Abu-Akel A, S Shamay-Tsoory. 2013. "Characteristics of theory of mind impairments in schizophrenia." In *Social Cognition in Schizophrenia*. Edited by D Roberts, D Penn. 196–214. Oxford: Oxford University Press.

Adams R, N Ambady, K Nakaya, S Shimojo, eds. 2011. *The Science of Social Vision*. Oxford: Oxford University Press.

Adams R, R Franklin, K Kveraga, N Ambady, R Kleck, P Whalen, N Hadjikhani, A Nelson. 2012. "Amygdala responses to averted vs. direct gaze fear vary as a function of presentation speed." *Social Cognitive and Affective Neuroscience* 7: 568–77.

Addington J. April 25, 2008. "Early identification and intervention: strategies in schizophrenia." Talk given at NYU Schizophrenia Conference: Applying New Research Findings to Clinical Practice.

Addington J, D Piskulic. 2013. "Social cognition early in the course of the illness." In *Social Cognition in Schizophrenia*. Edited by D Roberts, D Penn, 245–62. Oxford: Oxford University Press.

Adolphs R, F Gosselin, T Buchanan, D Tranel, P Schyns, A Damasio. 2005. "A mechanism for impaired fear recognition after amygdala damage." *Nature* 433: 68–72.

Adolphs R, D Tranel, A Damasio. 1998. "The human amygdala in social judgment." *Nature* 393: 470–74.

Adolphs R, D Tranel, H Damasio, A Damasio. 1994. "Impaired recognition of emotion in facial expressions following bilateral damage to the human amygdala." *Nature* 372: 669–72.

Aiello G, M Horowitz, N Hepgul, C Pariante, V Mondelli. 2012. "Stress abnormalities in individuals at risk for psychosis: a review of studies in subjects with familial risk or with 'at risk' mental state." *Psychoneuroendocrinology* 37: 1600–13.

BIBLIOGRAPHY

Allardyce J, H Gilmour, J Atkinson, T Rapson, J Bishop, R McCreadie. 2005. "Social fragmentation, deprivation and urbanicity: relation to first-admission rates for psychoses." *British Journal of Psychiatry* 187: 401–6.

Amador X, A David, eds. 2004. *Insight and Psychosis,* 2nd ed. Oxford: Oxford University Press.

Ames D, S Fiske, A Todorov. 2011. "Impression formation: a focus on others' intents." In *The Oxford Handbook of Social Neuroscience.* Edited by J Decety, J Cacioppo. 419–33. New York: Oxford University Press.

Amminger G, M Schäfer, K Papageorgiou, C Klier, M Schlögelhofer, N Mossaheb, S Werneck-Rohrer, B Nelson, P McGorry. 2012. "Emotion recognition in individuals at clinical high-risk for schizophrenia." *Schizophrenia Bulletin* 38: 1030–39.

Anderson B. 2006. *Imagined Communities.* London: Verso.

Andreasen N. 1999. "A unitary model of schizophrenia: Bleuler's 'fragmented phrene' as schizencephaly." *Archives of General Psychiatry* 56: 781–87.

Andreasen N. 2001. *Brave New Brain: Conquering Mental Illness in the Era of the Genome.* New York: Oxford University Press.

Andreasen N. 2011. "Concept of schizophrenia: past, present, and future." In *Schizophrenia*, 3rd ed. Edited by D Weinberger, P Harrison. 3–8. Oxford: Wiley-Blackwell.

Andreasen N, P Nopoulos, D O'Leary, D Miller, T Wassink, M Flaum. 1999. "Defining the phenotype of schizophrenia: cognitive dysmetria and its neural mechanisms." *Biological Psychiatry* 46: 908–20.

Andrews J, A Briggs, R Porter, P Tucker, K Waddington. 1997. *The History of Bethlem.* London: Routledge.

Angwin J, J Valentino-Devries. "Apple, Google collect user data." *Wall Street Journal,* April 22, 2011. Consulted August 12, 2013. http://online.wsj.com/article/SB10001 424052748703983704576277101723453610.html.

Antonovsky A. 1967. "Social class, life expectancy, and overall mortality." *Milbank Memorial Quarterly* 45: 31–73.

Appelbaum P, P Robbins, J Monahan. 2000. "Violence and delusions: data from the MacArthur Violence Risk Assessment Study." *American Journal of Psychiatry* 157: 566–72.

Apperly I. 2011. *Mindreaders.* Hove: Psychology Press.

Arseneault L, M Cannon, H Fisher, G Polanczyk, T Moffitt, A Caspi. 2011. "Childhood trauma and children's emerging psychotic symptoms: A genetically sensitive longitudinal cohort study." *American Journal of Psychiatry* 168: 65–72.

Asp E, D Tranel. 2013. "False tagging theory: toward a unitary account of prefrontal cortex function." In *Principles of Frontal Lobe Function.* Edited by D Stuss, R Knight. 383–416. Oxford: Oxford University Press.

Auchincloss E, E Samberg, eds. 2012. *Psychoanalytic Terms and Concepts,* 4th ed. New Haven: Yale University Press.

Bacon J, W Welch. "Security clearances held by millions of Americans." *USA Today.* June 10, 2013. Consulted August 8, 2013. http://www.usatoday.com/story/ news/2013/06/09/government-security-clearance/2406243.

BIBLIOGRAPHY

Ball K, K Haggerty, D Lyon, eds. 2012. *Routledge Handbook of Surveillance Studies*. London: Routledge.

Ballew C, A Todorov. 2007. "Predicting political elections from rapid and unreflective face judgments." *Proceedings of the National Academy of Sciences of the United States of America* 104: 17948–53.

Bar M, M Neta, H Linz. 2006. "Very first impressions." *Emotion* 6: 269–78.

Bar-El Y, R Durst, G Katz, J Zislin, Z Strauss, H Knobler. 2000. "Jersualem syndrome." *British Journal of Psychiatry* 176: 86–90.

Baron-Cohen S, A Leslie, U Frith. 1985. "Does the autistic child have a 'theory of mind'?" *Cognition* 2: 37–46.

Baron-Cohen S, A Riviere, M Fukushima, D French, J Hadwin, P Cross, C Bryant, M Sotillo. 1996. "Reading the mind in the face: a cross-cultural and developmental study." *Visual Cognition* 3: 39–59.

Baron-Cohen S, S Wheelwright, J Hill, Y Raste, I Plumb. 2001. "The 'Reading the Mind in the Eyes' test revised version: A study with normal adults, and adults with Asperger syndrome or high-functioning autism." *Journal of Child Psychology and Psychiatry* 42: 241–51.

Barrett D. "One surveillance camera for every 11 people in Britain, says CCTV survey." *Telegraph*. July 10, 2013. Consulted January 30, 2014. http://www.telegraph.co.uk/technology/10172298/One-surveillance-camera-for-every-11-people-in-Britain-says-CCTV-survey.html.

Barton R. 1996. "Neocortex size and behavioural ecology in primates." *Proceedings of the Royal Society of London* B 263: 173–77.

Battle Y, B Martin, J Dorfman, L Miller. 1999. "Seasonality and infectious disease in schizophrenia: the birth hypothesis revisited." *Journal of Psychiatric Research* 33: 501–9.

Bauman M, E Bliss-Moreau, C Machado, D Amaral. 2011. "The neurobiology of primate social behavior." In *The Oxford Handbook of Social Neuroscience*. Edited by J Decety, J Cacioppo. 683–701. New York: Oxford University Press.

Bauman M, P Lavenex, W Mason, J Capitanio, D Amaral. 2004. "The development of social behavior following neonatal amygdala lesions in rhesus monkeys." *Journal of Cognitive Neuroscience* 16: 1388–411.

Bebbington P, D Bhugra, T Brugha, N Singleton, M Farrell, R Jenkins, G Lewis, H Meltzer. 2004. "Psychosis, victimisation and childhood disadvantage: evidence from the second British National Survey of Psychiatric Morbidity." *British Journal of Psychiatry* 185: 220–26.

Bebbington P, L Kuipers. 1994. "The predictive utility of expressed emotion in schizophrenia: an aggregate analysis." *Psychological Medicine* 24: 707–18.

Bell V, E Grech, C Maiden, P Halligan, H Ellis. 2005. " 'Internet delusions': a case series and theoretical integration." *Psychopathology* 38: 144–50.

Bentall R. 2009. *Doctoring the Mind*. New York: New York University Press.

Bentall R, R Corcoran, R Howard, N Blackwood, P Kinderman. 2001. "Persecutory delusions: a review and theoretical integration." *Clinical Psychology Review* 21: 1143–92.

BIBLIOGRAPHY

Bentall R, C Fernyhough. 2008. "Social predictors of psychotic experiences: specificity and psychological mechanisms." *Schizophrenia Bulletin* 34: 1012–20.

Bentall R, S Kaney. 1989. "Content specific information processing and persecutory delusions: an investigation using the emotional Stroop test." *British Journal of Medical Psychology* 62: 355–64.

Bentall R, S Kaney, K Bowen-Jones. 1995. "Persecutory delusions and recall of threat-related, depression-related, and neutral words." *Cognitive Therapy and Research* 19: 445–57.

Bentall R, P Kinderman, S Kaney. 1994. "The self, attributional processes and abnormal beliefs: towards a model of persecutory delusions." *Behaviour Research and Therapy* 32: 331–41.

Bentall R, A Udachina. 2013. "Social cognition and the dynamics of paranoid ideation," in *Social Cognition in Schizophrenia*. Edited by D Roberts, D Penn. 215–44. Oxford: Oxford University Press.

Bentham J. 1843. "Panopticon; or the Inspection House." In *The Works of Jeremy Bentham*, v. 4. Edited by J Bowring. 36–248. Edinburgh: William Tait.

Bentham J. 1891. *A Fragment on Government,* edited by F Montague. Oxford: Clarendon.

Bentsen H, T Notland, O Munkvold, B Boye, I Ulstein, H Bjørge, G Uren, A Lersbryggen, K Oskarsson, R Berg-Larsen, O Lingjærde, UF Malt. 1998. "Guilt proneness and expressed emotion in relatives of patients with schizophrenia or related psychoses." *British Journal of Medical Psychology* 71: 125–38.

Berrios G. 2008. "Descriptive psychiatry and psychiatric nosology during the nineteenth century." In *History of Psychiatry and Medical Psychology*. Edited by E Wallace, J Gach, 353–79. New York: Springer.

Berrios E, Luque R. 1995. "Cotard's syndrome: analysis of 100 cases." *Acta Psychiatrica Scandinavica* 91: 185–88.

Berrios G, R Luque R, J Villagrán. 2003. "Schizophrenia: a conceptual history." *International journal of psychology and psychological therapy* 3: 111–40.

Berson R. 1983. "Capgras' syndrome." *American Journal of Psychiatry* 140: 969–78.

Bickart K, M Hollenbeck, L Barrett, B Dickerson. 2012. "Intrinsic amygdala-cortical functional connectivity predicts social network size in humans." *Journal of Neuroscience* 32: 14729–41.

Bickart K, C Wright, R Dautoff, B Dickerson, L Feldman Barrett. 2011. "Amygdala volume and social network size in humans." *Nature Neuroscience* 14: 163–64.

Bickle J. 1998. *Psychoneural Reduction.* Cambridge: MIT Press.

Blackwood N, R Howard, R Bentall, R Murray. 2001. "Cognitive neuropsychiatric models of persecutory delusions." *American Journal of Psychiatry* 158: 527–39.

Blanchard D, G Griebel, R Pobbe, R Blanchard. 2011. "Risk assessment as an evolved threat detection and analysis process." *Neuroscience and Biobehavioral Reviews* 35: 991–98.

Bleuler E. 1950. *Dementia Praecox: or, the Group of Schizophrenias.* Translated by J Zinkin. New York: International Universities Press.

BIBLIOGRAPHY

Bloomfield S, M Booth. 2013. "Top of the world." *Monocle* 7: 32–51.

Bolwig T. 2011. "How does electroconvulsive therapy work? Theories on its mechanism." *Canadian Journal of Psychiatry* 56: 13–18.

Bora E, M Yucel, C Pantelis. 2009. "Theory of mind impairment in schizophrenia: meta-analysis." *Schizophrenia Research* 109: 1–9.

Bosch F, L Rosich. 2008. "The contributions of Paul Ehrlich to pharmacology: a tribute on the occasion of the centenary of his Nobel Prize." *Pharmacology* 82: 171–79.

Boschan P. 2011. "Transference and countertransference in Sandor Ferenczi's clinical diary." *American Journal of Psychoanalysis* 71: 309–20.

Bourque F, E van der Ven, A Malla. 2011. "A meta-analysis of the risk for psychotic disorders among first- and second-generation immigrants." *Psychological Medicine* 41: 897–910.

Boydell J, K McKenzie. 2008. "Society, place and space." In *Society and Psychosis*. Edited by C Morgan, K McKenzie, P Fearon, 77–94. Cambridge: Cambridge University Press.

Boydell J, J van Os, K McKenzie, J Allardyce, R Goel, R McCreadie, R Murray. 2001. "Incidence of schizophrenia in ethnic minorities in London: ecological study into interactions with environment." *BMJ* 323: 1–4.

Boyer P. 2001. *Religion Explained*. New York: Basic Books.

Boyer P, P Liénard. 2006. "Why ritualized behavior? Precaution Systems and action parsing in developmental, pathological and cultural rituals." *Behavioral and Brain Sciences* 29: 595–613.

Brakoulias V, V Starcevic. 2008. "A cross-sectional survey of the frequency and characteristics of delusions in acute psychiatric wards." *Australasian Psychiatry* 16: 87–91.

Bresnahan M, M Begg, A Brown, C Schaefer, N Sohler, B Insel, L Vella, E Susser. 2007. "Race and risk of schizophrenia in a US birth cohort: another example of health disparity?" *International Journal of Epidemiology* 36: 751–58.

Brooks M, C Reiner. 2009. "The fig leaf." In *The 2000 Year Old Man: The Complete History*. Shout! Factory

Brown A, M Begg, S Gravenstein, C Schaefer, R Wyatt, M Bresahan, V Babulas, E Susser. 2004. "Serologic evidence of prenatal influenza in the etiology of schizophrenia." *Archives of General Psychiatry* 61:774–80.

Brüne M. 2008. *Textbook of Evolutionary Psychiatry*. Oxford: Oxford University Press.

Bryan C, trans. 1931. *The Papyrus Ebers*. New York: Appleton.

Buchan J. 1927. *Mr. Standfast*. London: Hodder and Stoughton.

Buchanan T, D Tranel, R Adolphs. 2009. "The human amygdala in social function." In *The Human Amygdala*. Edited by P Whalen, E Phelps. 289–318. New York: Guilford Press.

Buckle C, Y Chuah, C Fones, A Wong. 2007. "A conceptual history of Koro." *Transcultural Psychiatry* 44: 27–43.

Bürgy M. 2008. "The concept of psychosis: historical and phenomenological aspects." *Schizophrenia Bulletin* 34: 1200–10.

Burns J, A Tomita, A Kapadia. 2014. "Income inequality and schizophrenia: increased schizophrenia incidence in countries with high levels of income inequality." *International Journal of Social Psychiatry* 60: 185–96.

BIBLIOGRAPHY

Burton R. 2001. *The Anatomy of Melancholy.* New York: New York Review of Books.

Buss D. 2000. *The Dangerous Passion.* New York: Free Press.

Buss D. 2012. *Evolutionary Psychology,* 4th ed. Boston: Allyn & Bacon.

Buss D, J Duntley. 2008. "Adaptations for exploitation." *Group Dynamics: Theory, Research, and Practice* 12: 53–62.

Byrne R, N Corp. 2004. "Neocortex size predicts deception rate in primates." *Proceedings of the Royal Society of London* B: 1693–99.

Byrne R, A Whiten A, eds. 1988. *Machiavellian Intelligence.* Oxford: Oxford University Press.

Callard F, D Rose, E Hanif, J Quigley, K Greenwood, T Wykes. 2012. "Holding blame at bay? 'Gene talk' in family members' accounts of schizophrenia aetiology." *Bio-Societies* 7: 273–93.

Capgras J, J Reboul-Lachaux. 1923. "L'illusion des 'sosies' dans un délire systématisé chronique." *Bulletin de la Société Clinique de Médicine Mentale* 11: 6–16.

Capgras J, J Reboul-Lachaux. 1994. "L'illusion des 'sosies' dans un délire systématisé chronique." *History of Psychiatry* 5: 119–33.

Carpenter P. 1989. "Descriptions of schizophrenia in the psychiatry of Georgian Britain: John Haslam and James Tilly Matthews." *Comprehensive Psychiatry* 30: 332–38.

Cermolacce M, L Sass, J Parnas. 2010."What is bizarre in bizarre delusions? A critical review." *Schizophrenia Bulletin* 36: 667–79.

Chadwick P, M Birchwood, P Trower. 1996. *Cognitive Therapy for Delusions, Voices and Paranoia.* Chichester: John Wiley & Sons.

Chance M, A Mead. 1953. "Social behaviour and primate evolution." *Symposia of the Society for Experimental Biology* 7: 395–439.

Chomsky N. 1988. *Language Problems of Knowledge.* Cambridge: MIT Press.

Chowdhury A, H Mukherjee, K Ghosh, S Chowdhury. 2003. "Puppy pregnancy in humans: a culture-bound disorder in rural West Bengal, India." *International Journal of Social Psychiatry* 49: 35–42.

Churchland P, P Churchland. 1994. "Interthreoretic reduction: a neuroscientist's field guide." In *The Mind-Body Problem.* Edited by R Warner, T Szubka. 41–54. Cambridge: Blackwell.

Cohen N. "It's tracking your every move and you may not even know." *New York Times.* March 26, 2011. Consulted August 13, 2013. http://www.nytimes.com/2011/03/26/business/media/26privacy.html?_r=0.

Coid J, J Kirkbride, D Barker, F Cowden, R Stamps, M Yang, P Jones. 2008. "Raised incidence rates of all psychoses among migrant groups: findings from the East London first episode psychosis study." *Archives of General Psychiatry* 65: 1250–59.

Coid J, S Ullrich, C Kallis, R Keers, D Barker, F Cowden, R Stamps. 2013. "The relationship between delusions and violence: findings from the East London first episode psychosis study." *JAMA Psychiatry* 70: 465–71.

Colbert S, E Peters, P Garety. 2010. "Delusions and belief flexibility in psychosis." *Psychology and Psychotherapy: Theory, Research and Practice* 83: 45–57.

Collins J, R David, A Handler, S Wall, S Andes. 2004. "Very low birth weight in African-

BIBLIOGRAPHY

American infants: the role of maternal exposure to interpersonal racial discrimination." *American Journal of Public Health* 94: 2132–38.

Collins J, A Herman, R David. 1997. "Very-low-birthweight infants and income incongruity among African American and white parents in Chicago." *American Journal of Public Health* 87: 414–17.

Coltheart M. 1999. "Modularity and cognition." *Trends in Cognitive Science* 3: 115–20.

Coltheart M. 2007. "The 33rd Sir Frederick Bartlett lecture: cognitive neuropsychiatry and delusional belief." *The Quarterly Journal of Experimental Psychology* 60: 1041–62.

Coltheart M. 2013. "On the distinction between monothematic and polythematic delusions." *Mind & Language* 28: 103–12.

Coltheart M, R Langdon, R McKay. 2007. "Schizophrenia and monothematic delusions." *Schizophrenia Bulletin* 33: 642–47.

Coltheart M, R Langdon, R McKay. 2011. "Delusional belief." *Annual Review of Psychology* 62: 271–98.

Condon S. "Poll: one in four Americans think Obama was not born in U.S." CBS News, April 21, 2011. Consulted January 30, 2014. http://www.cbsnews.com/news/poll-one-in-four-americans-think-obama-was-not-born-in-us.

Connor S. 2008. "Pregnable of eye: X-rays, vision and magic." In *The Girl with X-Ray Eyes*. Edited by P Warnell. 73–88. Leamington Spa: Leamington Spa Art Gallery and Warwick Arts Centre.

Corcoran C, M Perrin, S Harlap, L Deutsch, S Fennig, O Manor, D Nahon, D Kimhy, D Malaspina, E Susser. 2009a. "Effect of socioeconomic status and parents' education at birth on risk of schizophrenia in offspring." *Social Psychiatry and Psychiatric Epidemiology* 44: 265–71.

Corcoran C, M Perrin, S Harlap, L Deutsch, S Fennig, O Manor, D Nahon, D Kimhy, D Malaspina, E Susser. 2009b. "Incidence of schizophrenia among second-generation immigrants in the Jerusalem perinatal cohort." *Schizophrenia Bulletin* 35: 596–602.

Corcoran R, G Mercer, C Frith. 1995. "Schizophrenia, symptomatology and social inference: investigating 'theory of mind' in people with schizophrenia." *Schizophrenia Research* 17: 5–13.

Corlett P, J Krystal, J Taylor, P Fletcher. 2009. "Why do delusions persist?" *Frontiers in Human Neuroscience* 3: doi: 10.3389/neuro.09.012.2009.

Cotard J. 1882. "Du délire des negations." In *Archives de Neurologie*, 4:152–70, 282–96.

Cougnard A, M Marcelis, I Myin-Germeys, R De Graaf, W Vollebergh, L Krabbendam, R Lieb, H Wittchen, C Henquet, J Spauwen, J van Os. 2007. "Does normal developmental expression of psychosis combine with environmental risk to cause persistence of psychosis? A psychosis proneness-persistence model." *Psychological Medicine* 37: 513–27.

Couture S, D Penn. 2013. "Introduction." In *Social Cognition in Schizophrenia*. Edited by D Roberts, D Penn. 1–16. Oxford: Oxford University Press.

Coy A, S Hutton. 2013. "The influence of hallucination proneness and social threat on time perception." *Cognitive Neuropsychiatry* 18: 463–76.

BIBLIOGRAPHY

Cutajar M, P Mullen, J Ogloff, S Thomas, D Wells, J Spataro. 2010. "Schizophrenia and other psychotic disorders in a cohort of sexually abused children." *Archives of General Psychiatry* 67: 1114–19.

Daniels N, B Kennedy, I Kawachi. 1999. "Why justice is good for our health: the social determinants of health inequalities." *Daedalus* 128: 215–51.

Dauncey K, J Giggs, K Baker, G Harrison. 1993. "Schizophrenia in Nottingham: lifelong residential mobility of a cohort." *British Journal of Psychiatry* 163: 613–19.

David R, J Collins. 1997. "Differing birth weight among infants of U.S.-born blacks, African-born blacks, and U.S.-born whites." *New England Journal of Medicine* 337: 1209–14.

Davies H, I Crombie, M Tavakoli. 1998. "When can odds ratios mislead?" *BMJ* 316: 989–91.

Davies M, M Coltheart, R Langdon, N Breen. 2001. "Monothematic delusions: towards a two-factor account." *Philosophy, Psychiatry, & Psychology* 8: 133–58.

Davis M, P Whalen. 2001. "The amygdala: vigilance and emotion." *Molecular Psychiatry* 6: 13–34.

Derovan D, G Scholem, M Idel. 2007. "Gematria." In *Encyclopedia Judaica*. Edited by M Berenbaum, F Skolnik. 424–27. Detroit: Macmillan Reference.

Devinsky O. 2009. "Delusional misidentifications and duplications." *Neurology* 72: 80–87.

de Waal F. 1998. *Chimpanzee Politics*. Baltimore: Johns Hopkins University Press.

Diagnostic and Statistical Manual: Mental Disorders, 1st ed. 1952. Washington: American Psychiatric Publishing.

Diagnostic and Statistical Manual of Mental Disorders, 2nd ed. 1968. Washington: American Psychiatric Publishing.

Diagnostic and Statistical Manual of Mental Disorders, 3rd ed. 1980. Washington: American Psychiatric Publishing.

Diagnostic and Statistical Manual of Mental Disorders, 4th ed. 1994. Washington: American Psychiatric Publishing.

Diagnostic and Statistical Manual of Mental Disorders, 4th ed., text revision, 2000. Washington: American Psychiatric Publishing.

Diagnostic and Statistical Manual of Mental Disorders, 5th ed. 2013. Washington: American Psychiatric Publishing.

Dick P. 2002. *Time Out of Joint.* New York: Vintage.

Dicks D, R Myers, A Kling. 1969. "Uncus and amygdala lesions: effects on social behavior in the free-ranging rhesus monkey." *Science* 165: 69–71.

Dixon L, F Dickerson, A Bellack, M Bennett, D Dickinson, R Goldberg, A Lehman, W Tenhula, C Calmes, R Pasillas, J Peer, J Kreyenbuhl. 2010. "The 2009 schizophrenia PORT psychosocial treatment recommendations and summary statements." *Schizophrenia Bulletin* 36: 48–70.

Dobson K. 2010. *Handbook of Cognitive-Behavioral Therapies,* 3rd ed. New York: Guilford Press.

Dobzhansky T. 1973. "Nothing in biology makes sense except in the light of evolution." *The American Biology Teacher* 35: 125–29.

BIBLIOGRAPHY

Docherty N, L Cutting, S Bers. 1998. "Expressed emotion and differentiation of self in the relatives of stable schizophrenia outpatients." *Psychiatry* 61: 269–78.

Dolnick E. 1998. *Madness on the Couch.* New York: Simon & Schuster.

Dominguez M, M Wichers, R Lieb, H Wittchen, J van Os. 2011. "Evidence that onset of clinical psychosis is an outcome of progressively more persistent subclinical psychotic experiences: an 8-year cohort study." *Schizophrenia Bulletin* 37: 84–93.

Dunbar R. 1988. *Primate Social Systems.* Ithaca: Cornell University Press.

Dunbar R. 1993. "Coevolution of neocortical size, group size and language in humans." *Behavioral and Brain Sciences* 16: 681–94.

Dunbar R. 1998. "The social brain hypothesis." *Evolutionary Anthropology* 6: 178–90.

Dunbar R. 2004. "Gossip in evolutionary perspective." *Review of General Psychology* 8: 100–10.

Dunbar R. 2013. "An evolutionary basis for social cognition." In *The Infant Mind: Origins of the Social Brain.* Edited by M Legerstee, D Haley, M Bornstein. 3–18. New York: Guilford Press.

Dunbar R, S Shultz. 2007. "Evolution in the social brain." *Science* 317: 1344–47.

Dunkel Schetter C, L Glynn. 2011. "Stress in pregnancy: empirical evidence and theoretical issues to guide interdisciplinary research." In *Handbook of Stress Science.* Edited by R Contrada, A Baum. 321–43. New York: Springer.

Dunlop A, H Salihu, G Freymann, C Smith, A Brann. 2011. "Very low birth weight births in Georgia, 1994–2005: trends and racial disparities." *Maternal and Child Health Journal* 15: 890–98.

Dupont J. 1988. "Ferenczi's 'madness.'" *Contemporary Psychoanalysis* 24: 250–61.

Durà-Vilà G, R Littlewood, G Leavey. 2013. "Depression and the medicalization of sadness: conceptualization and recommended help-seeking." *International Journal of Social Psychiatry* 59: 165–75.

Ebbinghaus H. 1908. *Psychology: An Elementary Text-Book.* Translated by M Meyer. Boston: D. C. Heath.

Edwards J. 2014. "Ghana's mental health patients confined to prayer camps." *The Lancet* 383: 15–6.

Eggert G, trans. 1977. *Wernicke's Works on Aphasia.* The Hague: Mouton.

Eibl-Eibesfeldt I. 1970. *Ethology: The Biology of Behavior.* Translated by E Kinghammer. New York: Holt, Rinehart, and Winston.

Elliott R. 2003. "Executive functions and their disorders." *British Medical Bulletin* 65: 49–59.

Ellis H, A Young. 1990. "Accounting for delusional misidentifications." *British Journal of Psychiatry* 157: 239–48.

Ellis H, A Young, A Quayle, K De Pauw. 1997. "Reduced autonomic responses to faces in Capgras delusion." *Proceedings of the Royal Society of London* B 264: 1085–92.

Emery N. 2000. "The eyes have it: The neuroethology, function and evolution of social gaze." *Neuroscience and Biobehavioral Reviews* 24: 581–604.

Enoch D, H Ball. 2001. *Uncommon Psychiatric Syndromes,* 4th ed. London: Arnold.

Enquist M, O Leimar. 1993. "The evolution of cooperation in mobile organisms." *Animal Behaviour* 45: 747–57.

BIBLIOGRAPHY

Eraña A. 2012. "Dual process theories versus massive modularity hypotheses." *Philosophical Psychology* 25: 855–72.

Evans F. 1996. *Harry Stack Sullivan*. London: Routledge.

Evans J. 2008. "Dual-processing accounts of reasoning, judgment, and social cognition." *Annual Review of Psychology* 59: 255–78.

Evans J. 2010. *Thinking Twice*. Oxford: Oxford University Press.

Eysenck H. 1985. "Behaviourism and clinical psychiatry." *International Journal of Social Psychiatry* 31: 163–69.

Eytan A, C Liberek, I Graf, J Golaz. 2002. "Electronic chips implant: a new culture-bound syndrome?" *Psychiatry* 65: 72–74.

Falloon I, J Boyd, C McGill, M Williamson, J Razani, H Moss, A Gilderman, G Simpson. 1985. "Family management in the prevention of morbidity of schizophrenia: clinical outcome of a two-year longitudinal study." *Archives of General Psychiatry* 42: 887–96.

Faris R, H W Dunham. 1965. *Mental Disorders in Urban Areas*. Chicago: University of Chicago.

Fearon P, J Kirkbride, C Morgan, P Dazzan, K Morgan, T Lloyd, G Hutchinson, J Tarrant, W Fung, J Holloway, R Mallett, G Harrison, J Leff, P Jones, R Murray. 2006. "Incidence of schizophrenia and other psychoses in ethnic minority groups: results from the MRC ÆSOP Study." *Psychological Medicine* 36: 1541–50.

Federn P. 1932. "Ego feeling in dreams." *Psychoanalytic Quarterly* 1: 511–42.

Federn P. 1934. "The analysis of psychotics." *International Journal of Psycho-Analysis* 15: 209–14.

Feinberg T, J Deluca, J Giacino, D Roane, M Solms. 2005. "Right-hemisphere pathology and the self: delusional misidentification and reduplication." In *The Lost Self*. Edited by T Feinberg, J Keenan. 100–130. Oxford: Oxford University Press.

Feinstein J, R Adolphs, A Damasio, D Tranel. 2011. "The human amygdala and the induction and experience of fear." *Current Biology* 21: 34–38.

Ferenczi S. 1911. "Letter from Sándor Ferenczi to Sigmund Freud, June 19, 1911." *The Correspondence of Sigmund Freud and Sándor Ferenczi*, v. 1. 1908–1914, 291–92.

Fiddick L. 2011. "There is more than the amygdala: potential threat assessment in the cingulate cortex." *Neuroscience and Biobehavioral Reviews* 35: 1007–18.

Fine C, J Craigie, I Gold. 2005. "Damned if you do; damned if you don't: The impasse in cognitive accounts of the Capgras delusion." *Philosophy, Psychiatry & Psychology* 12: 143–51.

Finlay B, R Darlington. 1995. "Linked regularities in the development and evolution of mammalian brains." *Science* 268: 1578–84.

Fisher D. "Detroit tops the 2012 list of America's most dangerous cities." *Forbes*, October 18, 2012. Consulted August 7, 2013. http://www.forbes.com/sites/daniel fisher/2012/10/18/detroit-tops-the-2012-list-of-americas-most-dangerous-cities.

Fisher H, P Jones, P Fearon, T Craig, P Dazzan, K Morgan, G Hutchinson, G Doody, P McGuffin, J Leff, R Murray, C Morgan. 2010. "The varying impact of type, timing and frequency of exposure to childhood adversity on its association with adult psychotic disorder." *Psychological Medicine* 40: 1967–78.

Flannelly K, H Koenig, K Galek, C Ellison C. 2007. Beliefs, mental health, and evolutionary threat assessment systems in the brain. *Journal of Nervous and Mental Disease* 195: 996–1003.

Fodor J. 1974. "Special sciences (or: the disunity of science as a working hypothesis)." *Synthese* 28: 97–115.

Fodor J. 1983. *The Modularity of Mind*. Cambridge: MIT Press.

Fodor J. 1997. "Special sciences: still autonomous after all these years." *Noûs* 31: 149–63.

Fortune C. 1993. "The case of 'RN': Sándor Ferenczi's radical experiment in psychoanalysis." In *The Legacy of Sándor Ferenczi*. Edited by L Aron, A Harris. 101–20. Hillsdale: Analytic Press.

Foster P, R Sanchez. "Washington Navy Yard shooting: Aaron Alexis 'had history of violence.'" *Telegraph*, September 16, 2013. Consulted October 13, 2013. http://www.telegraph.co.uk/news/worldnews/northamerica/usa/10314110/Washington-Navy-Yard-shooting-Aaron-Alexis-had-history-of-violence.html.

Foucault M. 1988. *Madness and Civilization*. Translated by R Howard. New York: Vintage.

Foucault M. 1995. *Discipline and Punish*, 2nd ed. Translated by A Sheridan. New York: Vintage.

Francescani C, Davis L. "Brave mother fights off psychotic psychiatrist." ABC News, July 26, 2007. Consulted August 14, 2013. http://abcnews.go.com/TheLaw/story?id=3416296&page=1.

Frankish K, J Evans. 2009. "The duality of mind: an historical perpective." In *In Two Minds*. Edited by J Evans, K Frankish. 1–29. Oxford: Oxford University Press.

Freeman D, P Garety. 2004. *Paranoia*. Hove: Psychology Press.

Freeman D, P Garety, E Kuipers, D Fowler, P Bebbington, G Dunn. 2007. "Acting on persecutory delusions: the importance of safety seeking." *Behaviour Research and Therapy* 45: 89–99.

Freeman D, M Gittins, K Pugh, A Antley, M Slater, G Dunn. 2008. "What makes one person paranoid and another person anxious? The differential prediction of social anxiety and persecutory ideation in an experimental situation." *Psychological Medicine* 38: 1121–32.

Freud A. 1937. *The Ego and the Mechanisms of Defence*. Translated by C Baines. London: Hogarth Press and the Institute of Psycho-Analysis.

Freud S. 1893/1955. "The psychotherapy of hysteria." In *The Standard Edition of the Complete Psychological Works of Sigmund Freud*, v. II. Translated by J Strachey. 253–305. London: Hogarth Press and the Institute of Psycho-Analysis.

Freud S. 1896/1962. "Further remarks on the neuro-psychoses of defence." In *The Standard Edition of the Complete Psychological Works of Sigmund Freud*, v. III. Translated by J Strachey. 157–85. London: Hogarth Press and the Institute of Psycho-Analysis.

Freud S. 1911/1958. "Psycho-analytic notes on an autobiographical case of paranoia (*dementia paranoides*)." In *The Standard Edition of the Complete Psychological*

BIBLIOGRAPHY

Works of Sigmund Freud, v. XII. Translated by J Strachey. 1–82. London: Hogarth Press and the Institute of Psycho-Analysis.

Freud S. 1913/1955. "The claims of psycho-analysis to scientific interest." In *The Standard Edition of the Complete Psychological Works of Sigmund Freud*, v. XIII. Translated by J Strachey. 163–90. London: Hogarth Press and the Institute of Psycho-Analysis.

Freud S. 1919/1955. "Lines of advance in psycho-analytic therapy." In *The Standard Edition of the Complete Psychological Works of Sigmund Freud*, v. XVII. Translated by J Strachey. 157–68. London: Hogarth Press and the Institute of Psycho-Analysis.

Freud S. 1920/1955. "Beyond the pleasure principle." *The Standard Edition of the Complete Psychological Works of Sigmund Freud*, v. XVIII. Translated by J Strachey. 1–64. London: Hogarth Press and the Institute of Psycho-Analysis.

Freud S. 1923/1955. "Two encyclopaedia articles." In *The Standard Edition of the Complete Psychological Works of Sigmund Freud*, v. XVIII. Translated by J Strachey. 233–60. London: Hogarth Press and the Institute of Psycho-Analysis.

Freud S. 1924/1961a. "Neurosis and psychosis." In *The Standard Edition of the Complete Psychological Works of Sigmund Freud*, v. XIX. Translated by J Strachey. 147–53. London: Hogarth Press and the Institute of Psycho-Analysis.

Freud S. 1924/1961b. "A short account of psycho-analysis." *The Standard Edition of the Complete Psychological Works of Sigmund Freud*, v. XIX. Translated by J Strachey. 189–210. London: Hogarth Press and the Institute of Psycho-Analysis.

Freud S. 1933/1964. "New introductory lectures on psycho-analysis." In *The Standard Edition of the Complete Psychological Works of Sigmund Freud*, v. XXII. Translated by J Strachey. 1–182. London: Hogarth Press and the Institute of Psycho-Analysis.

Freud S. 1938/1964. "An outline of psycho-analysis." In *The Standard Edition of the Complete Psychological Works of Sigmund Freud*, v. XXIII. Translated by J Strachey. 139–208. London: Hogarth Press and the Institute of Psycho-Analysis.

Frith C. 1992. *Cognitive Neuropsychology of Schizophrenia*. Hove: Lawrence Erlbaum.

Fromm-Reichmann F. 1948. "Notes on the development of treatment of schizophrenics by psychoanalytic psychotherapy." *Psychiatry* 11: 263–73.

Fuchs T. 2012. "Are mental illnesses diseases of the brain?" In *Critical Neuroscience*. Edited by S Choudhury, J Slaby. 331–44. Chichester: Wiley-Blackwell.

Gabriel T, J Goldstein, M Schmidt. "Suspect's past fell just short of raising alarm." *New York Times*, September 17, 2013. Consulted October 13, 2013. www.nytimes.com/2013/09/18/us/washington-navy-yard-shootings.html?hp&_r=0.

Gach J. 2008. "Biological psychiatry in the nineteenth and twentieth centuries." In *History of Psychiatry and Medical Psychology*. Edited by E Wallace, J Gach. 381–418. New York: Springer.

Galea S, J Ahern, S Rudenstine, Z Wallace, D Vlahov. 2005. "Urban built environment and depression: a multilevel analysis." *Journal of Epidemiology and Community Health* 59: 822–27.

Galea S, M Uddin, K Koenen. 2011. "The urban environment and mental disorders." *Epigenetics* 6: 400–4.

BIBLIOGRAPHY

Garber D. 2013. "Remarks on the pre-history of the mechanical philosophy." In *The Mechanization of Natural Philosophy*. Edited by D Garber, S Roux. 3–26. Dordrecht: Springer.

Garety P, D Freeman. 1999. "Cognitive approaches to delusions: a critical review of theories and evidence." *British Journal of Clinical Psychology* 38: 113–54.

Garety P, D Freeman, S Jolley, G Dunn, P Bebbington, D Fowler, E Kuipers, R Dudley. 2005. "Reasoning, emotions, and delusional conviction in psychosis." *Journal of Abnormal Psychology* 114: 373–84.

Garrett M, D Stone, D Turkington. 2006. "Normalizing psychotic symptoms." *Psychology and Psychotherapy: Theory, Research and Practice* 79: 595–610.

Gecici O, M Kuloglu, O Guler, O Ozbulut, E Kurt, S Onen, O Ekinci, D Yesilbas, A Caykoylu, M Emül, G Alatas, Y Albayrak. 2010. "Phenomenology of delusions and hallucinations in patients with schizophrenia." *Bulletin of Clinical Psychopharmacology* 20: 204–12.

Giggs J. 1986. "Mental disorders and ecological structure in Nottingham." *Social Science & Medicine* 23: 945–61.

Gilbert P. 1993. Defence and safety: their function in social behaviour and psychopathology. *British Journal of Clinical Psychology* 32: 131–53.

Gilman S. 2008. "Constructing schizophrenia as a category of mental illness." In *History of Psychiatry and Medical Psychology*. Edited by E Wallace, J Gach. 461–83. New York: Springer.

Glover E. 1931. "The therapeutic effect of inexact interpretation: a contribution to the theory of suggestion." *International Journal of Psychoanalysis* 12: 397–411.

Gold I. Forthcoming. *A Theory of Delusion*. Oxford: Oxford University Press.

Gold I. Forthcoming. "Outline of a theory of delusion." *Frontiers in Human Neuroscience*.

Gold J, I Gold. 2012. "The 'Truman Show' delusion: psychosis in the global village." *Cognitive Neuropsychiatry* 17: 455–72.

Gold I, Stoljar D. 1999. "A neuron doctrine in the philosophy of neuroscience." *Behavioral and Brain Sciences* 22: 809–30.

Goldberg A, C Allis, E Bernstein. 2007. "Epigenetics: a landscape takes shape." *Cell* 128: 635–38.

Goldstone E, J Farhall, B Ong. 2011. "Synergistic pathways to delusions: enduring vulnerabilities, proximal life stressors and maladaptive psychological coping." *Early Intervention in Psychiatry* 5: 122–31.

Gould S. 1978. "Sociobiology: the art of storytelling." *New Scientist* 80: 530–33.

Green H. 1964. *I Never Promised You a Rose Garden*. New York: Holt, Rinehart and Winston.

Green M, M Phillips. 2004. "Social threat perception and the evolution of paranoia." *Neuroscience and Biobehavioral Reviews* 28: 333–42.

Green M, L Williams, D Davidson. 2003a. "Visual scanpaths and facial affect recognition in delusion-prone individuals: increased sensitivity to threat?" *Cognitive Neuropsychiatry* 8: 19–41.

Green M, L Williams, D Davidson. 2003b. "Visual scanpaths to threat-related faces in deluded schizophrenia." *Psychiatry Research* 119: 271–85.

BIBLIOGRAPHY

Greenberg J, S Mitchell. 1983. *Object Relations in Psychoanalytic Theory.* Cambridge: Harvard University Press.

Griesinger W. 1882. *Mental Pathology and Therapeutics.* Translated by C Robertson, J Rutherford. New York: William Wood.

Haddock G, W Spaulding. 2011. "Psychological treatment of psychosis." In *Schizophrenia*, 3rd ed. Edited by D Weinberger, P Harrison. 666–86. Oxford: Wiley-Blackwell.

Hagen E. 2008. "Nonbizarre delusions as strategic deception." In *Medicine and Evolution.* Edited by S Elton, P O'Higgins. 181–216. Boca Raton: CRC.

Haigh J. 2012. *Probability: A Very Short Introduction.* Oxford: Oxford University Press.

Hall L. "Waterlow 'shattered by the reality' of killings." *Sydney Morning Herald.* April 13, 2011a. Consulted May 11, 2011. http://www.smh.com.au/nsw/waterlow-shattered-by-the-reality-of-killings-20110412-1dcpz.html.

Hall L. "Waterlow found not guilty of murdering father and sister." April 19, 2011b. Consulted May 11, 2011. *Sydney Morning Herald.* http://www.smh.com.au/nsw/waterlow-found-not-guilty-of-murdering-father-and-sister-20110419-1dmfd.html.

Halligan P, J Marshall. 1996. "The wise prophet makes sure of the event first: hallucinations, amnesia, and delusions." In *Method in Madness.* Edited by P Halligan, J Marshall. 237–64. Hove: Psychology Press.

Hamilton J. "Why is psychiatry's new manual so much like the old one?" National Public Radio. May 16, 2013. Consulted June 20, 2013. http://www.npr.org/blogs/health/2013/05/16/184454931/why-is-psychiatrys-new-manual-so-much-like-the-old-one.

Hanoeman M, Selten J, Kahn R. 2002. "Incidence of schizophrenia in Surinam." *Schizophrenia Research* 54: 219–21.

Harrington A. 2012. "The fall of the schizophrenogenic mother." *Lancet* 379: 1292–93.

Hart B. 1912. *The Psychology of Insanity.* Cambridge: Cambridge University Press.

Haselton M, D Nettle. 2006. "The paranoid optimist: an integrative evolutionary model of cognitive biases." *Personality and Social Psychology Review* 10: 47–66.

Haslam J. 1988. *Illustrations of Madness.* Edited by R Porter. London: Routledge.

Hastorf A, H Cantril. 1954. "They saw a game: a case study." *Journal of Abnormal and Social Psychology* 49: 129–34.

Havens, L. 1976. *Participant Observation.* New York: Aronson.

Havens L, J Frank. 1971. "Review of *Psychoanalysis and Interpersonal Psychiatry* by P Mullahy." *American Journal of Psychiatry* 127: 1704–5.

Healy D. 2002. *The Creation of Psychopharmacology.* Cambridge: Harvard University Press.

Heinlein R. 1941 (April). "They." Unknown: 84–95.

Heins M, C Simons, T Lataster, S Pfeifer, D Versmissen, M Lardinois, M Marcelis, P Delespaul, L Krabbendam, J van Os, I Myin-Germeys. 2011. "Childhood trauma and psychosis: a case-control and case-sibling comparison across different levels of genetic liability, psychopathology, and type of trauma." *American Journal of Psychiatry* 168: 1286–94.

BIBLIOGRAPHY

Hermann P, A Marimow. "Navy Yard shooter Aaron Alexis driven by delusions." *Washington Post.* September 25, 2013. Consulted October 13, 2013. http://www.washingtonpost.com/local/crime/fbi-police-detail-shooting-navy-yard-shooting/2013/09/25/ee321abe-2600-11e3-b3e9-d97fb087acd6_story.html.

Hippocrates. 1849. *The Genuine Works of Hippocrates,* v. 2. Translated by F Adams. London: Sydenham Society.

Hirjak D, T Fuchs. 2010. "Delusions of technical alien control: a phenomenological description of three cases." *Psychopathology* 43: 96–103.

Hollingshead A, F Redlich. 1958. *Social Class and Mental Illness.* New York: Wiley.

Holt A, M Albert. 2006. "Cognitive neuroscience of delusions in aging." *Neuropsychiatric Disease and Treatment* 2: 181–89.

Homer. 1996. *The Odyssey.* Translated by R Fagles. New York: Viking.

Hopcroft R. 2006. "Sex, status, and reproductive success in the contemporary United States." *Evolution and Human Behavior* 27: 104–20.

Horan W, J Lee, M Green. 2013. "Social cognition and functional outcome in schizophrenia." In *Social Cognition in Schizophrenia.* Edited by D Roberts, D Penn. 151–72. Oxford: Oxford University Press.

Hotchner A. "Hemingway, hounded by the Feds." *New York Times.* July 1, 2011. Consulted July 18, 2013. http://www.nytimes.com/2011/07/02/opinion/02hotchner.html?pagewanted=all&_r=0.

Howes O, S Kapur. 2009. "The dopamine hypothesis of schizophrenia: version III—the final common pathway." *Schizophrenia Bulletin* 35: 549–62.

Humphrey N. 1976. "The social function of intellect." In *Growing Points in Ethology.* Edited by P Bateson, R Hinde. 303–17. Cambridge: Cambridge University Press.

Humphrey N. 2007. "The society of selves." *Philosophical Transactions of the Royal Society B.* 362: 745–54.

Ibanez-Casas I, J Cervilla. 2012. "Neuropsychological research in delusional disorder: a comprehensive review." *Psychopathology* 45: 78–95.

"Incident report from Aaron Alexis's 2010 arrest." *Wall Street Journal.* September 16, 2013. Consulted October 13, 2013. http://blogs.wsj.com/washwire/2013/09/16/incident-report-from-aaron-alexiss-2010-arrest.

Ingraham L, S Kety. 2000. "Adoption studies of schizophrenia." *American Journal of Medical Genetics* 97: 18–22.

Insel T, R Quirion. 2005. "Psychiatry as a clinical neuroscience discipline." *JAMA* 294: 2221–24.

Jamison K. 1993. *Touched with Fire.* New York: Free Press.

Jamison K. 1995. *An Unquiet Mind.* New York: Vintage.

Janssen I, M Hanssen, M Bak, R Bijl, R de Graaf, W Vollebergh, K McKenzie, J van Os. 2003. "Discrimination and delusional ideation." *British Journal of Psychiatry* 182: 71–76.

Janssen I, L Krabbendam, M Bak, M Hanssen, W Vollebergh, R de Graaf, J van Os. 2004. "Childhood abuse as a risk factor for psychotic experiences." *Acta Psychiatrica Scandinavica* 109: 38–45.

BIBLIOGRAPHY

Jaspers K. 1997. *General Psychopathology,* v. 1. Translated by J Hoenig, M Hamilton. Baltimore: Johns Hopkins University Press.

Javitt D, J Kantrowitz. 2009. *Handbook of Neurochemistry and Molecular Neurobiology: Schizophrenia.* New York: Springer.

Jay M. 2014. *A Visionary Madness.* Berkeley: North Atlantic Books.

Johnson S, A Riley, D Granger, J Riis. 2013. "The science of early life toxic stress for pediatric practice and advocacy." *Pediatrics* 131: 319–27.

Jolly A. 1966. "Lemur social behavior and primate intelligence." *Science* 153: 501–6.

Kafka J. 2011. "Chestnut Lodge and the psychoanalytic approach to psychosis." *Journal of the American Psychoanalytic Association* 59: 27–47.

Kahneman D. 2011. *Thinking, Fast and Slow.* New York: Farrar, Straus & Giroux.

Kaney S, R Bentall. 1989. "Persecutory delusions and attributional style." *British Journal of Medical Psychology* 62: 191–98.

Kaney S, M Wolfenden, M Dewey, R Bentall. 1992. "Persecutory delusions and recall of threatening propositions." *British Journal of Clinical Psychology* 31: 85–87.

Kanner A, J Coyne, C Schaefer, R Lazarus. 1981. "Comparison of two modes of stress measurement: daily hassles and uplifts versus major life events." *Journal of Behavioral Medicine* 4: 1–39.

Kantrowitz J, D Javitt. 2009. "Glutamatergic approaches to the conceptualization and treatment of schizophrenia." In *Handbook of Neurochemistry and Molecular Neurobiology: Schizophrenia.* Edited by D Javitt, J Kantrowitz. 39–89. New York: Springer.

Kapur S. 2003. "Psychosis as a state of aberrant salience: a framework linking biology, phenomenology, and pharmacology in schizophrenia." *American Journal of Psychiatry* 160: 13–23.

Kawachi I, B Kennedy, R Wilkinson. 1999. *The Society and Population Health Reader,* v. 1. New York: New Press.

Kee K, W Horan, J Mintz, M Green. 2004. "Do the siblings of schizophrenia patients demonstrate affect perception deficits?" *Schizophrenia Research* 67: 87–94.

Kelleher I, M Harley, F Lynch, L Arseneault, C Fitzpatrick, M Cannon. 2008. "Associations between childhood trauma, bullying and psychotic symptoms among a school-based adolescent sample." *British Journal of Psychiatry* 193: 378–82.

Kelleher I, H Keeley, P Corcoran, H Ramsay, C Wasserman, V Carli, M Sarchiapone, C Hoven, D Wasserman, M Cannon. 2013. "Childhood trauma and psychosis in a prospective cohort study: cause, effect, and directionality." *American Journal of Psychiatry* 170: 734–41.

Kelly C. 1996. "Advertising, politicians, and delusions in the mentally vulnerable." *The Lancet* 348: 1385.

Kendell R, J Cooper, A Gourlay, J Copeland, L Sharpe, B Gurland. 1971. "Diagnostic criteria of American and British psychiatrists." *Archives of General Psychiatry* 25: 123–30.

Kendell R, E Juszcak, S Cole. 1996. "Obstetric complications and schizophrenia: a case control study based on standardised obstetric records." *British Journal of Psychiatry* 168: 556–61.

BIBLIOGRAPHY

Kendler K, A Gruenberg, D Kinney. 1994. "Independent diagnoses of adoptees and relatives as defined by DSM-III in the provincial and national samples of the Danish Adoption Study of Schizophrenia." *Archives of General Psychiatry* 51: 456–68.

Kendler K, Schaffner K. 2011. "The dopamine hypothesis of schizophrenia: an historical and philosophical analysis." *Philosophy, Psychiatry & Psychology* 18: 41–63.

Kety S, P Wender, B Jacobsen, L Ingraham, L Jansson, B Faber, D Kinney. 1994. "Mental illness in the biological and adoptive relatives of schizophrenic adoptees. Replication of the Copenhagen Study in the rest of Denmark." *Archives of General Psychiatry* 51: 442–55.

Kim K, H Hwu, L Zhang, M Lu, K Park, T Hwang, D Kim, Y Park. 2001. "Schizophrenic delusions in Seoul, Shanghai and Taipei: a transcultural study." *Journal of Korean Medical Science* 16: 88–94.

King M, E Coker, G Leavey, A Hoare, E Johnson-Sabine. 1994. "Incidence of psychotic illness in London: comparison of ethnic groups." *BMJ* 309: 1115–19.

Kingdon D, D Turkington. 2005. *Cognitive Therapy of Schizophrenia*. New York: Guilford Press.

Kirkbride J, D Barker, F Cowden, R Stamps, M Yang, P Jones, J Coid. 2008. "Psychoses, ethnicity and socio-economic status." *British Journal of Psychiatry* 193: 18–24.

Kirkbride J, P Fearon, C Morgan, P Dazzan, K Morgan, R Murray, P Jones. 2007. "Neighbourhood variation in the incidence of psychotic disorders in Southeast London." *Social Psychiatry and Psychiatric Epidemiology* 42: 438–45.

Kirkbride J, P Fearon, C Morgan, P Dazzan, K Morgan, J Tarrant, T Lloyd, J Holloway, G Hutchinson, J Leff, R Mallett, G Harrison, R Murray, P Jones. 2006. "Heterogeneity in incidence rates of schizophrenia and other psychotic syndromes: findings from the 3-center ÆSOP study." *Archives of General Psychiatry* 63: 250–58.

Kirkbride J, P Jones. 2008. "The mental ill-health of people who migrate and their descendants: risk factors, associated disability and wider consequences." *Mental Capital and Wellbeing Foresight State of Science Review SR-B13.* http://www.bis.gov.uk/assets/foresight/docs/mental-capital/sr-b13_mcw.pdf.

Kirkbride J, P Jones, S Ullrich, J W Coid. 2014. "Social deprivation, inequality, and the neighborhood-level incidence of psychotic syndromes in East London." *Schizophrenia Bulletin* 40: 169–80.

Kirkbride J, C Morgan, P Fearon, P Dazzan, R Murray, P Jones. 2007. "Neighbourhood-level effects on psychoses: re-examining the role of context." *Psychological Medicine* 37: 1413–25.

Kirmayer L, A Young. 1998. "Culture and somatization: clinical, epidemiological, and ethnographic perspectives." *Psychosomatic Medicine* 60: 420–30.

Klein M. 1932. *The Psycho-Analysis of Children*. Translated by A Strachey. London: The Hogarth Press.

Klein M. 1948. "A contribution to the theory of anxiety and guilt." *International Journal of Psycho-Analysis* 29: 114–23.

Klein M. 1960. "Symposium on 'depressive illness'—V. A note on depression in the schizophrenic." *International Journal of Psycho-Analysis* 41: 509–11.

BIBLIOGRAPHY

Klopfer P, D Rubenstein. 1977. "The concept *privacy* and its biological basis." *Journal of Social Issue* 33: 52–65.

Knobel A, A Heinz, M Voss. 2008. "Imaging the deluded brain." *European Archives of Psychiatry and Clinical Neuroscience* 258: 76–80.

Knowles R, S McCarthy-Jones, G Rowse. 2011. "Grandiose delusions: a review and theoretical integration of cognitive and affective perspectives." *Clinical Psychology Review* 31: 684–96.

Kohler C, E Hanson, M Marsh. 2013. "Emotion processing in schizophrenia." In *Social Cognition in Schizophrenia*. Edited by D Roberts, D Penn. 173–95. Oxford: Oxford University Press.

Kohler C, J Walker, E Martin, K Healey, P Moberg. 2010. "Facial emotion perception in schizophrenia: a meta-analytic review." *Schizophrenia Bulletin* 36: 1009–19.

Kojima Y, R Soetedjo, A Fuchs. 2010. "Behavior of the oculomotor vermis for five different types of saccade." *Journal of Neurophysiology* 104: 3667–76.

Kopytoff I. 1971. "Ancestors as elders in Africa." *Africa* 41: 129–42.

Kraepelin E. 1902. *Clinical Psychiatry,* 6th ed. Translated by A Diefendorf. New York: Macmillan.

Krauß F. *Nothschrei eines Magnetisch-Vergifteten* (1852) und *Nothgedrungene Fortsetzung meines Nothschrei* (1867). 1967. Edited by H Ahlenstiel, J Meyer. Leverkusen: Bayer.

Kroeze Y, H Zhou, J Homberg. 2012. "The genetics of selective serotonin reuptake inhibitors." *Pharmacology & Therapeutics* 136: 375–400.

Kuepper R, J van Os, R Lieb, H Wittchen, C Henquet. 2011. "Do cannabis and urbanicity co-participate in causing psychosis? Evidence from a 10-year follow-up cohort study." *Psychological Medicine* 41: 2121–29.

Labrie V, S Pai, A Petronis. 2012. "Epigenetics of major psychosis: progress, problems and perspectives." *Trends in Genetics* 28: 427–35.

Lataster T, J van Os, M Drukker, C Henquet, F Feron, N Gunther, I Myin-Germeys. 2006. "Childhood victimisation and developmental expression of non-clinical delusional ideation and hallucinatory experiences: victimisation and non-clinical psychotic experiences." *Social Psychiatry and Psychiatric Epidemiology* 41: 423–28.

Lawrie S, B Olabi, J Hall, A McIntosh. 2011. "Do we have any solid evidence of clinical utility about the pathophysiology of schizophrenia?" *World Psychiatry* 10: 19–31.

Lederbogen F, P Kirsch, L Haddad, F Streit, H Tost, P Schuch, S Wüst, J Pruessner, M Rietschel, M Deuschle, A Meyer-Lindenberg. 2011. "City living and urban upbringing affect neural social stress processing in humans." *Nature* 474: 498–501.

Leff J, L Kuipers, R Berkowitz, D Sturgeon. 1985. "A controlled trial of social intervention in the families of schizophrenic patients: two year follow-up." *British Journal of Psychiatry* 146: 594–600.

Lepore J. 2013. "The Prism." *The New Yorker* 89 (18): 32–36.

Levine M, Goldman R. "Capitol suspect Miriam Carey believed Obama electronically monitored her." ABC News. October 4, 2013. Consulted October 13, 2013. http://abcnews.go.com/US/capitol-suspect-miriam-carey-believed-obama-electronically-monitored/story?id=20470498.

BIBLIOGRAPHY

Lewis P, R Rezaie, R Brown, N Roberts, R Dunbar. 2011. "Ventromedial prefrontal volume predicts understanding of others and social network size." *Neuroimage* 57: 1624–29.

Lewis S, N Tarrier, G Haddock, R Bentall, P Kinderman, D Kingdon, R Siddle, R Drake, J Everitt, K Leadley, A Benn, K Grazebrook, C Haley, S Akhtar, L Davies, S Palmer, B Faragher, G Duun. 2002. "Randomised controlled trial of cognitive-behavioural therapy in early schizophrenia: acute-phase outcomes." *British Journal of Psychiatry* 181: s91–97.

Lin F, Y Zhou, Y Du, L Qin, Z Zhao, J Xu, H Lei. 2012. "Abnormal white matter integrity in adolescents with internet addiction disorder: a tract-based spatial statistics study." *PLoS One* 7: doi: 10.1371/journal.pone.0030253.

Link B, A Stueve. 1994. "Psychotic symptoms and the violent/illegal behavior of mental patients compared to the community." In *Violence and Mental Disorder*. Edited by J Monahan, H Steadman. 137–59. Chicago: University of Chicago Press.

Linn L. 1958. "Some comments on the origin of the influencing machine." *Journal of the American Psychoanalytic Association* 6: 305–8.

Locher P, R Unger, P Sociedade, J Wahl. 1993. "At first glance: accessibility of the physical attractiveness stereotype." *Sex Roles* 28: 729–43.

Locke J. 1975. *An Essay Concerning Human Understanding*. Edited by P Nidditch. Oxford: Clarendon Press.

Lofors J, K Sundquist. 2007. "Low-linking social capital as a predictor of mental disorders: a cohort study of 4.5 million Swedes." *Social Science & Medicine* 64: 21–34.

Lothane Z. 1992. *In Defense of Schreber*. Hillsdale: Analytic Press.

Lothane Z. 2011. "The partnership of psychoanalysis and psychiatry in the treatment of psychosis and borderline states: its evolution in North America." *Journal of the American Academy of Psychoanalysis and Dynamic Psychiatry* 39: 499–523.

Luhrmann T. 2007. "Social defeat and the culture of chronicity: or, why schizophrenia does so well over there and so badly here." *Culture, Medicine and Psychiatry* 31: 135–72.

Macdonald G, J Higgins, P Ramchandani, J Valentine, L Bronger, P Klein, R O'Daniel, M Pickering, B Rademaker, G Richardson, M Taylor. 2012. "Cognitive-behavioural interventions for children who have been sexually abused." *Cochrane Database Systematic Review* 5: CD001930.

Magnusson C, D Rai, A Goodman, M Lundberg, S Idring, A Svensson, I Koupil, E Serlachius, C Dalman. 2012. "Migration and autism spectrum disorder: population-based study." *British Journal of Psychiatry* 201: 109–15.

Maher B. 1974. "Delusional thinking and perceptual disorder." *Journal of Individual Psychology* 30: 98–113.

Maher B. 1992. "Delusions: contemporary etiological hypotheses." *Psychiatric Annals* 22: 260–68.

Maher B. 1999. "Anomalous experience in everyday life: its significance for psychopathology." *The Monist* 82: 547–70.

Manschreck T. 1979. "The assessment of paranoid features." *Comprehensive Psychiatry* 20: 370–77.

BIBLIOGRAPHY

March D, C Morgan, M Bresnahan, E Susser. 2008. "Conceptualising the social world." In *Society and Psychosis*. Edited by C Morgan, K McKenzie, P Fearon. 41–57. Cambridge: Cambridge University Press.

Marmot M. 2004. *The Status Syndrome*. New York: Holt.

Marneros A. 2008. "Psychiatry's 200th birthday." *British Journal of Psychiatry* 193: 1–3.

Martin C. 2006. "Ernest Hemingway: a psychological autopsy of a suicide." *Psychiatry* 69: 351–61.

Marx O. 2008. "German romantic psychiatry: Part I. Earlier, including more-psychological orientations." In *History of Psychiatry and Medical Psychology*. Edited by E Wallace, J Gach. 313–33. New York: Springer.

Masserman J. 1959. "Preface and dedication." In *Biological Psychiatry*. Edited by J Masserman. xiv–xvi. New York: Grune & Stratton.

Mathiesen T. 1997. "The viewer society: Michel Foucault's 'Panopticon' revisited." *Theoretical Criminology* 1: 215–34.

Maudlin T. 1996. "On the unification of physics." *Journal of Philosophy* 93: 129–44.

May M, M Wendt. 2013. "Visual perspective taking and laterality decisions: problems and possible solutions." *Frontiers in Human Neuroscience* 7: doi: 10.3389/fnhum.2013.00549.

May-Chahal C, P Cawson. 2005. "Measuring child maltreatment in the United Kingdom: a study of the prevalence of child abuse and neglect." *Child Abuse & Neglect* 29: 969–84.

Mayors Against Illegal Guns. "Analysis of recent mass shootings." September 2013. Consulted October 13, 2013. http://s3.amazonaws.com/s3.mayorsagainstillegalguns.org/images/analysis-of-recent-mass-shootings.pdf.

McCreadie R, A Robinson. 1987. "The Nithsdale Schizophrenia Survey. VI. Relatives' expressed emotion: prevalence, patterns, and clinical assessment." *British Journal of Psychiatry* 150: 640–4.

McCutcheon L, D Ashe, J Houran, J Maltby. 2003. "A cognitive profile of individuals who tend to worship celebrities." *Journal of Psychology* 137: 309–22.

McGillivray G, S Skull, G Davie, S Kofoed, A Frydenberg, J Rice, R Cooke, J Carapetis. 2007. "High prevalence of asymptomatic vitamin D and iron deficiency in East African immigrant children and adolescents living in a temperate climate." *Archives of Disease in Childhood* 92: 1088–93.

McGlashan T. 1984a. "The Chestnut Lodge follow-up study. I. Follow-up methodology and study sample." *Archives of General Psychiatry* 41: 573–85.

McGlashan T. 1984b. "The Chestnut Lodge follow-up study. II. Long-term outcome of schizophrenia and the affective disorders." *Archives of General Psychiatry* 41: 586–601.

McGowan P, A Sasaki, A D'Alessio, S Dymov, B Labonté, M Szyf, G Turecki, M Meaney. 2009. "Epigenetic regulation of the glucocorticoid receptor in human brain associates with childhood abuse." *Nature Neuroscience* 12: 342–48.

McGrath J. 1999. "Hypothesis: is low prenatal vitamin D a risk-modifying factor for schizophrenia?" *Schizophrenia Research* 40: 173–77.

BIBLIOGRAPHY

McGrath J, O El-Saadi, S Cardy, B Chapple, D Chant, B Mowry. 2001. "Urban birth and migrant status as risk factors for psychosis: an Australian case-control study." *Social Psychiatry and Psychiatric Epidemiology* 36: 533–36.

McGrath J, S Saha, J Welham, O El Saadi, C MacCauley, D Chant. 2004. "A systematic review of the incidence of schizophrenia: the distribution of rates and the influence of sex, urbanicity, migrant status and methodology." *BMC Medicine* 2: 13.

McKay R, D Dennett. 2009. "The evolution of misbelief." *Behavioral and Brain Sciences* 32: 493–510.

McKenzie K, P Fearon, G Hutchinson. 2008. "Migration, ethnicity and psychosis." In *Society and Psychosis*. Edited by C Morgan, K McKenzie, P Fearon. 143–60. Cambridge: Cambridge University Press.

McNaughton N, P Corr. 2004. "A two-dimensional neuropsychology of defense: fear/anxiety and defensive distance." *Neuroscience and Biobehavioral Reviews* 28: 285–305.

McNeil T, E Schubert, E Cantor-Graae, M Brossner, P Schubert, K Henriksson. 2009. "Unwanted pregnancy as a risk factor for offspring schizophrenia-spectrum and affective disorders in adulthood: a prospective high-risk study." *Psychological Medicine* 39: 957–65.

Mednick S, R Machon, M Huttunen, D Bonett. 1988. "Adult schizophrenia following prenatal exposure to an influenza epidemic." *Archives of General Psychiatry* 45: 189–92.

Miller R. 2009. "Mechanisms of action of antipsychotic drugs of different classes, refractoriness to therapeutic effects of classical neuroleptics, and individual variation in sensitivity to their actions: Part I." *Current Neuropharmacology* 7: 302–14.

Mitchell R, N Thompson, eds. 1986. *Deception: Perspectives on Human and Nonhuman Deceit*. Albany: SUNY Press.

Mittal V, D Dean, A Pelletier. 2013. "Internet addiction, reality substitution and longitudinal changes in psychotic-like experiences in young adults." *Early Intervention in Psychiatry* 7: 261–69.

Mojtabai R. 1994. "Fregoli syndrome." *Australian and New Zealand Journal of Psychiatry* 28: 458–62.

Mora G. 2008a. "Mental disturbances, unusual mental states, and their interpretation during the middle ages." In *History of Psychiatry and Medical Psychology*. Edited by E Wallace, J Gach. 199–226. New York: Springer.

Mora G. 2008b. "Renaissance conceptions and treatments of madness." In *History of Psychiatry and Medical Psychology*. Edited by E Wallace, J Gach. 227–54. New York: Springer.

Morgan C, H Fisher. 2007. "Environment and schizophrenia: environmental factors in schizophrenia: childhood trauma—a critical review." *Schizophrenia Bulletin* 33: 3–10.

Morgan C, J Kirkbride, J Leff, T Craig, G Hutchinson, K McKenzie, K Morgan, P Dazzan, G Doody, P Jones, R Murray, P Fearon. 2007. "Parental separation, loss and psychosis in different ethnic groups: a case-control study." *Psychological Medicine* 37: 495–503.

BIBLIOGRAPHY

Mortensen P, C Pedersen, T Westergaard, J Wohlfahrt, H Ewald, O Mors, P Andersen, M Melbye. 1999. "Effects of family history and place and season of birth on the risk of schizophrenia." *New England Journal of Medicine* 340: 603–8.

Moutoussis M, J Williams, P Dayan, R Bentall. 2007. "Persecutory delusions and the conditioned avoidance paradigm: towards an integration of the psychology and biology of paranoia." *Cognitive Neuropsychiatry* 12: 495–510.

Muchembled R. 2012. *A History of Violence*. Translated by J Birrell. Cambridge: Polity Press.

Müller-Lyer F. 1889. "Optische Urtheilstäuschungen." *Archiv für Physiologie* Supplement: 263–70.

Mullins S, S Spence. 2003. "Re-examining thought insertion: semi-structured literature review and conceptual analysis." *British Journal of Psychiatry* 182: 293–98.

Munro A. 1999. *Delusional Disorder*. Cambridge: Cambridge University Press.

Murray C, C Michaud, M McKenna, J Marks. 1998. "US patterns of mortality by county and race: 1965–1994." Cambridge: Harvard Center for Population and Development Studies.

Murray G. 2011. "The emerging biology of delusions." *Psychological Medicine* 41: 7–13.

Nagel E. 1979. *The Structure of Science*, 2nd ed. Indianapolis: Hackett Publishing.

National Institute of Mental Health Strategic Plan. 2008. Consulted January 30, 2014. http://www.nimh.nih.gov/about/strategic-planning-reports/index.shtml#strategic-objective1.

Ndetei D, A Vadher. 1984. "Frequency and clinical significance of delusions across cultures." *Acta Psychiatrica Scandinavica* 70: 73-76.

Nederlof A, P Muris, J Hovens. 2011. "Threat/control-override symptoms and emotional reactions to positive symptoms as correlates of aggressive behavior in psychotic patients." *Journal of Nervous & Mental Disease* 199: 342–47.

Neighbors H, S Trierweiler, B Ford, J Muroff. 2003. "Racial differences in DSM diagnosis using a semi-structured instrument: the importance of clinical judgment in the diagnosis of African Americans." *Journal of Health and Social Behavior* 44: 237–56.

Neill J. 1990. "Whatever became of the schizophrenogenic mother?" *American Journal of Psychotherapy* 44: 499–505.

Neuberg S, D Kenrick, M Schaller. 2011. "Human threat management systems: self-protection and disease avoidance." *Neuroscience and Biobehavioral Reviews* 35: 1042–51.

Neurath O. 1983. "Protocol Statements." In *Philosophical Papers 1913–1946*. Edited by R Cohen, M Neurath. 91–99. Dordrecht: Reidel.

Newman Taylor K, L Stopa. 2013. "The fear of others: a pilot study of social anxiety processes in paranoia." *Behavioural and Cognitive Psychotherapy* 41: 66–88.

Niccol A. 1998. *The Truman Show*. London: Nick Hern Books.

Nickerson R. 1998. "Confirmation bias: a ubiquitous phenomenon in many guises." *Review of General Psychology* 2: 175–220.

Nielson J, G Thompson. 1947. *The Engrammes of Psychiatry*. Springfield: Charles C. Thomas.

BIBLIOGRAPHY

Nietzsche F. 1968. *The Will to Power*. Edited by W Kaufmann. Translated by W Kaufmann, R Hollingdale. New York: Vintage.

Nitzan U, E Shoshan, S Lev-Ran, S Fennig. 2011. "Internet-related psychosis—a sign of the times." *Israel Journal of Psychiatry & Related Sciences* 48: 207–11.

North C, R Cadoret. 1981. "Diagnostic discrepancy in personal accounts of patients with 'schizophrenia'." *Archives of General Psychiatry* 38: 133–37.

Nunn C, S Altizer. 2006. *Infectious Diseases in Primates*. Oxford: Oxford University Press.

Onishi K, R Baillargeon. 2005. "Do 15-month-old infants understand false beliefs?" *Science* 308: 255–58.

Oosterhof N, A Todorov. 2008. "The functional basis of face evaluation." *Proceedings of the National Academy of Sciences* 105: 11087–92.

Palmer B. "Big Apple is watching you." Slate.com. May 3 2010. Consulted July 14, 2012. http://www.slate.com/articles/news_and_politics/explainer/2010/05/big_apple_is_watching_you.html.

Paracelsus. 1941. *Four Treatises of Theophrastus von Hohenheim, Called Paracelsus*. Edited by H Sigerist. Baltimore: Johns Hopkins University Press.

Paris J. 2005. *The Fall of an Icon*. Toronto: University of Toronto.

Patton K. 2004. "'A great and strange correction': intentionality, locality, and epiphany in the category of dream incubation." *History of Religions* 43: 194–223.

Pedersen C, P Mortensen. 2001. "Evidence of a dose-response relationship between urbanicity during upbringing and schizophrenia risk." *Archives of General Psychiatry* 58: 1039–46.

Peierls R. 1960. "Wolfgang Ernst Pauli. 1900–1958." *Biographical Memoirs of Fellows of the Royal Society* 5: 175–92.

Persons J. 1986. "The advantages of studying psychological phenomena rather than psychiatric diagnoses." *American Psychologist* 41: 1252–60.

Peters E, S Joseph, S Day, P Garety. 2004. "Measuring delusional ideation: the 21-item Peters et al. Delusions Inventory (PDI)." *Schizophrenia Bulletin* 30: 1005–22.

Phelan J, B Link, P Tehranifar. 2010. "Social conditions as fundamental causes of health inequalities: theory, evidence, and policy implications." *Journal of Health and Social Behavior* 51: S28–40.

Pinker S. 2011. *The Better Angels of Our Nature*. New York: Viking.

Pinkham A, C Brensinger, C Kohler, R Gur, R Gur. 2011. "Actively paranoid patients with schizophrenia over attribute anger to neutral faces." *Schizophrenia Research* 125: 174–78.

Plato. 1997. "Phaedrus." Translated by A Nehamas, P Woodruff. In *Plato: Complete Works*. Edited by J Cooper, D Hutchinson. 506–56. Indianapolis: Hackett.

Porter R. 1985. "'Under the influence': Mesmerism in England." *History Today* 35: 22–29.

Porter R. 1991. "Reason, madness, and the French Revolution." *Studies in Eighteenth Century Culture* 20: 55–79.

Porter R. 2002. *Madness: A Brief History*. Oxford: Oxford University Press.

BIBLIOGRAPHY

Powell N, A Tarr, J Sheridan. 2013. "Psychosocial stress and inflammation in cancer." *Brain, Behavior, and Immunity* 30: S41–47.

Puce A, D Perrett. 2003. "Electrophysiology and brain imaging of biological motion." *Philosophical Transactions of the Royal Society B* 358: 435–45.

Raedler T, R Freedman. 2009. "Cholinergic mechanisms in schizophrenia." In *Handbook of Neurochemistry and Molecular Neurobiology: Schizophrenia*. Edited by D Javitt, J Kantrowitz. 17–38. New York: Springer.

Raichle M, D Gusnard. 2002. "Appraising the brain's energy budget." *Proceedings of the National Academy of Science of the United States of America* 99: 10237–39.

Read J, J van Os, A Morrison, C Ross. 2005. "Childhood trauma, psychosis and schizophrenia: a literature review with theoretical and clinical implications." *Acta Psychiatrica Scandinavica* 112: 330–50.

Rector N, A Beck. 2012. "Cognitive behavioral therapy for schizophrenia: an empirical review." *Journal of Nervous and Mental Disease* 200: 832–39.

Regan P. 2004. "Old issues, new context: privacy, information collection, and homeland security." *Government Information Quarterly* 21: 481–97.

"Rehtaeh Parsons, Canadian girl, dies after suicide attempt; parents allege she was raped by 4 boys." Huffington Post. May 11, 2013. Consulted October 4, 2013. http://www.huffingtonpost.com/2013/04/09/rehtaeh-parsons-girl-dies-suicide-rape-canada_n_3045033.html.

Rennie J, ed. 2008. "The future of privacy." *Scientific American* 299: 46–106.

Ripke S, C O'Dushlaine, K Chambert, J Moran, A Kähler, S Akterin, S Bergen, A Collins, J Crowley, M Fromer et al. 2013. "Genome-wide association analysis identifies 13 new risk loci for schizophrenia." *Nature Genetics* 45: 1150–59.

Rivolta D, R Palermo, L Schmalzl. 2013. "What is overt and what is covert in congenital prosopagnosia?" *Neuropsychology Review* 23: 111–16.

Roberts D, D Penn, eds. 2013. *Social Cognition in Schizophrenia*. Oxford: Oxford University Press.

Rose G, M Marmot. 1981. "Social class and coronary heart disease." *British Heart Journal* 45: 13–19.

Rosenthal D, S Kety. 1968. *The Transmission of Schizophrenia*. Oxford: Pergamon Press.

Rossini N. 2011. "Deception cues in political speeches: verbal and non-verbal traits of prevarication." In *Analysis of Verbal and Nonverbal Communication and Enactment*. Edited by A Esposito, A Vinciarelli, K Vicsi, C Pelachaud, A Nijholt. 406–18. Berlin: Springer.

Rowley D. 1994. "Research issues in the study of very low birthweight and preterm delivery among African-American women." *Journal of the National Medical Association* 86: 761–64.

Sacks O, R Wasserman. 1987. "The case of the colorblind painter." *New York Review of Books* 34: 25–34.

Saks E. 2007. *The Center Cannot Hold: My Journey Through Madness*. New York: Hyperion.

Saks E. 2011. "Psychoanalysis and the psychoses: commentary on Kafka." *Journal of the American Psychoanalytic Association* 59: 59–70.

BIBLIOGRAPHY

Sapolsky R. 2004. "Social status and health in humans and other animals." *Annual Review of Anthropology* 33: 393–418.

Sartre J. 1956. *No Exit, and Three Other Plays*. New York: Vintage.

Schaller M. 2011. "The behavioural immune system and the psychology of human sociality." *Philosophical Transactions of the Royal Society B* 366: 3418–26.

Schipper L, J Easton, T Shackelford. 2007. "Morbid jealousy as a function of fitness-related life-cycle dimensions." *Behavioral and Brain Sciences* 29: 630.

Schlund M, C Hudgins, S Magee, S Dymond. 2013. "Neuroimaging the temporal dynamics of human avoidance to sustained threat." *Behavioural Brain Research* 257: 148–55.

Schmidt M. "Gunman said electronic brain attacks drove him to violence, F.B.I. says." *New York Times*. September 16, 2013. Consulted October 13, 2013. http://www.nytimes.com/2013/09/26/us/shooter-believed-mind-was-under-attack-official-says.html.

Schomerus G, D Heider, M Angermeyer, P Bebbington, J Azorin, T Brugha, M Toumi. 2008. "Urban residence, victimhood and the appraisal of personal safety in people with schizophrenia: results from the European Schizophrenia Cohort (EuroSC)." *Psychological Medicine* 38: 591–97.

Schreber D. 1955. *Memoirs of My Nervous Illness*. Translated by I Macalpine, R Hunter. New York: New York Review of Books.

Schreier A, D Wolke, K Thomas, J Horwood, C Hollis, D Gunnell, G Lewis, A Thompson, S Zammit, L Duffy, G Salvi, G Harrison. 2009. "Prospective study of peer victimization in childhood and psychotic symptoms in a nonclinical population at age 12 years." *Archives of General Psychiatry* 66: 527–36.

Selten J, E Cantor-Graae. 2005. "Social defeat: risk factor for schizophrenia?" *British Journal of Psychiatry* 187: 101–2.

Selten J, E Cantor-Graae, R Kahn. 2007. "Migration and schizophrenia." *Current Opinion in Psychiatry* 20: 111–15.

Selten J, E Cantor-Graae, J Slaets, R Kahn. 2002. "Ødegaard's selection hypothesis revisited: schizophrenia in Surinamese immigrants to the Netherlands." *American Journal of Psychiatry* 159: 669–71.

Semple J. 1992. "Foucault and Bentham: a defence of panopticism." *Utilitas* 4: 105–20.

Seth. 2003. *It's a Good Life, if You Don't Weaken*. Montreal: Drawn and Quarterly.

Sharp T, P Cowen. 2011. "5-HT and depression: is the glass half-full?" *Current Opinion in Pharmacology* 11: 45–51.

Sher L. 2000. "Social events and scientific innovations may affect the content of delusions." *Southern Medical Journal* 93: 440–41.

Shorter E. 1997. *A History of Psychiatry*. New York: John Wiley & Sons.

Shrivastava A, M Johnston, K Terpstra, Y Bureau. 2013. "Pathways to psychosis in cannabis abuse." *Clinical Schizophrenia & Related Psychoses*. doi: 10.3371/csrp.shjo.030813.

Siena K. 2013. "The moral biology of 'the itch' in eighteenth-century Britain." In *A Medical History of Skin*. Edited by J Reinarz, K Siena. 71–83. London: Pickering and Chatto.

Signer S. 1987. "Capgras' syndrome: the delusion of substitution." *Journal of Clinical Psychiatry* 48: 147–50.

Silva J, G Leong, R Weinstock, C Boyer. 1989. "Capgras syndrome and dangerousness." *Bulletin of the American Academy of Psychiatry and the Law* 17: 5–14.

Silver E, E Mulvey, J Swanson. 2002. "Neighborhood structural characteristics and mental disorder: Faris and Dunham revisited." *Social Science & Medicine* 55: 1457–70.

Simion F, L Regolin, H Bulf. 2008. "A predisposition for biological motion in the newborn baby." *Proceedings of the National Academy of Science* 105: 809–13.

Simon B. 2008. "Mind and madness in classical antiquity." In *History of Psychiatry and Medical Psychology*. Edited by E Wallace, J Gach. 175–97. New York: Springer.

Simon H. 1957. *Models of Man, Social and Rational*. New York: Wiley.

Simons R, C Hughes. 1985. *The Culture-Bound Syndromes*. Dordrecht: Reidel.

Sledge W. 1992. "Introduction to Tausk, 'On the origin of the "influencing machine" in schizophrenia.'" *Journal of Psychotherapy Practice and Research* 1: 184.

Smith G, J Boydell, R Murray, S Flynn, K McKay, M Sherwood, W Honer. 2006. "The incidence of schizophrenia in European immigrants to Canada." *Schizophrenia Research* 87: 205–11.

So S, D Freeman, G Dunn, S Kapur, E Kuipers, P Bebbington, D Fowler, P Garety. 2012. "Jumping to conclusions, a lack of belief flexibility and delusional conviction in psychosis: a longitudinal investigation of the structure, frequency, and relatedness of reasoning biases." *Journal of Abnormal Psychology* 121: 129–39.

Soyka M, G Naber, A Völcker. 1991. "Prevalence of delusional jealousy in different psychiatric disorders. An analysis of 93 cases." *British Journal of Psychiatry* 158: 549–53.

Speechley W, E Ngan. 2008. "Dual-stream modulation failure: a novel hypothesis for the formation and maintenance of delusions in schizophrenia." *Medical Hypotheses* 70: 1210–14.

Spielberg S. 1971. "Columbo: By the Book." Universal TV: Los Angeles.

Spielberg S. 2002. *Catch Me If You Can*. DreamWorks Pictures: Universal City.

Stanovich K. 2009. "Distinguishing the reflective, algorithmic, and autonomous minds: is it time for a tri-process theory?" In *In Two Minds*. Edited by J Evans, K Frankish. 55–88. Oxford: Oxford University Press.

Steadman P. 2007. "The contradictions of Jeremy Bentham's panopticon penitentiary." *Journal of Bentham Studies* 9.

Stiller J, R Dunbar. 2007. "Perspective-taking and memory capacity predict social network size." *Social Networks* 29: 93–104.

Stompe T, G Ortwein-Swoboda, K Ritter, H Schanda. 2003. "Old wine in new bottles? Stability and plasticity of the contents of schizophrenic delusions." *Psychopathology* 36: 6–12.

Stompe T, G Ortwein-Swoboda, H.Schanda. 2004. "Schizophrenia, delusional symptoms, and violence: the threat/control-override concept reexamined." *Schizophrenia Bulletin* 30: 31–44.

Suhail K. 2003. "Phenomenology of delusions in Pakistani patients: effect of gender and social class." *Psychopathology* 36: 195–99.

BIBLIOGRAPHY

Suhail K, R Cochrane. 2002. "Effect of culture and environment on the phenomenology of delusions and hallucinations." *International Journal of Social Psychiatry* 48: 126–38.

Sullivan H. 1962. *Schizophrenia as a Human Process*. New York: Norton.

Sullivan H. 1976. *A Harry Stack Sullivan Case Seminar*. Edited by R Kvarnes, G Parloff. New York: Norton.

Swanson J. 1994. "Mental disorder, substance abuse, and community violence: an epidemiological approach." In *Violence and Mental Disorder*. Edited by J Monahan, H Steadman. 101–36. Chicago: University of Chicago Press.

Swanson J. 2008. "Preventing the unpredicted: managing violence risk in mental health care." *Psychiatric Services* 59: 191–3.

Swanson J. June 7, 2013. "Violence and delusion." Talk given at the International Symposium on Controversies in Psychiatry, Cancun.

Swanson J, R Borum, M Swartz, J Monahan. 1996. "Psychotic symptoms and disorders and the risk of violent behaviour in the community." *Criminal Behaviour and Mental Health* 6: 309–29.

Swanson J, M Swartz, R Van Dorn, E Elbogen, H Wagner, R Rosenheck, T Stroup, J McEvoy, J Lieberman. 2006. "A national study of violent behavior in persons with schizophrenia." *Archives of General Psychiatry* 63: 490–99.

Swazey J. 1974. *Chlorpromazine in Psychiatry*. Cambridge: MIT Press.

Szasz T. 1974. *The Myth of Mental Illness*. New York: Harper and Row.

Takei N, P Sham, E O'Callaghan, R Murray. 1992. "Cities, winter birth, and schizophrenia." *Lancet* 340: 558–59.

Tarrier N, C Kinney, E McCarthy, L Humphreys, A Wittkowski, J Morris. 2000. "Two-year follow-up of cognitive-behavioral therapy and supportive counseling in the treatment of persistent symptoms in chronic schizophrenia." *Journal of Consulting and Clinical Psychology* 68: 917–22.

Tateyama M, M Asai, M Hashimoto, M Bartels, S Kasper. 1998. "Transcultural study of schizophrenic delusions." *Psychopathology* 31: 59–68.

Tausk V. 1919. "Über die Entstehung des Beeinflussungsapparates." *Internationale Zeitschrift für Ärztliche Psychoanalyse* 5: 1–33.

Tausk V. 1933. "On the origin of the 'influencing machine' in schizophrenia." *Psychoanalytic Quarterly* 2: 519–56.

Taylor C, trans. 1999. *The Atomists, Leucippus and Democritus*. Toronto: University of Toronto Press.

Taylor M, E Shorter, N Vaidya, M Fink. 2010. "The failure of the schizophrenia concept and the argument for its replacement by hebephrenia: applying the medical model for disease recognition." *Acta Psychiatrica Scandinavica* 122: 173–83.

Tessari A, G Ottoboni, A Mazzatenta, A Merla, R Nicoletti. 2012. "Please don't! The automatic extrapolation of dangerous intentions." *PLoS One* 7: e49011.

Tidey J, K Miczek. 1996. "Social defeat stress selectively alters mesocorticolimbic dopamine release: an in vivo microdialysis study." *Brain Research* 721: 140–49.

Tienari P, K Wahlberg. 2008. "Family environment and psychosis." In *Society and Psycho-*

sis. Edited by C Morgan, K McKenzie, P Fearon. 112–26. Cambridge: Cambridge University Press.

Tienari P, L Wynne, A Sorri, I Lahti, K Läksy, J Moring, M Naarala, P Nieminen, K Wahlberg. 2004. "Genotype-environment interaction in schizophrenia-spectrum disorder: long-term follow-up study of Finnish adoptees." *British Journal of Psychiatry* 184: 216–22.

Todorov A. 2008. "Evaluating faces on trustworthiness: an extension of systems for recognition of emotions signaling approach/avoidance behaviors." *Annals of the New York Academy of Science* 1124: 208–24.

Todorov A, A Mandisodza, A Goren, C Hall. 2005. "Inferences of competence from faces predict election outcomes." *Science* 308: 1623–26.

Todorov A, M Pakrashi, N Oosterhof. 2009. "Evaluating faces on trustworthiness after minimal time exposure." *Social Cognition* 27: 813–33.

Tooby J, L Cosmides. 2005. "Conceptual foundations of evolutionary psychology." In *The Handbook of Evolutionary Psychology.* Edited by D Buss. 5–67. Hoboken: John Wiley & Sons.

Torrey E, A Bowler, K Clark. 1997. "Urban birth and residence as risk factors for psychoses: an analysis of 1880 data." *Schizophrenia Research* 25: 169–76.

Toyokawa S, M Uddin, K Koenen, S Galea. 2012. "How does the social environment 'get into the mind'? Epigenetics at the intersection of social and psychiatric epidemiology." *Social Science & Medicine* 74: 67–74.

The Tragically Hip. 2002. "It's a good life if you don't weaken." *In Violet Light.* Burlington: Zoë Records.

Tranel D, B Hyman. 1990. "Neuropsychological correlates of bilateral amygdala damage." *Archives of Neurology* 47: 349–55.

Tseng W. 2001. *Handbook of Cultural Psychiatry.* San Diego: Academic Press.

Tuke S. 1813. *Description of the Retreat.* York: W. Alexander.

Tversky A, D Kahneman. 1981. "The framing of decisions and the psychology of choice." *Science* 211: 453–58.

Ullman S, D Harari, N Dorfman. 2012. "From simple innate biases to complex visual concepts." *Proceedings of the National Academy of Science* 109: 18215–20.

van Os J, G Driessen, N Gunther, P Delespaul. 2000. "Neighbourhood variation in incidence of schizophrenia: evidence for person-environment interaction." *British Journal of Psychiatry* 176: 243–48.

van Os J, M Hanssen, R Bijl, A Ravelli. 2000. "Strauss (1969) revisited: a psychosis continuum in the general population?" *Schizophrenia Research* 45: 11–20.

van Os J, M Hanssen, R Bijl, W Vollebergh. 2001. "Prevalence of psychotic disorder and community level of psychotic symptoms: an urban-rural comparison." *Archives of General Psychiatry* 58: 663–68.

van Rossum J. 1966. "The significance of dopamine-receptor blockade for the mechanism of action of neuroleptic drugs." *Archives Internationales de Pharmacodynamie et de Thérapie* 160: 492–94.

van Winkel R, N Stefanis, I Myin-Germeys. 2008. "Psychosocial stress and psychosis. A

BIBLIOGRAPHY

review of the neurobiological mechanisms and the evidence for gene-stress interaction." *Schizophrenia Bulletin* 34: 1095–105.

Varese F, F Smeets, M Drukker, R Lieverse, T Lataster, W Viechtbauer, J Read, J van Os, R Bentall. 2012. "Childhood adversities increase the risk of psychosis: a meta-analysis of patient-control, prospective- and cross-sectional cohort studies." *Schizophrenia Bulletin* 38: 661–71.

Vargas T, S Hendrix, M Fisher. "Aaron Alexis, 34, is dead gunman in Navy Yard shooting, authorities say." *Washington Post*. September 16, 2013. Consulted October 13, 2013. http://articles.washingtonpost.com/2013-09-16/local/42106919_1_buddhist-temple-seattle-police-navy-reserve.

Vassos E, C Pedersen, R Murray, D Collier, C Lewis. 2012. "Meta-analysis of the association of urbanicity with schizophrenia." *Schizophrenia Bulletin* 38: 1118–23.

Veen N, J Selten, H Hoek, W Feller, Y van der Graaf, R Kahn. 2002. "Use of illicit substances in a psychosis incidence cohort: a comparison among different ethnic groups in the Netherlands." *Acta Psychiatrica Scandinavica* 105: 440–43.

Veling W, H Hoek, J Selten, E Susser. 2011. "Age at migration and future risk of psychotic disorders among immigrants in The Netherlands: a 7-year incidence study." *American Journal of Psychiatry* 168: 1278–85.

Veling W, J Selten, J Mackenbach, H Hoek. 2007. "Symptoms at first contact for psychotic disorder: comparison between native Dutch and ethnic minorities." *Schizophrenia Research* 95: 30–38.

Vos T, A Flaxman, M Naghavi, R Lozano, C Michaud, M Ezzati, K Shibuya, J Salomon, S Abdalla, V Aboyans et al. 2012. "Years lived with disability (YLDs) for 1160 sequelae of 289 diseases and injuries 1990–2010: a systematic analysis for the Global Burden of Disease Study 2010." *Lancet* 380: 2163–96.

Walker E, D Diforio. 1997. "Schizophrenia: a neural diathesis-stress model." *Psychological Review* 104: 667–85.

Walker E, V Mittal, K Tessner. 2008. "Stress and the hypothalamic pituitary adrenal axis in the developmental course of schizophrenia." *Annual Review of Clinical Psychology* 4: 189–216.

Wallace E. 2008. "Contextualizing the history of psychiatry/psychology and psychoanalysis." In *History of Psychiatry and Medical Psychology*. Edited by E Wallace, J Gach. 117–69. New York: Springer.

Wallerstein R. 2002. "The growth and transformation of American ego psychology." *Journal of the American Psychoanalytic Society* 50: 135–69.

Walston F, R Blennerhassett, B Charlton. 2000. "Theory of mind," persecutory delusions and the somatic marker mechanism. *Cognitive Neuropsychiatry* 5: 161–74.

Walston F, A David, B Charlton. 1998. Sex differences in the content of persecutory delusions: a reflection of hostile threats in the ancestral environment? *Evolution and Human Behavior* 19: 257–60.

Watts J, W Freeman. 1948. "Prefrontal lobotomy: indications and results in schizophrenia." *American Journal of Surgery* 75: 227–30.

Weaver I, N Cervoni, F Champagne, A D'Alessio, S Sharma, J Seckl, S Dymov, M Szyf,

BIBLIOGRAPHY

M Meaney. 2004. "Epigenetic programming by maternal behavior." *Nature Neuroscience* 7: 847–54.

Weich S, G Holt, L Twigg, K Jones, G Lewis. 2003. "Geographic variation in the prevalence of common mental disorders in Britain: a multilevel investigation." *American Journal of Epidemiology* 157: 730–37.

Weich S, J Nazroo, K Sproston, S McManus, M Blanchard, B Erens, S Karlsen, M King, K Lloyd, S Stansfeld, P Tyrer. 2004. "Common mental disorders and ethnicity in England: the EMPIRIC study." *Psychological Medicine* 34: 1543–51.

Weinberger D, P Harrison, eds. 2011. *Schizophrenia*, 3rd ed. Oxford: Wiley-Blackwell.

Weiner D. 2008a. "The madman in the light of reason. Enlightenment psychiatry. Part I. Custody, therapy, theory, and the need for reform." In *History of Psychiatry and Medical Psychology*. Edited by E Wallace, J Gach. 255–77. New York: Springer.

Weiner D. 2008b. "The madman in the light of reason. Enlightenment psychiatry. Part II. Alienists, treatises, and the psychologic approach in the era of Pinel." In *History of Psychiatry and Medical Psychology*. Edited by E Wallace, J Gach. 281–303. New York: Springer.

Weiser M, N Werbeloff, T Vishna, R Yoffe, G Lubin, M Shmushkevitch, M Davidson. 2008. "Elaboration on immigration and risk for schizophrenia." *Psychological Medicine* 38: 1113–19.

Werbeloff N, S Levine, J Rabinowitz. 2012. "Elaboration on the association between immigration and schizophrenia: a population-based national study disaggregating annual trends, country of origin and sex over 15 years." *Social Psychiatry and Psychiatric Epidemiology* 47: 303–11.

Wheaton K, G Aranda, A Puce. 2002. "ERPs elicited to combined emotional and gestural movements of the face as a function of congruency." Abstract no. 14186. Academic Press OHBM Annual Scientific Meeting.

Whiten A, R Byrne, eds. 1997. *Machiavellian Intelligence II*. Cambridge: Cambridge University Press.

Whitney W, trans. 1905. *Atharva-Veda Saṁhitā*. Cambridge: Harvard University.

Wible C. 2012. "Schizophrenia as a disorder of social communication." *Schizophrenia Research and Treatment*: doi: 10.1155/2012/920485.

Wicks S, A Hjern, D Gunnell, G Lewis, C Dalman. 2005. "Social adversity in childhood and the risk of developing psychosis: a national cohort study." *American Journal of Psychiatry* 162: 1652–57.

Wilkinson R. 1997. "Health inequalities: relative or absolute material standards?" *BMJ* 314: 591–95.

Wilkinson R. 1999. "Health, hierarchy, and social anxiety." *Annals of the New York Academy of Sciences* 896: 48–63.

Wilkinson R. 2001. *Mind the Gap*. New Haven: Yale University Press.

Wilkinson R, M Marmot, eds. 2003. *Social Determinants of Health*, 2nd ed. Copenhagen: World Health Organization.

Wimmer H, J Perner. 1983. "Beliefs about beliefs: representation and constraining function of wrong beliefs in young children's understanding of deception." *Cognition* 13: 103–28.

Winnicott D. 1960. "The theory of the parent-infant relationship." *International Journal of Psycho-Analysis.* 41: 585–595

Winnicott D. 1963. "Dependence in infant care, in child care, and in the psycho-analytic setting." *International Journal of Psycho-Analysis* 44: 339–44.

Winston A, R Rosenthal, H Pinsker. 2012. *Learning Supportive Psychotherapy.* Washington: American Psychiatric Publishing.

Woodward T, S Moritz, C Cuttler, J Whitman. 2006. "The contribution of a cognitive bias against disconfirmatory evidence (BADE) to delusions in schizophrenia." *Journal of Clinical and Experimental Neuropsychology* 28: 605–17.

Woody E, H Szechtman. 2011. "Adaptation to potential threat: the evolution, neurobiology, and psychopathology of the security motivation system." *Neuroscience and Biobehavioral Reviews* 35: 1019–33.

Wykes T, C Steel, B Everitt, N Tarrier. 2008. "Cognitive behavior therapy for schizophrenia: effect sizes, clinical models, and methodological rigor." *Schizophrenia Bulletin* 34: 523–37.

Yang B, H Zhang, W Ge, N Weder, H Douglas-Palumberi, F Perepletchikova, J Gelernter, J Kaufman. 2013. "Child abuse and epigenetic mechanisms of disease risk." *American Journal of Preventive Medicine* 44: 101–7.

Yip K. 2003. "Traditional Chinese religious beliefs and superstitions in delusions and hallucinations of Chinese schizophrenic patients." *International Journal of Social Psychiatry* 49: 97–111.

Yorifuji T, S Kashima, T Tsuda, K Ishikawa-Takata, T Ohta, K Tsuruta, H Doi. 2013. "Long-term exposure to traffic-related air pollution and the risk of death from hemorrhagic stroke and lung cancer in Shizuoka, Japan." *Science of the Total Environment* 443: 397–402.

Young L, D Dodell-Feder, R Saxe. 2010. "What gets the attention of the temporo-parietal junction? An fMRI investigation of attention and theory of mind." *Neuropsychologia* 48: 2658–64.

Young-Bruehl E. 2002. "A visit to the Budapest school." *Psychoanalytic Study of the Child* 57: 411–32.

Yuan K, W Qin, G Wang, F Zeng, L Zhao, X Yang, P Liu, J Liu, J Sun, K von Deneen, Q Gong, Y Liu, J Tian. 2011. "Microstructure abnormalities in adolescents with internet addiction disorder." *PLoS One* 6: e20708.

Yung A, P McGorry. 1996. "The initial prodrome in psychosis: descriptive and qualitative aspects." *Australian and New Zealand Journal of Psychiatry* 30: 587–99.

Zammit S, G Lewis, J Rasbash, C Dalman, J Gustafsson, P Allebeck. 2010. "Individuals, schools, and neighborhood: a multilevel longitudinal study of variation in incidence of psychotic disorders." *Archives of General Psychiatry* 67: 914–22.

Zernike K, M Thee-Brenan. "Poll finds Tea Party backers wealthier and more educated." *New York Times.* April 14, 2010. Consulted June 13, 2013. http://www.nytimes.com/2010/04/15/us/politics/15poll.html?_r=1&.

BIBLIOGRAPHY

Zilboorg G. 1941. *A History of Medical Psychology.* New York: W.W. Norton.

Zimmermann G, J Favrod, V Trieu, V Pomini. 2005. "The effect of cognitive behavioral treatment on the positive symptoms of schizophrenia spectrum disorders: a meta-analysis." *Schizophrenia Research* 77: 1–9.

Zolkowska K, E Cantor-Graae, T McNeil. 2001. "Increased rates of psychosis among immigrants to Sweden: is migration a risk factor for psychosis?" *Psychological Medicine* 31: 669–78.

Zolotova J, M Brüne. 2006. "Persecutory delusions: reminiscence of ancestral hostile threats?" *Evolution and Human Behavior* 27: 185–92.

Zubin J, B Spring. 1977. "Vulnerability—a new view of schizophrenia." *Journal of Abnormal Psychology* 86: 103–26.

Ødegaard Ø. 1932. "Emigration and insanity." *Acta Psychiatrica et Neurologica Scandinavica* 7: 9–206.

FIGURE SOURCES

FIGURE SOURCES

210 Figure 22: From Bentham, 1843; the plate follows p. 172. McGill University Library, Rare Books and Special Collections.

242 Figure 23: Amanda Hall, 2014. Reproduced with permission.

PAGE

64 Table 1: Redrawn from Brakoulias and Starcevic, 2008, p. 90; Gecici et al., 2010, p. 207; Kim et al., 2001, p. 90; Ndetei and Vadher, 1984, p. 74; Suhail and Cochrane, 2002, pp. 130-1; and Tateyama et al., 1998, p. 62.

97 Table 2: Redrawn from Frith, 1992, p. 127.

183 Table 3: Redrawn from Evans, 2008, p. 257.

INDEX

Note: Page numbers in *italics* refer to illustrations or charts. Patient names are changed.

INDEX

INDEX

and social group size, 158, *159*
and stress, 133, 150
brain lesions, studies of, 87–88, *87*
Bresnahan, Michaeline, 136
Brian (Truman Show patient), 5–6
British civil servants:
　life expectancy of, 142, *142*
　stress of, 206
Brooks, Mel, 157
Bullard, William, 26
bullying, 123–24, 132, 180, 220
Burton, Robert, *Anatomy of Melancholy*,
　21
Byrne, Richard, 162

Cade, John, 42
Calvin: Othello in New York, 185–90
Campion, Jane, 179
cannabis, 134, 147
Cantor-Graae, Elizabeth, 136, 137, 204,
　206
Capgras, Joseph, 63
Capgras delusion, 63, 75–78, 82, 92
Carey, Miriam, 178–79
Carlsson, Arvid, 48
Caro, Heinrich, 43
Carrey, Jim, 4, 7
Catch Me If You Can (film), 161
Cathy (New York resident), 204–5
cell phones, 207
cerebellum, 88
Chantimoine tower, Caen, 22
Charcot, Jean-Martin, 33
Charley (Truman Show patient), 6, 103–7
charms, to ward off madness, 17, 19
Charpentier, Paul, 43, 44
Chestnut Lodge, Maryland, 37, 38, 39–40
Chiarugi, Vincenzio, 24
childhood:
　abuse in, 122–23, 134, 146, 150, 204,
　　205, 206
　adopted into dysfunctional family
　　environment, 125

bullying in, 123–24, 180
and death of parent, 124
children:
　core identity of, 37
　parents as responsible for, 125
　"unwanted," 124
chlorpromazine (4560 RP), 44–48, 52
Chomsky, Noam, 233
cities, 131–33
　imagined, 219–21
　and social drift hypothesis, 132–33
　social factors in, 134, 204–5, 206
Clark, Kitty, 132
Clarke, Arthur C., Three Laws, 111
clozapine, 48
Clutterbuck, Henry, 27
cognition:
　dual process, 182, *183*, 200
　modularity or modular,
　　182–84, *183*, 200
　and Suspicion System, 163
cognitive behavioral therapy (CBT),
　224–25
cognitive distortions, threat-related,
　121
cognitive dysmetria, 88
cognitive function:
　decline in, 32
　social, 118, 158, 182
　systems for handling of, 181–84
Collins, James, 140, 141
Coltheart, Max, 81, 82
"Columbo: By the Book" (TV), 161–62
community:
　electronic, 219–21
　shared culture in, 135
　and social cohesion, 135
　and Truman Show delusion, 11–12
　voter participation in, 135
competence, judging, 171
competition, 159, 160
computer-mediated communication,
　221

307

INDEX

INDEX

polythematic, 60, 82
reasoning hypothesis of, 81
of reference, 8
reluctance to give them up, 80
Ruby: All Dressed Up, 83–85
and strange experiences, 76–79, 92
and Suspicion System breakdown,
191–97, 199–201, 203, 206
taken as true, 202
theory of, 73, 76–79, 91, 95, 195–96,
199
two-factor approach to, 83, 90
two senses of, 65
types of, 62–63, 64
understanding, 199–204
and violence, 178–81
dementia, 87
dementia praecox, 32, 122
Deniker, Pierre, 45–46, 47
depression, 132
and delusion, 60
Donald: Depression and Damnation,
40–41
electroconvulsive therapy for, 52, 231
depressive position, 37
Devil, battle between Holy Ghost and, 19
diagnosis:
biological model, 51, 53
medical model, 51
psychiatric, 49–51
*Diagnostic and Statistical Manual of
Mental Disorders (DSM)*, 49–51,
52–53, 61–62
dialectical method, 20
diathesis-stress model, 147
Dick, P. K., *Time Out of Joint*, 101, 108
Dickinson, Rod, *The Air Loom, A Human
Influencing Machine*, 29
Dicks, Dennis, 172
discrimination:
and birth weight, 141
in ethnic communities, 129
and ethnic fragmentation, 135

and immigration, 128, 135
medical consequences of, 145
and psychosis, 129
racial, 135
and socio-economic status, 135,
139–45
dissociation, 139
DNA, and epigenetics, 149–50
DNA structure, 231–32
Dobzhansky, Theodosius, 243
dominance hierarchies, 143–44
Dominguez, Maria-de-Gracia, 148
Donald: Depression and Damnation,
40–41
dopamine, 87, 90–92, 148, 206
dopamine receptors, 48, 52
dream interpretation, 20
drug abuse, 134
dual process theories, 182, 200
Dunham, Warren, 131
duplicity, 162
dyes:
alizarin, 43
methylene blue, 43
synthetic, 42–43
dysfunctional family environment, 125

earthquakes, 232–33
Easton, Judith, 196
Ebbinghaus, Hermann, 21
ego, 34, 35–36
Ehrlich, Paul, 43
elaboration, 203
electroconvulsive therapy (ECT), 52,
231
Ellis, Hayden, 77, 82, 92
Ellul, Jacques, *The Technological Society*,
168
emotion:
and body language, 177–78
deficits in, 118
expressed (EE), 125–26, 224
recognition of, 173–74

INDEX

INDEX

INDEX

Stoljar, Margaret Mahony, 67
Stompe, Thomas, 180
Stopa, Luisa, 121
straitjackets, 26
strange experiences, 76–79, 81, 92
stress:
    biological, 146–47
    and the brain, 133, 150
    and HPA axis, 148, 149
    in primates, 144
    and psychosis, 149, 204
    sensitization to, 149
    and social status, 144–45, 146
    and vigilance, 205–6
    and vulnerability, 145–50, *146, 149*
striatum, 148
Study of Cognitive Re-alignment Therapy
    for Early Schizophrenia (SoCRATES),
    225
Stueve, Ann, 179
substance abuse, 134, 148
suicide, studies of, 150
Sullivan, Harry Stack, 37–39
    Schizophrenia as a Human Process,
    37–38
superego, 36
surveillance, 209, 210–13
suspicion:
    of being exploited, 163
    and deception, 176
    and paranoia, 192
    sources of, 175–78
Suspicion System, 163–66
    breakdown of, 191–97, 199–201,
    203, 206
    Calvin Moore, 201–2
    damage to, 174
    evidence for the existence of, 172
    and face perception, 169–72
    and indirect evidence, 178, 205
    and loyalty card discounts, 165–66
    modularity of, 184
    purpose of, 166, 182, 184, 194

and Reflective System, 200, 202–3
as special-purpose mechanism,
    181–84, *183*
and uncertainty, 200
vigilance in, 204–6
Swanson, Jeffrey, 179
synopticism, 212, 213
Szasz, Thomas, 53

tactical deception, 162
Tausk, Victor, 71–72
technology:
    Air Loom, 27–28, *29*, 63, 66
    control via, 70–73
    and delusion, 181
    exploitation via, 219–21
    and fear, 208
    John: The Academic, 167–69
    Lawrence: Artificial Intelligence,
    213–18
    and surveillance, 211–13
    and *The Truman Show,* 207–9, 211–13
temporal lobe, 87, *87*
temporal-parietal junction (TPJ), 197
thalamus, 88
Theodosius, 21
Theory of Mind (ToM), 95–98, *97*
    and brain size, 162
    and cooperation, 159–60
    and deception, 160–62
    and delusions of thought, 193
    and false belief task, 118
    and group size, 206
    and hinting task, 118–19
    Reading the Mind in the Eyes test,
    119, *119*
    in schizophrenia, 118
Thorazine, 47
thought:
    and social life, 116
    thinking about, 95–98
    thinking about others, 117–22
thought insertion, 59, 62, 193

INDEX

White, William Alanson, 26
Whitehall Studies (Britain), 142, 144, *145*
Whiten, Andrew, 162
Winnicott, Donald, 37
witchcraft, 19
women, status of, 195

"word salad," 88–90
workplace autonomy, 144, *145*

Young, Andrew, 77, 82, 92

Zubin, Joseph, 146

ABOUT THE AUTHORS

Joel Gold, MD, is Clinical Associate Professor of Psychiatry at the NYU School of Medicine. Dr. Gold is on the faculty of the Institute for Psycho-analytic Education and has a psychotherapy practice in Manhattan. He lives with his family in Brooklyn.

Ian Gold is Associate Professor of Philosophy and Psychiatry at McGill University. He lives with his family in Montreal.